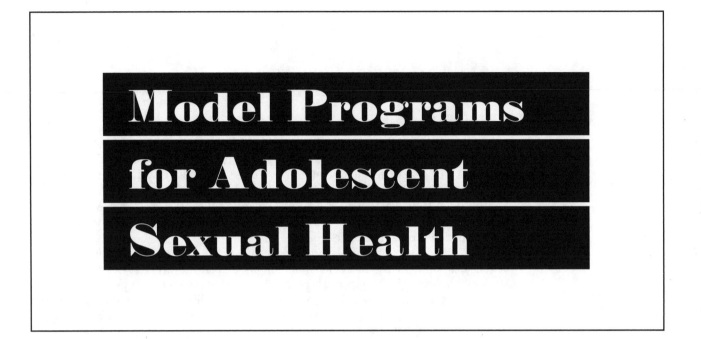

Model Programs for Adolescent Sexual Health

Josefina J. Card, PhD, is Founder and President of Sociometrics Corporation. Card is a nationally recognized social scientist and an expert in the establishment and operation of research-based social science resources, products, and services for population researchers and health practitioners. She has served as Principal Investigator of over 70 grants and contracts funded by the National Institutes of Health and the National Science Foundation, including the AIDS/STI Data Archive, Program Archive on Sexuality, Health, and Adolescence (PASHA), and the HIV/AIDS Prevention Program Archive.

Card has established a solid track record as a health and population scientist. She has authored over 80 books, monographs, and journal articles. Her work is noted for its integration of behavioral, psychological, and demographic perspectives.

Card has served as a member of many federal advisory committees, including the NIH (National Institutes of Health) Study Section for Social Sciences and Population, the NICHD (National Institute on Child Health and Human Development) Population Research Committee, and the NICHD Advisory Council.

Tabitha A. Benner, MPA, is a Research Associate at Sociometrics Corporation and currently the project director of two projects related to STI/HIV/AIDS prevention for at-risk youth and/or adults: Program Archive on Sexuality, Health, and Adolescence (PASHA); and Computer-Based HIV Prevention Interventions for African American Women (SAHARA).

As program director of PASHA, she oversees researching new and innovative effective interventions in the areas of primary/secondary pregnancy prevention and STI/HIV/AIDS prevention for youth and works with the original program developers to create user-friendly replication kits. As project director for the SAHARA program, she developed the storyboards and scripts for two interactive, new media interventions—one for African American women, and the second for Hispanic women.

Prior to joining Sociometrics, Benner completed a masters of public administration at the American University in Washington, DC, with an emphasis on the impact of state and local regulations on minors' access to family planning and reproductive health services without parental consent. She is also a full-time Yoga instructor and hypnotherapist.

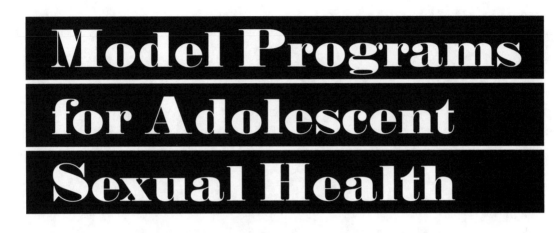

Model Programs for Adolescent Sexual Health

Evidence-Based HIV, STI, and Pregnancy Prevention Interventions

EDITORS Josefina J. Card, PhD   Tabitha A. Benner, MPA

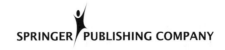

SPRINGER PUBLISHING COMPANY

New York

Springer Publishing Company, LLC
11 West 42nd Street
New York, NY 10036
www.springerpub.com

Acquisitions Editor: Jennifer Perillo
Production Editor: Julia Rosen
Cover design: Mimi Flow
Composition: Apex Publishing, LLC.

08 09 10 11/ 5 4 3 2 1

Library of Congress Cataloging-in-Publication Data

Model programs for adolescent sexual health : evidence-based HIV, STI, and pregnancy
prevention interventions/Josefina J. Card, Tabitha A. Benner, editors.
    p. ; cm.
  Includes bibliographical references and index.
  ISBN 978-0-8261-3824-8 (alk. paper)
 1. Sex instruction for teenagers.   2. Sexually transmitted diseases—Prevention.
3. Preventive health services for teenagers.   I. Card, Josefina J.   II. Benner, Tabitha.
  [DNLM: 1. Adolescent Health Services.   2. School Health Services.   3. Adolescent
Behavior.   4. Adolescent.   5. Pregnancy in Adolescence—prevention & control.
6. Sexually Transmitted Diseases—prevention & control.   WA 330 M689 2008]
HQ35.M595   2008
373.17'14—dc22   2007051941

Printed in Canada by Transcontinental.

Dedication

For Dr. Susan Newcomer of the National Institute of Child
Health and Human Development, staunch supporter of
developing and disseminating model programs for adolescent
sexual health

Contents

P A R T I

PRIMARY PREGNANCY PREVENTION PROGRAMS

P A R T   I I

SECONDARY PREGNANCY PREVENTION

P A R T   I I I

STI/HIV/AIDS PREVENTION

Acknowledgments

The development of this compilation of model programs for adolescent sexual health was funded by the National Institute of Child Health and Human Development under a series of grants and contracts to Sociometrics Corporation (Dr. Josefina J. Card, Principal Investigator).

Introduction

Funders and lawmakers are increasingly requiring that adolescent pregnancy and STI/HIV prevention programs be based on effective prevention strategies to be considered for funding. Moreover, for funding to continue, programs are now generally expected to document their own effectiveness in preventing adolescent pregnancy or STI/HIV or in changing the risky sexual behaviors antecedent to these problems. Behavioral change, as opposed to knowledge or attitudinal change alone, is the standard criterion of effectiveness. Included in the list of behaviors to be changed are those known to lead to adolescent pregnancy and sexually transmitted infections, such as early age at first intercourse, numerous sex partners, frequent intercourse, failure to use contraception and/or an STI-prophylactic (e.g., a condom) at first intercourse, and inconsistent use of effective contraception and/or a condom at every intercourse.

Originally established in the early 1990s and continuing to grow through the present day, the Program Archive on Sexuality, Health & Adolescence (PASHA) is a resource aimed at assisting teachers and health educators around the country in meeting the field's demands by: (1) facilitating access to proven effective adolescent pregnancy and adolescent STI/HIV prevention programs, and (2) encouraging rigorous re-evaluation of these programs at sites different from the ones in which they were developed. The PASHA collection includes program and evaluation materials from intervention programs judged by a Scientist Expert Panel to have demonstrated salutary impact on one or more of the fertility- or STI-related behaviors listed previously, in at least one subgroup of adolescents and/or young adults ages 10–19 (10–21 for STI/HIV prevention programs) in at least one site in the United States.

For each program in the PASHA collection, we prepare a box (henceforth called the PASHA program package or replication kit) containing all the materials required to replicate the promising intervention. We encourage rigorous re-evaluation of the program by including in each box two evaluation instruments: the original instrument used to demonstrate the program's effectiveness, as well as a generic Prevention Minimum Evaluation Data Set. Finally, a PASHA staff-prepared user's guide gives the program's history, rationale, the evidence for the program's effectiveness, and program implementation tips. Each PASHA program package can be used as a stand-alone intervention. Two or more program packages can also be creatively combined, or used in tandem, by communities engaged in coordinated, community-wide adolescent pregnancy or STI/HIV prevention initiatives.

This book describes the model programs comprising PASHA. Bridging research and practice, the model programs in the book pull together scientific research findings on the effectiveness of existing adolescent pregnancy prevention and STI/HIV prevention programs, highlighting the most promising of the lot for national attention and scrutiny. Readers interested in replicating or adapting any of the model programs in this book can acquire the program and evaluation materials from www.socio.com/pasha.htm.

PART I

Primary Pregnancy

Prevention Programs

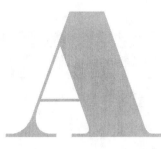

Programs Designed for Youths in Middle School or Junior High School

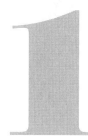

Reach for Health: A School-Sponsored Community Youth Service Intervention for Middle School Students

Diana Dull Akers, Tabitha A. Benner, and the Education Development Center Staff

Original Program Developers and Evaluators

Lydia O'Donnell, EdD
Alexi San Doval, MPH
Richard Duran, MSW
Deborah Haber, MEd
Rebecca Atnafou, MPH
Renée F. Wilson-Simmons, DrPH
    Education Development Center
    Newton, MA

Ann Stueve, PhD
    Division of Epidemiology
    Columbia University School of Public Health
    New York, NY

Reach for Health was supported by grants from the National Institute of Child Health and Human Development (Grants HD30101 and 1RO1HD35378) and the National Institute for Nursing Research (Grant NR03633).

3

Norma Johnson, MS, RN
Uda Grant, MS, RN
Helen Murray, MS, RN
   Department of Nursing
   Medgar Evers College
   City University of New York
   New York, NY

PROGRAM ABSTRACT

Summary

Originally implemented in two middle schools in Brooklyn, New York, in the mid-1990s, *Reach for Health* (RFH-CYS) is a service-learning intervention that combines community field placements with classroom health instruction to help middle school students develop the knowledge, attitudes, and skills that will keep them safe and healthy. Through field placements in various health and social service settings, students have the opportunity to experience the sense of empowerment and accomplishment that comes from being asked to do something meaningful, and doing it well. Back in the classroom, they are provided with the information, skills, and support they need to reinforce their community service experiences through health instruction that focuses on reducing risks related to early and unprotected sex as well as other health-compromising behaviors.

Several key features of *RFH-CYS* increase the likelihood of success and enhance ease of implementation:

 RFH-CYS is based on a theoretical model of behavior change. The program is grounded in the theories of social development and social learning, which help explain why young adolescents behave as they do. *RFH-CYS* also highlights four positive themes in young people's lives: protection, responsibility, interdependence, and affirmation of positive behaviors.

 RFH-CYS is designed for diverse student audiences. The program is based on research exploring the culture-, gender-, and developmental-based reasons why people engage in unhealthy behaviors. Community placements are tailored to the needs, interests, and developmental levels of students or groups of students. Lessons are active and geared toward diverse learning styles. Materials offer opportunities for creative thinking as well as for critical analysis.

 RFH-CYS is easily integrated into school health programs. Both the service learning and the curriculum are designed to supplement rather than replace existing health education programs offered in middle schools. *RFH-CYS* can be easily adapted to any health curriculum and will support these programs by providing clear, consistent prevention messages as well as the opportunity to practice important health-promoting skills.

Further, evaluation of *RFH-CYS* demonstrates that the program has a positive impact on reducing risky behaviors. Compared with students in control groups, students participating in the *RFH-CYS* program were

 significantly *less likely* to report recent intercourse at 6-month and 2-year follow-up;

- significantly *less likely* to report sexual initiation at 6-month and 2-year follow-up;
- *less likely* to report recent sex without a condom or other birth control at 6-month and 2-year follow-up;
- *less likely* to report violent behaviors at 6-month follow-up.

The National Campaign to Prevent Teen Pregnancy has recognized *RFH-CYS* as a model sexually transmitted infection (STI)/HIV/AIDS prevention and teen pregnancy prevention program (Kirby, 2001).

Focus

☑ Primary pregnancy prevention ☑ Secondary pregnancy prevention ☑ STI/HIV/AIDS prevention

Original Site

☑ School based ☑ Community based ☐ Clinic based

Suitable for Use In

RFH-CYS was designed to be implemented in middle schools and surrounding community health care and social service settings such as day-care centers (in the 7th grade), or nursing homes, health clinics, or senior centers (in the 8th grade).

Approach

- ☑ Abstinence
- ☑ Behavioral skills development
- ☑ Community outreach
- ☐ Contraceptive access
- ☑ Contraceptive education
- ☑ Life option enhancement
- ☑ Self-efficacy/Self-esteem
- ☑ Sexuality/HIV/AIDS/STI education

Original Intervention Sample

In the fall of 1994, 1,157 students completed the baseline survey. Of these, 1,061 completed the spring follow-up in 1995. At baseline, the average ages of 7th and 8th graders were 12.2 and 13.3, respectively. About half of all participants completing both surveys were 8th graders (48.4%), and slightly more than half of the sample was female (52.8%). Almost all students identified themselves as non-Hispanic African American (79.2%) or Latino (15.9%).

During spring 1998, 195 students completed a 10th-grade survey. Almost all students identified themselves as non-Hispanic African American (71%) or Latino (26%).

Program Components

- ☑ Adult involvement
- ☐ Case management
- ☑ Group discussion
- ☑ Lectures
- ☐ Peer counseling/instruction
- ☐ Public service announcements
- ☑ Role play

☐ ☑ Video
☐ ☑ Other: Service learning

Program Length

RFH-CYS is an intensive intervention, taught over the course of a full school year in 7th and 8th grades. During the year, students spend approximately 3 hours per week in a supervised community placement. In addition to that off-site work, students receive weekly health lessons—35 lessons in the 7th grade and 30 in the 8th grade—that supplement the traditional health class curriculum.

Staffing Requirements/Training

Implementation of *RFH-CYS* requires collaboration between middle schools and community service sites. In the original implementation of *RFH-CYS, a full-time, on-site coordinator* was hired to manage activities between school and community sites as well as communication among various agents and players, including students, parents, school administrators, teachers, field-site mentors, and other community site staff.

At the middle school, *health teachers* delivered the classroom component of *RFH-CYS*. Teachers participated in four training sessions designed to prepare them to deliver *RFH* lessons led by experienced health education trainers.

At the community sites, *nursing students* and *other agency staff* mentored students and crafted and supervised community experiences. Staff participated in program orientation.

BIBLIOGRAPHY

Kirby, D. (2001). *Emerging answers: Research findings on programs to reduce teen pregnancy.* Washington, DC: National Campaign to Prevent Teen Pregnancy.

O'Donnell, L., Duran, R., San Doval, A., Breslin, M., Juhn, G., & Stueve, A. (1997). Obtaining written parent permission for school-based health surveys of urban young adolescents. *Journal of Adolescent Health, 21*(6), 376–383.

O'Donnell, L., Myint-U, A., O'Donnell, C., & Stueve, A. (2003). Long-term influence of sexual norms and attitudes on timing of sexual initiation among urban minority youth: Implications for prevention programs. *Journal of School Health, 73*(2), 68–75.

O'Donnell, L., O'Donnell, C., & Stueve, A. (2001). Early sexual initiation and subsequent sex-related risks among urban minority youth: The Reach for Health study. *Family Planning Perspectives, 33*(6), 268–275.

O'Donnell, L., Stueve, A., O'Donnell, C., Duran, R., San Doval, A., Wilson, R. F., et al. (2002). Long-term reductions in sexual initiation and sexual activity among urban middle schoolers in the Reach for Health service learning program. *Journal of Adolescent Health, 31*(1), 93–100.

O'Donnell, L., Stueve, A., San Doval, A., Duran, R., Atnafou, R., Haber, D., et al. (1999). Violence prevention and young adolescents' participation in community youth service. *Journal of Adolescent Health, 24*(1), 28–37.

O'Donnell, L., Stueve, A., San Doval, A., Duran, R., Haber, D., Atnafou, R., et al. (1999). The effectiveness of the Reach for Health Community Youth Service learning program in reducing early and unprotected sex among urban middle school students. *American Journal of Public Health, 89*(2), 176–181.

Related References by the Developers of *Reach for Health*

O'Donnell, L., Stueve, A., Wardlaw, D. M., & O'Donnell, C. (2003). Adolescent suicidability and adult support: The Reach for Health Study of urban youth. *American Journal of Health Behavior, 27*(6), 633–644.

O'Donnell, L., Stueve, A., & Wilson-Simmons, R. (2005). Aggressive behaviors in early adolescence and subsequent suicidality among urban youth. *Journal of Adolescent Health, 517,* 15–517, e.25.

O'Donnell, L., Stueve, A., Wilson-Simmons, R., Dash, K., Agronick, A., & JeanBaptiste, V. (2006). Heterosexual risk behaviors among urban young adolescents. *Journal of Early Adolescence, 26*, 87–109.

THE PROGRAM

Program Rationale and History

RFH-CYS was originally implemented and evaluated in two middle schools in Brooklyn, New York, during the mid-1990s.[1] The program combined service learning with health instruction in order to provide low-income, inner-city students with the information, skills, and support they needed to stay healthy. Working with youths at a critical developmental stage in their lives, the *RFH-CYS* program sought to promote health and reduce sexual risk taking and other health-compromising behaviors.

RFH-CYS built upon a preexisting community services program in Brooklyn's School District 13. The existing program was a collaborative effort between the school district, Medgar Evers College Department of Nursing, and several community service organizations in the area. Program expansion involved increasing the number of participating organizations to accommodate a larger number of students, and incorporating a classroom component on health education—the companion *RFH* curriculum.

The original curriculum consisted of 40 lessons in 7th grade and 34 lessons in 8th grade and was designed to supplement rather than replace the existing New York City health education program. Lessons were designed to be culturally relevant to the needs of urban youths and focus on risks related to early and unprotected sex, violence, and substance use. Teachers, parents, and students contributed extensively to development of the curriculum content in a series of advisory meetings and focus groups.

Theoretical Framework

Theories of social development and social learning, which seek to explain why young people behave the way they do, guided intervention development. Social development theories provide a model for understanding how a young person's life course is influenced by the availability of prosocial and antisocial opportunities, the rewards reaped from involvement in such opportunities, and the bonding to those groups that provide the opportunities. In other words, to reduce the likelihood of risky or antisocial behavior, youths must have opportunities for prosocial involvement (in the family, in school, or in the neighborhood). They then have to get involved in these opportunities. (To some extent this involvement depends on the youth's academic and social skills.) If involvement is meaningful and rewarding, youths may form bonds to the prosocial groups that offer the opportunities and share their beliefs.

Social learning theories—including such theories as social influence, planned behavior, and social inoculation—complement social development theories and suggest that behavior is learned, influenced, or mediated by the following:

- How young people perceive social norms (at the neighborhood, school, family, and peer levels)
- How young people assess information (regarding the benefits and costs of different actions, the expectations of significant others to behave a certain way, and their ability to do the right thing)
- How much youths rehearse or practice prosocial ways of thinking about or responding to pressures and influences

Thus, to reduce the likelihood of early sexual involvement and other health-compromising behaviors, youths must learn to

- challenge or demystify social norms that promote risky behaviors while also recognizing and embracing those community standards that encourage health-promoting behaviors;
- think critically about behaviors that put them at risk, seek alternative solutions to risky behavior, and act in ways that promote their health and well-being;
- rehearse or practice ways to resist future peer pressure to engage in risky behaviors.

The following principles, which bind together the two main elements of the program—community service and school health education—also guided intervention development:

- *Protection:* We must take action, individually and as a society, to protect our health and well-being as well as to protect the health and well-being of others in our community.
- *Responsibility:* We each must act responsibly, respecting ourselves and others, and identifying the things we can change in ourselves and our surroundings.
- *Interdependence:* We are all connected; therefore, our actions, the actions of our peers, and the actions of the greater community matter to all of us.
- *Affirmation of positive behaviors:* Our efforts to promote health in ourselves and our community are supported by members of our community, and we can take pride in staying healthy.

Drawing on these perspectives, *RFH-CYS* developers worked with urban communities to design, implement, and evaluate an intervention that affirmed health-promoting patterns of thinking and acting among youths.

Program Elements

RFH-CYS included two core elements: community field placements and the *RFH* sexuality curriculum. These two elements combined a youth development approach with skills-based learning that specifically focused on reducing sexual risk taking. Of the two elements, the service-learning component was crucial.

Community Field Placements

Well-selected community field placements provided young people with opportunities to contribute to their communities in ways that were rewarding for both students and the agencies they served. At the beginning of each school term, students participated in an orientation that defined the goals of service learning, provided codes of conduct for being in community settings, and prepared them for specific responsibilities and situations (such as what they would be likely to see in a nursing home and how to be respectful of elders). During this time, they

- learned more about the organization where they might be assigned;
- set personal goals for what they wanted to achieve in the field;
- recognized the importance of their role in the site where they would be working;
- made predictions about what to expect on-site;
- considered and, as necessary, challenged their attitudes about the population with whom they would be working.

At the completion of the orientation lessons, students received an *RFH-CYS* jacket and an identification badge to wear to their field placements.

After orientation, 7th and 8th graders were assigned to two different field placements per academic year (to broaden exposure and maintain interest), for a total of approximately 90 hours (3 hours per week/30 sessions). This included both travel time to the sites and debriefing sessions back in the classroom. Unlike less-organized volunteer work in the community, *RFH-CYS* was a group experience. In most settings, classrooms were divided into two or three groups of students and then assigned to placements by group. Students then went to their field placements with their peers and accompanying teachers. Transportation was provided.

Within a field placement, students were assigned to a specific area where they could perform a variety of tasks under the direction of field-site staff who served as mentors. They also had the opportunity at the end of their visit for on-site informal interactions with adults. In the field, students provided service in health settings, such as nursing homes, senior centers, full-service clinics, and child day-care centers. In these settings, students performed a variety of tasks tailored to the needs and interests of individual students or groups of students and to students' maturity and developmental levels. Examples of tasks included reading to elders; assisting and observing doctors and dentists during medical examinations; clerical tasks; assisting with meals; and helping with exercise, recreation, and arts and crafts groups. Back in their classroom, students shared their experiences in debriefing sessions used to reinforce skills in decision making, communication, information seeking, health advocacy, and other areas.

Sexuality Curriculum

The *RFH* curriculum contains ten 7th-grade and ten 8th-grade lessons on healthy development and sexuality and was designed to supplement rather than supplant existing health curricula. The curriculum focused on sexual behaviors that could result in pregnancy, HIV infection, and other STIs. Using developmentally appropriate and culturally relevant situations and student-centered, hands-on, interactive classroom activities aimed at reaching all learners, the curriculum aimed to help students choose healthy options, communicate their needs effectively, and avoid risky behaviors.

The curriculum also offered opportunities for students to learn and practice health-enhancing skills, including self-assessment, risk assessment, communication, decision making, goal setting, healthy self-management, and resistance or refusal skills.

The *RFH* sexuality curriculum drew from the *Teenage Health Teaching Modules (THTM)*, a nationally recognized and independently evaluated comprehensive school health curriculum. It also drew from the *Michigan Model* and other research-based curricula, including *Reducing the Risk, Postponing Sexual Involvement,* and *Being Healthy.*

The curriculum gave clear messages about the importance of risk reduction and the consequences of early and unprotected sex. The behavior goals, teaching methods, and materials were appropriate to the age, sexual experience, and culture of the students. For example, greater attention was paid to refusal skills and reasons not to have sex than to the use of protection, although this also was addressed.

While the original intervention included lessons on violence and substance abuse prevention, the adolescent growth, development and sexuality lessons are the only ones included in this replication kit, given the intervention's predominant focus on reducing sexual risk taking. Should you opt to enhance the sexuality curriculum with lessons on substance use and/or violence prevention, there are many effective programs from which to choose—some of which are described in this book.

Program Implementation

Implementation of *RFH* requires advanced planning. While the objectives you set for your milieu (for example, the number of students, community sites, and how to integrate *RFH* into existing health education efforts) will influence the way your school implements *RFH-CYS*, there are some factors critical to its successful delivery. These factors include a team of well-prepared staff in the school and at community placement sites, parent involvement, well-vetted and well-selected community placement sites, and in-class time for reflection. Each of these factors is described in greater detail below.

Staff Involvement

At minimum, the *RFH-CYS* team consists of the following individuals at the school:

- *An administrator* (e.g., superintendent, principal, assistant principal) with the power to allocate human and material resources to the program.
- *Health education teachers* responsible for conducting the *RFH* curriculum lessons, selecting and working with community placement sites, and integrating service into the curriculum.

And at the community placement site, the team consists of these individuals:

- *A manager* with the power to allocate human and material resources to the program, oversee mentoring and supervision of students, and answer questions or problems as they arise;
- *Community agency staff* responsible for mentoring students as well as crafting and supervising community service experiences.[2]

Further, of critical importance to achieving buy-in at the community level as well as responding to local norms and concerns will be the establishment of an *advisory board*. These boards should be established early in the preparation process. The board should include several youth representatives, given that service learning is a youth development model. School administrators who sanction the program and teachers responsible for its day-to-day delivery should also sit on the advisory board, as should representatives from the field placement sites and *parents*.

Schools might also consider hiring or assigning a hands-on leader or *coordinator* to introduce the program and usher it through implementation. One of the biggest challenges to implementing the original *RFH-CYS* program was the coordination of activities across institutions. To deal with the challenges of creating field-visit schedules, field-site supervision, and transportation for students, *RFH-CYS* hired a full-time, on-site project coordinator. This person coordinated activities between school and community sites as well as communication among the various agents and players, including students, parents, school administrators, teachers, field-site mentors, and other community site staff. Specifically, this coordinator

- developed a protocol for student travel to and from field sites;
- reviewed teacher performance and provided feedback;
- recruited new field sites;
- conducted focus groups with students; and
- visited field sites to monitor activities.

Staff preparation was vital to the successful implementation of *RFH-CYS*. The training, delivered by the original developers, provided an overview and rationale for the program, as well as opportunities for participants to observe lessons, practice teaching, and receive feedback from their peers. Training was conducted in a workshop format, using interactive teaching techniques such as role-playing and small-group work to emphasize key points. Those attending the training included health and physical education teachers as well as teachers drawn from other subject areas and assigned to teach *RFH-CYS*. Thus, teachers had varying levels of expertise and experience with the health curriculum. The trainers also worked with small groups of teachers throughout the school year, as the different *RFH* curriculum units were delivered.

In addition to the primary focus on delivering the health curriculum, the training devoted time to describing and discussing the rationale of service learning and the teacher's role as facilitator of students' community placement experiences. Teachers practiced generating open-ended questions to promote student reflection. They generated ideas for leading students in debriefing and reflection activities as well as strategies for incorporating student self-assessment of their learning in the community.

Members of the community involved in the service-learning placements, including students and faculty from local community colleges, also attended the training sessions. Such support contributed to the strength of the school–community collaboration that was required to maintain a service-learning program.

Parent Involvement

If encouraged to participate, parents assist with a variety of tasks such as providing transportation to service sites and helping with fund-raising and public relations events. They play an important role in program planning. One way strong school–family partnerships can be forged is via a pledge or compact—a written agreement among the school, *RFH-CYS* students, and their parents to work together to enhance student learning and create effective school–family partnerships. School officials and parents collaborate to determine the feasibility and nature of such a pledge.

Although there are many benefits to strong school–family partnerships, there are also many challenges that must be addressed. These challenges may include

- conflicting values and beliefs, based in large part on social class and/or racial and ethnic differences;
- school concerns related to loss of control;
- family fears related to insufficient experience dealing with schools;
- the limited time available to working families for involvement in school activities;
- the difficulties of balancing school and program requirements with parental interests.

Parents are more likely to welcome service-learning programs in schools that open their doors to families and the larger community for after-hours recreational activities and parent education classes, and in schools where parents are viewed as true partners in their child's educational process. However, if only a small group of parents is currently involved in school activities, they can be called on to help develop parent support for community youth service. For example, parents can assist staff in forming an *RFH-CYS* parent advisory committee or identifying possible representatives to serve on the advisory board.

Whether serving as members of an advisory committee or planning team, parents are able to make significant contributions to the development, effective operation, and continued existence of *RFH-CYS*. Among other things, they can help identify student needs and assess community deficits and resources, explain potential parental concerns and expectations (as well as help address them), and assist in mapping out a role for parents and clarifying the roles of other participants. As with any program that addresses health-risk behaviors and, specifically, topics related to sexuality and HIV transmission, parental and community support for implementation is one of the best ways to ensure that the program will not meet with opposition once implemented.

Exhibits 1.1 and 1.2 offer samples of a parent information letter and parent permission form.

EXHIBIT 1.1 SAMPLE PARENT INFORMATION LETTER

Dear Parents:

Our school needs you! NAME OF SCHOOL is part of a special new program called *Reach for Health*. This program provides opportunities for your child to participate in community service activities at local day-care and senior centers as well as to receive a new health curriculum. The purpose of the program is to help make better school health programs for boys and girls who live in NAME OF COMMUNITY.

Through Reach for Health, NAME OF SCHOOL is committed to helping students learn to stay healthy by teaching them how to do the following:

- Choose healthy options
- Realize their potential
- Avoid risky behaviors
- Cope effectively in their school and community

As part of this special program, we are asking for your permission for your child to participate in the community service activities. If you grant permission, your child will spend about 3 hours a week at a community site such as a day-care center or senior citizen home. Some activities that students may participate in include reading to the elderly or to children, assisting with meals, and helping with arts and crafts. The school will provide transportation to and from the site, and students will have adult supervision at all times. In addition, all students will receive an orientation before they start their community service. This orientation will prepare your child for what to expect when he or she arrives at the community site for the first time. Finally, students will have a chance to talk about their experiences and ask questions or voice concerns when they are back in their health classes.

Whether or not you give permission for your child to participate in the community service activities, we need you to sign and return the enclosed consent form in the self-addressed, stamped envelope. If you have any questions or would like more information, please call the project coordinator at TELEPHONE NUMBER.

Sincerely,

NAME

Principal

EXHIBIT 1.2 SAMPLE PARENT PERMISSION FORM

REACH FOR HEALTH
Community Service Activities
PARENT PERMISSION FORM

Your Child's Name: _____

Your Child's Date of Birth: _____

Please circle YES or NO below.

YES, I give permission for my son/daughter to participate in the community service activities that are part of the **Reach for Health** program.

NO, I do not give permission for my son/daughter to participate in the community service activities that are part of the **Reach for Health** program.

_____   _____
Signature of Parent or Guardian   Date

_____   _____
Name of Parent or Guardian   Phone Number
(Please Print)

WHETHER OR NOT YOU GRANT PERMISSION FOR YOUR CHILD TO
PARTICIPATE IN THE COMMUNITY SERVICE ACTIVITIES, PLEASE SIGN
THIS FORM AND RETURN IT IMMEDIATELY IN THE SELF-ADDRESSED,
STAMPED ENVELOPE TO

Reach for Health Project Coordinator
Smith Junior High
55 Main Street
Any Town, USA 00001

Community Site Selection

Simply putting students in a community agency several times a week will not ensure that they have a meaningful experience. Assignments and placements need to be tailored to the needs and interests of individual students or groups of students and to students' maturity and developmental levels. When researching community placements and service-learning experiences, keep in mind that young adolescents

- can be involved in planning but need to be pushed to follow through;
- will discuss current events, so political and societal issues should be incorporated into reflection activities;

    ☐ are still forming their identities and developing relationships with peers, members of the opposite sex, family, siblings, and friends, so be flexible and give them the opportunity to interact with others of all ages and sexes;

    ☐ may evade difficult tasks and make unrealistic choices, so give them a lot of support and guidance around realistic choices, and push them to try new tasks.

The first step in selecting agencies that can cater to the developmental needs of middle school students is to learn as much as possible about them. Interested agencies are identified by working through the school and other community contacts, and then visited by school/program staff. During the initial information-seeking stage, school and community leaders can share the goals of the program; determine together whether the setting is appropriate for young adolescents; and decide whether the agency's mission, values, and goals are consistent with those of the school and the *RFH-CYS* program. This is the time to discuss the following questions:

    ☐ *Will students be safe?* Can the organization provide sufficient supervision and safety assurances? Is the agency in a safe location?

    ☐ *What staff members are available to help implement the program?* Is there a designated agency staff person present to assist the teacher with supervision as well as to answer questions and deal with any problems or issues that may arise? Are there staff members available to provide individual supervision and mentoring to students? Is there a sponsor willing to take on the responsibility of overseeing student placements?

    ☐ *Is the site easily accessible?* How close is the site? Can students get there by public transportation? Could they walk there?

    ☐ *Is there meaningful work to perform?* Would students be meeting an actual organizational need or just marking time? What knowledge and skills would the students be building? Is there an opportunity for students to see a tangible outcome as the result of their work? Is there some follow-through from the beginning of the assignment to the end?

    ☐ *Is that work compatible with the goals of* RFH-CYS? Does the agency's mission fit with the goals of the service-learning project?

Thus, selection of community agencies with both the commitment to youths and the capacity to oversee such an effort is important. There is no doubt that youths can provide valuable service to a variety of agencies, but it is also clear that the agencies are providing a service to youths. The matching of mutual needs is key to a successful community placement.

Once a site is selected for field placements, meetings between school and agency staff must be held to clarify roles and responsibilities. Agency staff members should be invited to attend some teacher-training events, as well as an orientation session at the school. During this session, agency staff can ask questions about the program as well as about important practical issues. School and agency staff can then review rules of conduct for student behavior and discuss what is reasonable to expect from youths of this age, including the types of guidance and support students might need in order to complete tasks successfully.

After identifying agencies whose missions and operating procedures match the goals and objectives of the service-learning program, it is necessary to establish lines of communication so that any potentially harmful issues can be discussed when and if they arise. Strong relationships with community agencies help make students' experiences more meaningful.

In-Class Reflection

Reflection is one of the most critical elements of a service-learning program. Indeed, it is what puts the "learning" in service learning and distinguishes it from community service. Service learning is guided by the principle that students do not learn solely by doing but rather from thinking about and reflecting upon what they are doing. Without reflection, students can still have a valuable experience, but may learn the wrong lessons or fail to build new skills. Providing in-class time to make observations, pose questions, and analyze their experiences provides students with a way to put their service experience into a context. The process gives students an opportunity to take an unstructured service activity and turn it into a constructive and productive learning experience.

RFH-CYS students went through a process of reflection before, during, and after service. Before service, students mentally and practically prepared for their field visits by learning more about the organization where they would be placed. In addition, with the help of teachers and nursing students, they set goals, thought about their role in the service environment, made predictions about what to expect, and looked at their current views of the population they would be helping. During the service experience, students highlighted problems they encountered, thought about solutions, posed questions, and shared feedback. All of these exercises were important for making the experience more real in a larger societal context. Finally, after the service experience was complete, students had the opportunity to step back and analyze what they learned. Having some distance from the project gave students time to think about how they made a difference, what they learned, and how to use their newly found knowledge and skills.

While some form of reflection was necessary at several stages during the service experience, the form it took varied from student to student. Each student experienced service in a different way and, therefore, needed to have a variety of options for expressing those lessons learned. Students reflected on their experiences, interactions, effectiveness of service provided, and the social problems leading to service by doing the following:

- Writing poems, letters, stories, and in journals
- Creating songs, dance, drawings, cartoons, and photographs
- Making scrapbooks that combined both writing and art
- Meeting face-to-face with teachers
- Getting together and talking with small groups of students

Keep in mind that students must choose reflection activities that are relevant and appropriate for their developmental stage and personality.

Although reflection activities should be led by students, this does not mean they should be disorganized or lack structure. Teachers must provide guidance and help students think about and understand the implications of their service experience. They are facilitators, asking questions and guiding discussion without injecting their own opinions or dominating the conversation. *RFH-CYS* teachers were trained in the curriculum and theoretical underpinnings of service learning, so they were aware of their role as facilitators. Teachers were encouraged to ask open-ended but pointed questions such as the following:

- What did you enjoy doing?
- What did you avoid doing?
- What did you learn about yourself or others?
- How did you feel about yourself and what you did?

These questions were designed to teach students how to think critically and creatively, make effective observations, analyze new experiences, and pose solutions to key problems. Students working in places like elder-care homes, day-care centers, and health clinics encountered illness, poverty, disabilities, and aging—all issues that raise key questions for young people. Finding unique and creative ways to tap into each student's thoughts on these issues and the service experience is the key to effective reflection activities.

PROGRAM EVALUATION

The Original Evaluation

Objective

RFH-CYS was originally conceived as a school-based, service-learning intervention designed to reduce sexual risk taking as well as other health-compromising behaviors among African American and Latino youths in urban areas. Key outcome indicators included reports of sexual initiation, recent sexual intercourse, and contraceptive use with recent sexual intercourse.

Intervention

Students participated in mentored community service activities in health care settings and then reflected upon and evaluated these experiences back in the classroom. Community field placements were also linked to comprehensive health instruction that focused on reducing risks related to early and unprotected sex, violence, and substance use.

Design

In 1994, two large middle schools in Brooklyn, New York, were recruited to participate in a service-learning intervention designed to reduce sexual risk taking as well as violence and substance abuse. One school was designated as the intervention school, the other as the control. A total of 68 classrooms participated in the initial implementation. In the control school, 33 classrooms (584 students) received the standard New York City health education program, which includes some mandated lessons on drugs and AIDS. Within the intervention school, 22 classrooms (222 students) were randomly assigned to receive the core *RFH* curriculum (classroom component only). The remaining 13 intervention classrooms (255 students) received the service learning *and* the *RFH* curriculum (community field placements and classroom component combined).

The sites were closely matched in terms of student-body size and ethnicity (more than 700 students in each school, 99% combined African American and Hispanic), a high-risk health profile (rates of violence-related injuries, HIV, STIs, teen pregnancy, etc.), a high-risk academic profile (below-grade standardized test scores, low attendance, low high school graduation rates), and limited access to resources (including a Title I poverty index above the New York City average, and limited school-based health programs). The majority of the students at the two sites scored substantially below the New York City average on standardized tests; fewer than a third scored above the 50th percentile in math, and fewer than 40% scored above the 50th percentile in reading.

Data Collection Procedures

The classroom health surveys were conducted in fall 1994 and spring 1995. Before students could participate, research staff obtained written informed consent from both students and parents. About 6 weeks before survey administration, parent consent letters (in both English and Spanish) were distributed to all students. The letters described the purpose and content of the survey, which

- was designed to help identify types of health programs that would work best for New York City students;
- asked questions about behaviors (e.g., fighting, taking drugs, and early sexual relationships) that place students' health at risk;
- included questions about behaviors (e.g., doing well in school and playing sports) that protect students' health.

Letters assured parents that survey responses would be confidential, and that students would be able to skip any question they chose not to answer or not take the survey at all. Consent packages also informed parents that neither they nor anyone else at the school would have access to the responses.

Research staff made multiple attempts to enlist student and teacher support in returning completed forms. They offered substantial incentives to encourage the return of signed forms, whether or not participation consent was granted. Schools received gift certificates ($250) when 90% of the forms were returned. Teachers received smaller gift certificates when their classes returned 90% of the signed forms. Students who returned their signed forms received an *RFH* T-shirt (each school held a design contest) with the winning design.

Approximately 20% of parents either did not give consent or did not return the survey. Although the surveys were available at school offices for parental review prior to making a decision, schools reported that no parents requested this option.

Research staff administered both baseline and follow-up surveys in group/classroom settings using pencil and paper format. Each survey contained approximately 250 items. Gender and school grade questions were asked directly. Ethnicity was assessed via separate questions. Other questions addressed the following topics:

- Lifetime experience with intercourse
- Recent intercourse
- Use of protection (condoms with or without other birth control) with recent intercourse
- Fighting
- Threatening to beat up, cut, stab, or shoot others
- Weapon carrying and use
- Social desirability issues

Final Sample Composition

In the fall of 1994, 1,157 students completed the baseline survey (74.7% of eligible students). Researchers conducted multiple survey sessions to ensure that all students who had parental consent were included in the survey. Of these, 94% were surveyed. In the spring of 1995, 1,061 students completed the follow-up survey (91.7% retention). Nearly all students who did not complete the spring survey were no longer students in the study sites.

At baseline, the average ages of 7th and 8th graders were 12.2 and 13.3, respectively; 48.4% were 8th graders, and 47.2% were male. Students self-identified as Hispanic (15.9%), non-Hispanic African American (79.2%), or other (4.9%, including missing data). Of the 1,061 students who completed both the fall and spring surveys, 255 participated in the *RFH-CYS* intervention, and 222 participated in the curriculum-only *RFH;* the remaining 584 served as controls.

Evaluation Results

Results of the evaluation demonstrated that the *RFH-CYS* program had a positive impact on reducing sexual behaviors of middle school students at risk for HIV, STIs, and unintended pregnancy. Those students who received the strongest intervention (curriculum plus service learning) showed the greatest gains. The evaluation also demonstrated that *RFH-CYS* had a positive impact on reducing violent behaviors, particularly among 8th-grade students.

Sexual Initiation and Recent Sex

Significant differences in sexual initiation rates were observed between baseline and follow-up among students reporting no sexual activity at baseline. At follow-up, 13.0% of the *RFH-CYS* group reported having had sex, compared with 17.3% of curriculum-only *RFH* participants and 21.2% of control group students. *RFH-CYS* students who were not virgins at baseline were less likely to report recent sex (within the last 3 months) (51.5%) at follow-up as compared to *RFH* students (60.9%) and their control group counterparts (59.4%).

A logistical regression analysis (controlling for recent sex at baseline, gender, and grade) revealed that students participating in the *RFH-CYS* program were significantly less likely ($p < .05$) to report recent intercourse at follow-up than were the students in either the control group or the *RFH* curriculum-only group. There was a positive trend ($p < .08$) for students in the curriculum-only condition versus their peers in the control condition.

The research team also found that the effect of participating in *RFH-CYS* was stronger among 8th graders than among 7th graders. It is worth noting that the 8th-grade *RFH-CYS* program was more intensive than the 7th-grade program. Eighth grade students had two separate field assignments during the year with higher levels of responsibility than their 7th-grade counterparts. They also had additional orientation sessions, which prepared them for their field assignments.

Recent Sex Without a Condom and Without Birth Control

When asked in the baseline survey about condom use during recent sex, 34.7% of the control group who had had recent sex reported doing so *without* a condom. By comparison, 48.3% of *RFH* curriculum-only students and 42.6% of *RFH-CYS* students reported recent sex without a condom. At follow-up, those numbers had changed to 37.7% control (an increase from 34.7%), 35.6% *RFH* curriculum-only (a decrease from 48.3%), and 26.7% *RFH-CYS* (a decrease from 42.6%).

At baseline, 38.1% of the sexually active control group members reported having had recent sex without a condom or other form of birth control. Among *RFH* curriculum-only students and *RFH-CYS* group members, the figures were 58.6% and 48.9%, respectively. At follow-up, the control group percentage had increased to 46.1%, while the *RFH* curriculum-only students and *RFH-CYS* group percentages decreased to 53.6% and 40.5%, respectively. These figures are summarized in Table 1.1.

Special Education Students

Among special education students, it appeared that the curriculum-only *RFH* was most effective in positively impacting sexual risk behaviors, as shown in Table 1.2.

Summary

Overall, the researchers concluded that a well-organized intervention program, of sufficient intensity, that includes a community youth services component can have

Baseline and Follow-Up Risk Behavior Percentages Among Intervention and Control Groups (All Participants)

	BASELINE PERCENTAGE	FOLLOW-UP PERCENTAGE	DELTA
Ever had sex			
Control	32.5	40.7	+8.2
RFH	34.3	37.7	+3.4
RFH-CYS	27.8	32.2	+4.4
Recent sex			
Control	22.9	28.2	+5.3
RFH	25.7	29.1	+3.4
RFH-CYS	21.0	20.6	−0.4
Recent sex without condom			
Control	34.7	37.7	+3.0
RFH	48.3	35.6	−12.7
RFH-CYS	42.6	26.7	−15.9
Recent sex without birth control			
Control	38.1	46.1	+9.0
RFH	58.6	53.6	−5.0
RFH-CYS	48.9	40.5	−8.4

Baseline and Follow-Up Risk Behavior Percentages Among Intervention and Control Groups (Special Education Students Only)

	BASELINE PERCENTAGE	FOLLOW-UP PERCENTAGE	DELTA
Ever had sex			
Control	34.4	60.5	+26.1
RFH	45.2	32.4	−12.8
RFH-CYS	26.9	31.3	+4.4
Recent sex			
Control	24.2	55.3	+31.1
RFH	38.1	27.0	−11.1
RFH-CYS	15.4	18.8	+3.4
Recent sex without condom			
Control	42.9	35.3	−7.6
RFH	57.1	30.0	−27.1
RFH-CYS	100.0	0.0	−100.0
Recent sex without birth control			
Control	33.3	55.6	+22.3
RFH	53.3	33.3	−22.0
RFH-CYS	50.0	0.0	−50.0

a positive effect on reducing sexual risk behaviors among middle school students. Such programs can also be effective in reducing violent behaviors among 8th graders.

The study also demonstrated that curriculum-only programs can be effective in reducing sexual risk behaviors among students in special education classes.

Parallel Study

Additional funding enabled the research team to follow a group of students from their baseline survey in fall 1994 (7th grade only, n = 1,287) through a follow-up survey at the completion of their 10th-grade year in spring 1998 (n = 970). These students were from three middle schools in Brooklyn, New York. They were tested at four data points: 7th grade, fall and spring; 8th grade, spring; and 10th grade, spring. The average age at baseline was 12.2, and 16.1 at final follow-up.

The core survey questions remained the same throughout the study, but some questions were added/modified to account for maturation and to prevent boredom. The study revealed that minority adolescents who initiate sexual activity early tend to engage in behaviors that place them at high risk for negative health outcomes. Early sexual initiators had an increased likelihood of having multiple partners, forcing a partner to have sex, having frequent intercourse, and having sex while drunk or high.

Long-Term Follow-Up Study

To evaluate the sustained effectiveness of *RFH-CYS* on reducing sexual initiation and recent sex, researchers at EDC conducted a follow-up survey in the spring of 1998, as they were completing their 10th-grade year (whether or not they continued to attend school regularly). This evaluation point was nearly 4 years after initial enrollment (fall 1994, 7th grade) and 2 years after completion of the middle school program. Self-reported sexual behaviors of youths who participated in *RFH-CYS* (combined service learning and health curriculum) were compared with those of controls receiving the *RFH* classroom curriculum alone.

Findings indicate that *RFH-CYS* participants were significantly less likely than controls to report sexual initiation. Those receiving 2 years of the intervention reported slightly better odds of delaying sexual initiation than those receiving 1 year of *RFH-CYS*. Among those who were virgins at 7th grade, 80% of males in the *RFH* curriculum-only condition had initiated sex, compared with 61.5% who received 1 year of *RFH-CYS*, and 50% who received 2 years. Among females, the figures were 65.2%, 48.3%, and 39.6%, respectively.

NOTES

1. A full set of program materials, including sample curricula, teacher's guide, videotape, evaluation materials, and more, is available for purchase from Sociometrics at http://www.socio.com/pasha.htm.
2. In the original implementation of *RFH-CYS*, nursing students from the same community and ethnic and cultural backgrounds as middle school students served as educators, mentors, and advocates for health promotion.

Human Sexuality— Values & Choices: A Values-Based Curriculum for 7th and 8th Grades

Starr Niego, Alisa Mallari, M. Jane Park, and Janette Mince

Original Program Developer and Evaluator

Michael Donahue, PhD
  The Search Institute
  Minneapolis, MN
  HealthStart Inc.
  St. Paul, MN

PROGRAM ABSTRACT

Summary

Developed for use in 7th- and 8th-grade classrooms, *Human Sexuality—Values & Choices* (hereafter referred to as *Values & Choices*) aims to reduce teenage pregnancy by promoting seven core values that support sexual abstinence and healthy social relationships. The curriculum—including 15 student lessons and 3 adult-only sessions—is distinguished by: (a) an emphasis on parent–child communication; and (b) the use of a standardized, video-assisted format. Participants gain

Human Sexuality—Values & Choices was supported by a contract from Office of Adolescent Pregnancy Programs, U.S. Department of Health and Human Services.

mastery through role plays, group discussions, and behavioral skills exercises. Following a field test in nine schools, program participants showed a greater understanding of the risks associated with early sexual involvement and expressed increased support for postponing sexual activity, as compared to a control group of their peers.

Focus

☑ Primary pregnancy   ☐ Secondary pregnancy   ☐ STI/HIV/AIDS
   prevention   prevention   prevention

Original Site

☑ School based   ☐ Community based   ☐ Clinic based

Suitable for Use In

This program is suitable for use in schools and any other community organization that provides education or services to 7th and 8th graders.

Approach

- ☑ Abstinence
- ☐ Behavioral skills development
- ☐ Community outreach
- ☐ Contraceptive access
- ☐ Contraceptive education
- ☑ Life option enhancement
- ☐ Self-efficacy/self-esteem
- ☑ Sexuality/HIV/STI education

Original Intervention Sample

Age   56% age 12, 33% age 13, 7% age 14.
Gender   48% male.
Race/ethnicity 62% White, 19% African American, 10% Hispanic, 9% Other (includes Asian and Native American).

Program Components

- ☑ Adult involvement
- ☐ Case management
- ☑ Group discussion
- ☑ Lectures
- ☐ Peer counseling/instruction
- ☐ Public service announcements
- ☑ Role play
- ☑ Video
- ☐ Other

Program Length

The 15 student lessons are designed to run 45–50 minutes each. The 3 parent sessions each last about 2 hours. The sequencing of the sessions is flexible.

Staffing Requirements/Training

There are no special requirements.

BIBLIOGRAPHY

Chilman, C. S. (Ed.). (1980). *Adolescent pregnancy and childbearing: Findings for research.* Washington, DC: Government Printing Office.

Donahue, M. J. (1987). *Technical report of the national demonstration project field test of human sexuality: Values & Choices.* Minneapolis, MN: Search Institute.

Search Institute. (1987). Educating youth about human sexuality: The case for a values-based approach. *Source, 3*(1).

Related References by the Developers of *Values & Choices*

Benson, P. L. (2002). Adolescent development in social and community context: a program of research. *New Directions for Youth Development, 95,* 123–147.

Leffert, N. (1997). Building assets: A positive approach to adolescent health. *Minnesota Medicine, 80*(12), 27–30.

Scales, P. C. (1999). Reducing risks and building developmental assets: Essential actions for promoting adolescent health. *Journal of School Health, 69*(3), 113–119.

THE PROGRAM

Program Rationale and History

HealthStart and the Search Institute initiated *Values & Choices* in 1983, as a 15-session curriculum for 7th- and 8th-grade students that included a three-session minicourse for parents.[1] The school-based program aimed to reduce teenage pregnancy by teaching not only "the facts" of human reproduction but also a core set of values supportive of sexual abstinence and healthy social relationships. Set in the context of a comprehensive sexuality education program, *Values & Choices* is distinguished by: (a) an emphasis on parental involvement across the curriculum; and (b) the use of a standardized, video-assisted format. The program, which targeted younger adolescents, measured changes in attitudes, knowledge, and intentions as indicators of future sexual behavior.

The intervention was developed under Title XX—Adolescent Family Life Demonstration Projects—a 1983 congressional amendment to the Public Health Service Act. As a national demonstration project, *Values & Choices* was sponsored by the Office of Adolescent Pregnancy Programs, U.S. Department of Health and Human Services, with additional private matching funds. Following the curriculum development process, researchers conducted an experimental field test and evaluation study in a diverse set of schools across five sites: Detroit, Michigan; Minneapolis and Grand Rapids, Minnesota; Denver, Colorado; and the San Francisco Bay area in California.

Since the original demonstration effort, *Values & Choices* has been implemented in more than 2,000 schools in the United States and Canada.

Seven Core Values

The program presented the following seven values as the basis for understanding human relationships in general, and sexuality in particular:

- Equality
- Honesty
- Respect
- Responsibility

- Promise keeping
- Self-control
- Social justice

The decision to emphasize values stemmed from research in social psychology demonstrating links between an individual's values and behavior. For example, research conducted during the 1970s found that college students who had been induced to change the relative importance they attached to particular values, including freedom and equality, later showed an increase in such behaviors as donating money to charitable organizations and enrolling in ethnic studies courses.

In 1996, the Search Institute slightly revised this list of values to reflect new research related to its *Healthy Communities–Healthy Youth* initiative. This revision had relatively minor implications for program implementation, which is described later in this section.

Theoretical Framework

Values & Choices applied Fishbein's Behavioral Intention Model, which argues that an action, such as the decision to have sex, results from an individual's intention to act. Such behavioral intentions, in turn, consist of four components:

1. *Beliefs* about the outcomes of actions
2. *Evaluations* of those outcomes
3. *Perceptions* of others' opinions about the act
4. *Motivation* to comply with others' opinions

In preliminary research for the program, 7th- and 8th-grade students expressed nine beliefs concerning the outcomes of sexual intercourse:

1. Getting pregnant (or getting someone pregnant)
2. Getting a sexually transmitted infection (STI)
3. Showing people that I love them
4. Pleasing my boyfriend/girlfriend
5. Being popular
6. Holding on to a boyfriend/girlfriend
7. Feeling worthwhile, feeling important
8. Feeling grown-up
9. Finding out what sex is like

Fishbein's Behavioral Intention Model recognizes that students' beliefs about intercourse may not be rational or logical. Nevertheless, these beliefs, in conjunction with evaluations, perceptions, and motivations, determine whether one will act. In addition, the program developers added values as a final component of their model.

Program Overview

In their field test of *Values & Choices,* researchers measured the relative importance of, and change over time in students' beliefs, evaluations, motivations, perceptions, and values regarding sexual decision making, as well as in students' overall intention to engage in sexual activity. The specific indicators and equations used to assess the program's effectiveness are described in greater detail later in this chapter.

The parental component of the program was tied to research associating positive parent–child communication on sexuality with both a delay in the onset of sexual intercourse and, among teens who did engage in intercourse, greater probability of effective contraception use (Chilman, 1980). The program developers reasoned that parental involvement could help reduce community opposition to sexuality education while enabling adults to reach informed decisions about their children's participation. In addition, it was hoped that the parental sessions would foster mutual support and encouragement among participants for discussing sexuality at home.

The program developers used video because of its convenience, perceived effectiveness, and popularity. Further, they believed that interviews with a racially, ethnically, and socioeconomically diverse sample of youths, as was feasible with prerecorded material, would carry greater significance for students. Finally, the standardized format could alleviate parents' concerns about the presentation of sensitive material to their children.

Program Objectives

The overall goal of the curriculum was to delay initial sexual involvement among 7th- and 8th-grade students. Three objectives supported this goal:

1. To decrease students' intention to engage in intercourse "while I am a teenager."
2. To strengthen values supporting sexual abstinence during adolescence.
3. To increase parent–child communication regarding sexuality.

Hypothesized Outcomes

For students participating in the *Values & Choices* program, the following outcomes were predicted:

Hypothesis 1: Effects on Students

- Increased support for sexual restraint during adolescence
- Decreased support for the idea that males have a stronger, less controllable sex drive
- Increased knowledge concerning human reproduction and the effects of adolescent pregnancy
- Increased frequency of conversations with parents concerning sexuality
- Decreased support for sexual coercion
- Increased support for values that will inhibit premature sexual involvement
- Decreased behavioral intention to engage in intercourse
- No change in overall attitude toward sexuality

Hypothesis 2: Effects of Parent Involvement

It was expected that the above effects would be stronger for those students whose parents also participated in the program.

Hypothesis 3: Effects of Other Important Variables

In their field test of the curriculum, researchers measured the influence of a number of background variables on program outcomes. Lacking sufficient information from previous investigations to predict the effects of these variables, the researchers hypothesized that the outcomes described above would be significant across different demographic categories regardless of students' gender, race, virginity status, or educational aspirations. Similarly, they predicted that the income and educational level of participants' parents would not affect the overall pattern of results.

Intervention Goals

Values & Choices aimed to promote sexual abstinence among adolescents, while addressing the full range of issues facing this age group. In addition, because youngsters tended to form their values during adolescence, the program encouraged students to incorporate values into sexual decision making and all social relationships.

Program Schedule

Program Outline

Each of the 15 student lessons was tied to one or more of the program's seven core values. Key concepts were defined and reinforced through in-class and at-home activities. Class sessions were designed to last approximately 45 to 50 minutes.

During the adult sessions, typically held on three weekday evenings, parents viewed the program videotape, met their child's teacher, and reviewed the course outline and homework activities for all 15 lessons. Parents received a manual (one per household) to assist them in discussing sexuality with their children, both in the context of the *Values & Choices* program, and in a more general way. Sessions were designed to last approximately 2 hours.

Listed below are the titles, goals, and original values for the student sessions.

Student Lessons

Lesson 1: Starting Out!

Goal: To introduce the program and establish a friendly atmosphere and basic ground rules for the course.

Values emphasized: Respect (primarily self-respect) (*Integrity*)

Lesson 2: What's Really Important?

Goals: (1) To increase students' understanding of the concept of values and the role of values in decision making. (2) To increase students' familiarity with the basic values promoted by this curriculum.

Values emphasized: All

Lesson 3: Changes

Goal: To promote an understanding of the physical changes in puberty and their relationships to sexuality.

Values emphasized: Respect, Responsibility (*Integrity*)

Lesson 4: More Changes

Goal: To promote an understanding of emotional changes in adolescence, especially sexual attraction, and to promote positive ways of dealing with emotions.

Values emphasized: Responsibility, Self-Control (*Restraint*)

Lesson 5: Equal Though Different

Goal: To promote equality and social justice for human beings, regardless of gender.

Values emphasized: Equality, Social Justice, Respect (*Integrity*)

Lesson 6: Making Choices

Goal: To help adolescents understand that choices are involved in most situations, and that in making choices, it helps to think about basic human values and possible consequences of choices.

Values emphasized: Honesty, Self-Control, Responsibility, Promise Keeping (*Restraint, Integrity, and Caring*)

Lesson 7: Going Out?

Goal: To explore various aspects of dating and to develop guidelines for acting in ways that will promote healthy development.

Values emphasized: Honesty, Self-Control, Equality, Responsibility, Respect (*Restraint, Integrity, and Caring*)

Lesson 8: Saying No

Goal: To help teens recognize sexual pressure and to present reasons and ways to say no to sexual pressure.

Values emphasized: Self-Control, Respect, Promise Keeping, Equality, Honesty (*Restraint, Integrity, and Caring*)

Lesson 9: Pregnancy and Birth

Goal: To promote an understanding of fetal growth and development, maternal changes, the process of labor and birth, and the influence of parents' health on the baby's well-being.

Values emphasized: Responsibility, Self-Control, Equality (*Restraint*)

Lesson 10: Planning

Goals: (1) To promote abstinence as the best method of avoiding pregnancy for teens. (2) To provide information on other available family planning methods.

Values emphasized: Responsibility, Respect, Equality (*Integrity*)

Lesson 11: Teenage Pregnancy—The Reality

Goal: To provide an understanding of the consequences of teenage pregnancy and the choices involved.

Values emphasized: Responsibility, Respect, Equality (*Restraint, Integrity, and Caring*)

Lesson 12: Teenage Pregnancy—The Choices

Goal: To provide an understanding of the consequences of teenage pregnancy and the choices involved.

Values emphasized: Responsibility, Respect, Equality (*Integrity*)

Lesson 13: Taking Chances

Goal: To promote awareness of STIs as a possible consequence of sexual activity, along with knowledge of treatment and prevention.

Values emphasized: Honesty, Responsibility, Self-Control, Social Justice (*Restraint and Integrity*)

Lesson 14: The Power of Touch

Goal: To promote an understanding of the difference between positive and abusive touch.

Values emphasized: Respect, Responsibility, Social Justice, Self-Control (*Restraint, Integrity, and Caring*)

Lesson 15: Moving On!

Goal: To apply the values and content of the course to practical situations faced by teens.

Values emphasized: All

Program Implementation

Prior to the first lesson, instructors should read all program materials and view the accompanying video. Included are current statistics on teen pregnancy, summaries of male and female sexual development, and additional resources to help prepare instructors to address questions from students and parents, as well as community concerns about the appropriateness of a sexuality education program. Issues concerning effective communication, personal disclosure, and the use of street versus slang language are discussed in the guide for effective teaching.

In addition, instructors will want to familiarize themselves with procedures for responding to three special issues likely to arise during the program: (a) confidentiality and mandated reporting of abuse, should students share personal experiences of such incidents; (b) laws and policies related to STIs, including testing, treatment, and reporting; and (c) student requests for counseling, family planning, and pregnancy testing, as well as parental notification laws regarding such services.

It is recommended that the first parent session take place before the student lessons begin. Teachers may wish to invite their principals to welcome participants.

Revised Values List

The Search Institute revised its values list slightly in 1996 to reflect research related to its *Healthy Communities–Healthy Youth* initiative. Specifically,

- *self-control* was renamed *restraint*;
- *equality* and *social justice* were combined;

- *promise keeping* and *respect* were folded into *integrity*;
- *caring* was added.

PROGRAM EVALUATION

The Original Evaluation

Design

The program's effectiveness was originally investigated in a field study conducted in nine schools across the country. The study compared the sexual attitudes of 7th- and 8th-grade students who completed the *Values & Choices* curriculum to those of a control group of teens selected from the same grades and schools. Data were collected with a self-report questionnaire administered to both groups of youths at three points in time:

- Time 1: before the start of *Values & Choices*
- Time 2: immediately following the lessons
- Time 3: 3 to 4 months following completion of the program

In addition, parents participating in the adult sessions were given brief questionnaires at Time 1 and Time 2.

The nine schools serving as study sites were located in five areas: Detroit, Michigan; Minneapolis and Grand Rapids, Minnesota; Denver, Colorado; and the San Francisco Bay area in California. The full sample included 657 students from rural, urban, and suburban communities, collectively representing a range of ethnic, racial, and socioeconomic characteristics.

Evaluation Questions

Three empirical questions guided the field study:

1. What effects does program participation have on 7th- and 8th-grade students? In particular, how effective is the course in
   - decreasing teenagers' intention to engage in intercourse "while I am a teenager"?
   - strengthening values supporting sexual restraint in adolescence?
   - increasing parent–child communication concerning sexuality?
2. What impact does parental participation have on student outcomes?
3. Do the effects of program participation vary with a student's gender, race, virginity status, family income, parental education, and personal educational aspirations?

All student data were gathered with a 100-item questionnaire developed and pilot tested for use with 7th- and 8th-grade populations. To assess students' attitudes toward sexual restraint, for example, respondents were asked whether they agreed or disagreed (on a 5-point Likert scale) with the following items: "Having sex is something that only adults should do" and "Even if I'm physically mature, that doesn't mean I'm ready to have sex." Individual items were combined into the following composite measures: Sexual Restraint Scale, Beliefs Concerning the Male Sex Drive, Sexual Knowledge Test, Parental Conversations Scale, Sexual Coercion Scale, Behavioral Intention to Engage in Intercourse, Perceptions and Motivations, Attitudes Toward Sexuality, and Values.

Parent data were gathered in a separate, shorter questionnaire assessing attitudes toward teen sexual involvement, frequency and scope of conversations with child concerning sex, and personal feelings about such conversations. Background data on the home environment and parents' age, marital status, and educational level were also collected. With the exception of the parental education variable, these measures were primarily used to address evaluation question #2, as listed above.

Data Collection Procedures

Prior to the start of the *Values & Choices* program, letters carrying the principal's endorsement were sent to the parents of all students enrolled in classes participating in the intervention. The research team explained the course's purpose and methods and requested consent for the child's participation. A preaddressed, stamped envelope addressed to the school was also enclosed.

Following a "school as its own control" strategy, a comparison group of students was constructed within each participating school. Parents of students enrolled in control classes received a separate letter and information packet. These materials highlighted both the importance of control groups to evaluation research and the potential for their child's later participation in the *Values & Choices* program.

Regional researchers administered the Time 1 questionnaire, in class and before the start of the lessons, to all students whose parents consented. Teens were assured that their questionnaire responses would be anonymous (e.g., school personnel and parents would not have access to them), and the phrase "Confidential—to be opened by Search Institute personnel only" was printed on the envelope containing each test booklet. After answering procedural questions, researchers asked students to respond the way they "really felt" to each of the test items. The remainder of the survey was self-administered.

Similar procedures were followed for the Time 2 and Time 3 administrations, as well as for the parent questionnaires.

Research Sample

Across field study sites, usable data from all three survey periods were gathered for 452 students in the treatment group and 205 control group students. With the exception of gender, for which the experimental group had a greater proportion of males (48% vs. 43%), few demographic differences were observed between the groups. Overall, 62% of respondents described themselves as White, 19% as African American, 8% as Hispanic, 3% as Asian or American Indian, and 4% as Other. The majority of students, approximately 70%, reported that they lived in two-parent families. More than half of the fathers and 40% of the mothers had completed college.

On measures of sexual behavior, 57% of students reported dating in the past year, and 20% described themselves as nonvirgins.

Evaluation Results

Analysis of the survey data revealed that the short-term intervention produced a number of immediate attitudinal changes in teens; long-term change, on the other hand, was far more difficult to sustain.

Effects on Student Attitudes

At Time 2, immediately following completion of the *Values & Choices* lessons, 7th- and 8th-grade participants showed

- increased support for sexual restraint;
- decreased belief that boys have stronger or more uncontrollable sex drives than girls;

■ increased knowledge of human reproduction;
■ increased belief that having intercourse can result in pregnancy;
■ increased belief that intercourse can result in STIs;
■ increased frequency of conversations concerning sexuality;
■ decreased intention to engage in intercourse while a teenager;
■ decreased support for the use of coercion in sexual relations.

The significance level for all effects was at least $p < .05$.

In the long term, as measured 3 to 4 months following participation in the program, *Values & Choices* students were still

■ less likely to believe that boys had stronger or more uncontrollable sex drives than girls;
■ more likely to believe that they could get an STI if they had teen sex;
■ more likely to believe that they could get pregnant if they had sex as a teenager.

Again, all effects were significant at least at the $p < .05$ level.

To illustrate one of the changes: Before *Values & Choices*, 33% of treatment group students believed it would be against their values to have sex as a teenager. Immediately following the program, 45% of treatment group students felt this way. Although the figure declined to 38% in the delayed posttest period, the proportion of students endorsing sexual restraint remained above the pretest level.

In evaluating their empirical model, the researchers compared students' behavioral intention to engage in sex across the three survey periods. Overall, on a 100-point intention scale, the control group showed no change over time, measuring 49.7 across all test periods. The treatment group, in contrast, showed a small but significant decline between Time 1 and Time 2 (from 50.7 to 46.5), followed by a small, significant increase to 48.4 at Time 3. Focusing on individual components of the model, the researchers found that values were most influential in determining whether a teenager would be likely to engage in sex.

Effects of Parental Participation

Only one significant effect was found for parental participation in the *Values & Choices* program. On measures of sexual knowledge, students whose parents attended the adult sessions showed a smaller decline in their scores over time, relative to their peers with nonparticipating parents. Yet the researchers' hypothesis was refuted, for parental participation had no effect on student attitudes toward sexual intercourse.

Effects of Other Important Variables

Three of the background variables—gender, virginity status, and race—showed consistent effects on the outcome measures. Compared to boys and nonvirgins, girls' and virgins' attitudes were less supportive of sexual activity during adolescence. Race showed consistent effects, and the other variables measured—income, parental education, and educational aspirations—appeared insignificant.

Summary

Overall, the researchers concluded that *Values & Choices* had a positive, short-term effect on the sexual attitudes and values of 7th- and 8th-grade students. As predicted, students completing the 15-session curriculum showed an increased understanding of human reproduction and the risks associated with early sexual activity, relative to their peers in the control group; they were also more likely to discuss such matters with their parents. In addition, these teens showed less support for the idea that boys' sexual drive is uncontrollable or that sexual coercion is acceptable. And they showed greater sexual restraint, expressing less intention to engage in intercourse as a teenager. Such effects were strongest for females and virgins.

However, in the follow-up survey taken 3 to 4 months after the program, only three effects remained significant. Compared with their control group peers, *Values & Choices* participants were still more likely to recognize the risks associated with sexual activity (e.g., STIs, pregnancy) and less likely to believe that boys' sex drives were uncontrollable. All other program effects had faded.

The researchers emphasized that their data fit the pattern typical of attitudinal change research, with significant short-term gains that weaken over time. Once the program ended, the researchers reasoned, students would have found little support in the media or their peer culture for the kinds of lessons promoted in the *Values & Choices* curriculum, notably sexual restraint in adolescence. Furthermore, in interpreting the small differences between many of the treatment and control group scores, the researchers suggested both maturation and spillover effects. First, some of the measures included in the study might be expected to change over time; for example, teenage students would become more knowledgeable about sex as they sought out new information. Second, with both groups of students attending the same schools, the attitudes and values of the control group might spill over to students in the treatment condition. The researchers noted that both processes would yield conservative measures of the program's effectiveness.

AWARDS AND RECOGNITION

Human Sexuality—Values & Choices: A Values-Based Curriculum of 7th and 8th Grades has received a number of awards, including the following:

- Certificate of Merit for Excellence in Education and Prevention for Adolescent Sexuality, American Medical Association
- Silver Apple, National Educational Film Video Festival
- Certificate of Merit, Chicago International Film Festival
- Award of Merit (Top 100 Products of the Year), Curriculum Product News
- Finalist, John Muir Medical Film Festival

VALUES & CHOICES IN THE COMMUNITY TODAY

In the past 3 years, *Values & Choices* has been implemented in communities in 17 states—ranging from Massachusetts to Oklahoma to Washington. It has also been implemented in Puerto Rico and Japan.

NOTE

1. A full set of program materials, including teacher's manual, curricula, activity masters, videotape, evaluation materials, parent guides, and more, is available for purchase from Sociometrics at http://www.socio.com/pasha.htm.

Project Taking Charge: A Pregnancy Prevention Program for Junior High School Youth

J. Barry Gurdin, Starr Niego, M. Jane Park, and Janette Mince

Original Program Developers

Carol Hunter-Geboy
  Prescott, AZ

Irene K. Lee
  Pine Bluff, AR

Janet Preston
  Logan, UT

Jerelyn B. Schultz
  College of Human Ecology
  Ohio State University
  Columbus, OH

Robin White
  Ankeny, IA

Project Taking Charge was supported by grants from the American Home Economics Association (now called the American Association of Family and Consumer Sciences) and the U.S. Office of Adolescent Pregnancy Programs, Department of Health and Human Services (APH 000817–04).

Original Program Evaluator

Stephen R. Jorgensen, PhD
Department of Human Development and Family Studies
Texas Tech University
Lubbock, TX

PROGRAM ABSTRACT

Summary

Project Taking Charge, developed for junior high school home economics classrooms, integrates family life education with lessons on vocational exploration, interpersonal relationships, decision making, and goal setting. A key premise of the intervention is that vocational planning can lead to attractive alternatives to early sexual involvement and parenthood. In a special job-shadowing exercise, for example, students observe and interview individuals working in a variety of occupations. In addition, placing a strong emphasis on values, *Project Taking Charge* emphasizes that equality, self-control, respect for others, responsibility, honesty, promise keeping, self-esteem, dependability, trustworthiness, justice, and fairness lead to good citizenship, fulfilling relationships, and sound personal ethics. Along with values, *Project Taking Charge* promotes abstinence as the correct choice for adolescents. No material on contraception is included.

The curriculum comprises five instructional units that are divided into 27 class lessons. There are also three parent–youth sessions during which adults are encouraged to communicate their own sexual standards and assist teens in defining and attaining occupational goals.

A field study was conducted with 136 youths from three low-income communities with elevated rates of teen pregnancy. Six months following the program, participants showed significant gains in knowledge of sexual development, sexually transmitted infections (STIs), and the risks of adolescent pregnancy, relative to a comparison group of students. There was also some evidence, falling just short of significance, that participation was associated with a delay in the initiation of sexual intercourse.

Focus

☑ Primary pregnancy prevention   ☐ Secondary pregnancy prevention   ☐ STI/HIV/AIDS prevention

Original Site

☑ School based   ☐ Community based   ☐ Clinic based

Suitable for Use In

Although it was originally implemented in school classrooms, the curriculum can also be presented by health educators in community-based organizations.

Approach

- ☑ Abstinence
- ☑ Behavioral skills development

- ■ ☐ Community outreach
- ■ ☐ Contraceptive access
- ■ ☑ Contraceptive education
- ■ ☑ Life option enhancement
- ■ ☑ Self-efficacy/self-esteem
- ■ ☑ Sexuality/HIV/STI education

Original Intervention Sample

Age, gender   The field study included 136 7th-grade students, evenly divided by gender; of this group, 60% were 12 years old, and 34% were 13.

Race/ethnicity   63% White, 29% African American, 4% Hispanic, 4% Other.

Program Components

- ■ ☑ Adult involvement
- ■ ☐ Case management
- ■ ☑ Group discussion
- ■ ☑ Lectures
- ■ ☐ Peer counseling/instruction
- ■ ☐ Public service announcements
- ■ ☑ Role play
- ■ ☑ Video
- ■ ☐ Other

Program Length

The curriculum contains five instructional units, with 27 class lessons. Scheduling is flexible—the full program may take between 6 and 9 weeks to complete.

Staffing Requirements/Training

Lessons are designed for family life educators to use in their 7th-grade classrooms. The national office of the American Association of Family and Consumer Services, one of the original funders of *Project Taking Charge*, offers materials to help prepare instructors (for details, call the national office toll free at 1-800-424-8080).

BIBLIOGRAPHY

Jorgensen, S. R. (1991). *Project Taking Charge:* An evaluation of an adolescent pregnancy prevention program. *Family Relations, 40*(4), 373–380.

Jorgensen, S. R., Potts, V., & Camp, B. (1993). *Project Taking Charge:* Six-month follow-up of a pregnancy prevention program for early adolescents. *Family Relations, 42*(4), 401–406.

THE PROGRAM

Program Rationale and History

Based on the idea that vocational planning could lead teens to attractive alternatives to premature sexual activity and parenthood, *Project Taking Charge* integrated sexuality and family life education with lessons on vocational development, interpersonal relationships, decision making, and goal setting.[1] The program presented sexuality as a lifelong process. The process involved knowledge acquisition and the development of attitudes, beliefs, and values about identity, relationships, and intimacy. Sexual maturation, human reproduction, interpersonal relationships, affection, intimacy, body image, and gender roles were all part of one's sexuality.

To provide junior high school home economics students with a comprehensive understanding of sexuality, *Project Taking Charge* included discussion of anatomy, physiology, family, parenthood, STIs, and HIV/AIDS. Throughout the program, abstinence from premature sexual intercourse was promoted as the most responsible choice for young teenagers. In addition, lessons and group activities were designed to help participants: (a) recognize that their current decisions would impact their future lives; (b) understand the physical and emotional sides of puberty; and (c) enhance their ability to speak about sexuality, education, and career development with their parents.

During the fall of 1989, a field study of the program was conducted with 136 low-income 7th-grade students and their parents in Delaware, Mississippi, and Ohio.

Theoretical Framework

Project Taking Charge was based on Robert J. Havighurst's concept of developmental tasks. These tasks, which arise at a particular stage of life, present a person with important psychological and social challenges. During adolescence, for example, youths must begin making decisions about (future) marriage and family life, as well as planning for a career. The resolution of such tasks brings a sense of well-being and confidence in meeting new challenges. Alternatively, failure to resolve tasks at one stage of development may lead to social disapproval, unhappiness, and difficulties in approaching future tasks.

Tasks Addressed in the Program

The *Project Taking Charge* curriculum introduced teens to the following developmental tasks:

- Learning to get along with friends of both genders
- Accepting one's physical body and keeping it healthy
- Becoming more self-sufficient
- Making decisions about (future) marriage and family life
- Preparing for a job or career
- Acquiring a set of values to guide behavior (including self-respect or self-esteem)
- Becoming socially responsible

As part of the sixth developmental task, the curriculum emphasized values that were generally regarded as basic tenets of good citizenship, fulfilling relationships, and sound personal ethics: equality, self-control, respect for others, responsibility, honesty, promise keeping, self-respect or self-esteem, dependability, trustworthiness, justice, and fairness.

Program Overview

Focusing on the values and developmental tasks described above, *Project Taking Charge* aimed to help young teens identify what they needed to accomplish in order to mature successfully, make healthy behavioral choices, gain self-esteem, and develop fulfilling relationships. Moreover, the program encouraged youths to take an active part in their own development ("taking charge") while clarifying personal values and abstaining from sexual involvement. Parent–child communication concerning sexual values, standards, and vocational planning was also promoted.

To help teens gain a deeper sense of the opportunities ahead, the curriculum encouraged collaboration among businesses, parents, and schools. In a special job-shadowing exercise, for example, students observed and interviewed individuals working in a variety of occupations.

Program Objectives

The objectives of *Project Taking Charge* were adapted from the goals and objectives of the Office of Adolescent Pregnancy Programs, Department of Health and Human Services, under the 1981 Adolescent Family Life Act (Title XX of the Public Health Services Act). Accordingly, the program aimed to help youths

- identify values, their sources and their impact on behavior;
- relate moral dimensions of values in goal setting to decision making;
- recognize the influence of gender-based roles, stereotypes, inequities, and discrimination;
- analyze the choices and challenges facing early adolescents;
- understand adolescent development and human reproduction;
- develop a more positive attitude about each individual's worth and about one's ability to "take charge" of one's own life;
- recognize the importance of relationships with family members and friends;
- develop and practice skills for communicating about sexual facts, personal values, and vocational-planning strategies;
- develop and practice conflict resolution skills;
- identify high-risk behaviors that can prevent one from reaching life goals;
- understand the importance of abstinence from high-risk behaviors, including sexual intercourse and the use of alcohol and other drugs;
- practice "saying no" to high-risk behaviors;
- gain knowledge of various occupational requirements (education and training), job-seeking strategies, and community vocational resources;
- identify personal interests;
- review community resources available to provide information about various occupations, occupational requirements (education and training), and job-seeking strategies.

Program Schedule

The *Project Taking Charge* curriculum included three main sections: "Who Am I?" "Where Am I Going?" and "How Do I Get There?" The curriculum was further divided into five units (with 27 lessons, total) and three parent–youth sessions. Each lesson could be completed in approximately 45 minutes, with individual activities requiring about 15 to 30 minutes. The curriculum was flexible enough to be completed in a 6- to 9-week time frame.

Unit 1: Who Am I? Making Healthy Choices

Four lessons were included in this unit:

- 1.1 Setting the Stage for Taking Charge of My Life
- 1.2 What's Really Important to Me?
- 1.3 Gender Roles and Stereotypes: Understanding My Choices
- 1.4 Diversity: Expanding Horizons

This unit introduced students to the idea that healthy choices were based on values, sound decision-making skills, and positive goal setting. After discussing the goals and expectations of the program, teens "took charge" of their development and futures at an exciting and important stage of their lives.

During the second half of the unit, students prepared a "Values Chart." They also investigated gender roles and stereotypes by videotaping 15 minutes of children's television, including commercials. The final lesson explored diversity as a way to expand one's horizons.

Unit 2: Where Am I Going? Taking Charge of My Life

Seven lessons were included in this unit:

- 2.1 Plan for the Future: A Time to Dream
- 2.2 Changes and Challenges
- 2.3 Human Sexuality
- 2.4 Human Reproduction
- 2.5 Dealing With Things We Can and Cannot Change
- 2.6 Setting Goals
- 2.7 Making Decisions

The goals of this unit were, first, to help students understand the experiences and challenges of early adolescence, including human reproductive development, and then, to begin to "take charge" of their futures. In a class activity, students videotaped a short segment of a current television program and interpreted the media's portrayal of teens. Next, the physical and emotional aspects of puberty were explored, and students sorted the myths from the facts about this stage of life. The last few lessons in the unit were devoted to setting goals and making decisions. These tasks were personalized in an exercise in which students developed individual plans for realizing a goal they had set for their futures.

Unit 3: How Do I Get There? Making the Most of Relationships

Six lessons were included in this unit:

- 3.1 A Closer Look at Relationships
- 3.2 Understanding Different Perspectives
- 3.3 Future Dating Relationships
- 3.4 The Basics of Communication
- 3.5 Practicing Communication Techniques
- 3.6 Sexual Abuse: Your Body Is Your Own

This unit covered family relationships, future dating relationships, and vocational planning. Students learned how families and friends served as support systems and provided assistance with decision making and developmental tasks. To help students achieve fulfilling relationships, both within and outside the family, successful communication techniques were explained and practiced. In one of the optional activities, the class videotaped several brief interactions between family members on television programs. In another activity, students interviewed several teachers about parenting or caregiving. Understanding sexual abuse was the focus of the last lesson in the unit.

Unit 4: How Do I Get There? Taking Charge of My Choices and Behaviors

Five lessons were included in this unit:

- 4.1 Risky Business: Knowing When to Say No
- 4.2 Abstinence: Saying No

- 4.3 Alcohol, Other Drugs & You: Resisting Peer Pressure
- 4.4 Sex Can Be Dangerous: Sexually Transmitted Infections (STIs) and Acquired Immune Deficiency Syndrome (AIDS)
- 4.5 Abstinence and the Costs of Early Parenthood

In this unit, students learn about risky behaviors, reasons why adolescents engage in them, and how to say "no." The benefits of abstinence are again affirmed in relation to avoiding STIs and early parenthood. One group activity, for example, used popcorn as a symbol for illustrating peer pressure to use drugs. Within each group of five to eight students, one member was instructed not to eat any popcorn, while the others were told both to eat and to encourage others to do so. The class observed how group members pressured the "abstinent" student to conform. Other activities in this unit encouraged students to contact community resources for information about STIs and to research laws regarding teenage fatherhood and welfare at Social Services and the Human Resources Department.

Unit 5: How Do I Get There? Taking Charge of My Vocational Future

Five lessons were included in this unit:

- 5.1 Getting and Keeping a Job
- 5.2 Planning for Career Exploration
- 5.3 The Career Exploration Experience
- 5.4 Career Exploration: Sharing Experiences
- 5.5 Taking Charge: Where Do I Go From Here?

In the final unit of the program, students began to take stock of themselves as future jobholders. They assessed their inherent talents and abilities, and they investigated areas providing challenges for growth. The heart of this unit was an introduction to the workplace, and the curriculum included three possible strategies. In Option 1, a job-shadowing exercise, students visited community members at work and interviewed them about job requirements, including education and training, as well as their feelings about the position, potential for advancement, and so forth. A similar activity, Option 2, allowed students to interview employees when visiting a work site. In Option 3, the class interviewed a panel of employees who visited the class. To increase the number of positions to which students were exposed, each option allowed for a full class period in which students discussed and compared what they had learned.

Parent–Youth Sessions

Three sessions were designed for students *and* their parents or guardians:

- 1. Understanding Adolescence (Unit 1)
- 2. Communicating Parent–Teen Concerns (Unit 4)
- 3. Career Planning: A Lifelong Process (Unit 5)

These sessions aimed to develop skills in communicating about sexual facts, personal values, and vocational-planning strategies. They also introduced participants to community agencies that provided information about various occupations, occupational requirements (education and training), and job-seeking strategies. The first parent–youth session, Understanding Adolescence, introduced the basic philosophy of *Project Taking Charge* and invited parents to preview course materials.

The second parent–youth session provided participants with opportunities to practice communicating feelings about sexuality, and the final session featured a job/education fair. The fair was designed to build parental support for and involvement in realistic educational and career planning. In the original field study, a video about working was also shown during this session. The video provided a basic overview about applying and interviewing for an entry-level position, and it emphasized the importance of hard work, dedication, and reliability. Although the video is no longer available, you can incorporate this information into your own intervention.

Supplemental Lesson

A supplemental lesson on sexual hygiene emphasized teens' responsibility to care for their developing bodies, and it covered such topics as daily bathing, masturbation, menstruation, STI testing, and regular medical care.

Program Implementation

Organizing the Parent Sessions

Instructors checked with parents to find the most convenient times to schedule the parent–youth sessions. During the field study, it was helpful to send home with students a survey that asked parents to select from a choice of times and probed barriers to their attendance, such as transportation and child care.

Organizing the Job-Shadowing Exercise

Regardless of the option selected, advance preparation was required for the job-shadowing exercise.

Establishing Ground Rules

Because the success of the program depended upon the comfort level of participants, the first program unit aimed to develop group cohesiveness and an open climate for discussion. The rules were based on the assumption that people felt comfortable when others listened, tried to understand what they were saying, and displayed a caring attitude toward them. Nevertheless, it was considered wise not to take big risks (e.g., disclose secrets) if one's level of trust in the group was not high.

Teachers conveyed the principles listed below and posted them on a bulletin board for the duration of the program.

1. Full participation is expected. The program will be fun and successful if everyone participates in class activities and discussions.
2. Any question is okay—no one should feel afraid to ask a question. It is likely that other students will want to ask the same question. Moreover, in each class period a few questions will be answered from the anonymous question box in the classroom.
3. Everyone has a right to "pass" on a question or activity. Similarly, no one has to share anything he or she does not want others to know. If a participant feels uncomfortable about answering a particular question, he or she can say "I pass." However, the person will still need to listen to others' answers and take part in the activity.
4. Respect others' points of view. It is okay to disagree, but not to put down or tease someone. It is all right to laugh with, but not at, someone. Everyone has the right to his or her ideas and opinions.
5. The sessions will be confidential. Participants should try not to repeat things said during a lesson outside of the class. Students may talk to each other and to family members or friends about the topics and issues discussed, but they should

try not to use names (for example, say, "Today in my class, someone said . . ." instead of "Mary said . . .").

PROGRAM EVALUATION

The Original Evaluation

Design

The effectiveness of *Project Taking Charge* was investigated in a field study conducted in 1989 with 136 teenagers in Delaware, Mississippi, and Ohio. Following a quasi-experimental design, the study compared program participants with a group of their peers who were selected from the same schools but received no intervention. The researchers compared the two groups of youths on a wide range of measures, including self-esteem, knowledge of sexual development, intentions regarding sexual activity, patterns of communication with parents, and educational aspirations. To assess the effectiveness of the program over time, surveys were administered to the teens at three points:

- Time 1: prior to the start of the program (pretest)
- Time 2: at the conclusion of the program (posttest)
- Time 3: 6 months following the conclusion of the program (follow-up)

Evaluation Questions

The evaluation was designed to measure the degree to which program participants developed the values and skills that would enable them to plan for their future occupations and abstain from sexual activity. In particular, the researchers predicted that program participants would show the following outcomes, relative to the comparison group of peers:

- Higher self-esteem
- Greater understanding of the consequences of early pregnancy on adolescents' educational and vocational plans
- Greater knowledge of human sexuality, sexual development, and STIs
- Greater clarity of sexual values
- Greater intention to postpone sexual intercourse
- More frequent and comfortable communication with parents about sexual issues
- More frequent and comfortable communication with parents about vocational planning
- Higher educational aspirations

Additionally, the researchers hypothesized similar positive outcomes for the parents who participated in *Project Taking Charge*. In particular, they predicted that parents would show an increased understanding of human sexuality and sexual development, greater frequency and comfort in communicating with their children about vocational planning and sexual issues, and stronger support for postponing early sexual activity.

Recruitment and Data Collection

The researchers recruited a set of family life education teachers at schools in Delaware, Mississippi, and Ohio; all had previously been recognized for their superior teaching skills. At the start of the study, one teacher in each site was randomly selected into the treatment group and asked to implement the curriculum and evaluation measures with one of their 7th-grade home economics classes. A second teacher in each participating school was randomly selected into the comparison group. These teachers were asked to administer the same set of evaluation instruments, at the same points in time, to one of their 7th-grade home economics classes. However, no intervention was given to these classes.

Sample

The research sample included 136 teens: 77 program participants and 59 comparison group members. Of the 126 parents who participated, 69 were included in the comparison group, and 57 in the comparison group. Across sites, the number of participants in the treatment and comparison groups varied, ranging from a low of 14 teenagers (and 13 parents) in the Delaware comparison group, to a high of 27 teenagers (and 27 parents) in the Mississippi treatment group. There was no attrition among the teens, and only 2 parents failed to complete the posttest assessment.

Approximately equal numbers of male and female students were included in the final research sample. On average, the youths were either 12 or 13 years of age, living with both parents, and White. However, more than one-third were minority group members, predominantly African American.

Evaluation Results

At the start of the study, less than 25% of the teens reported previous sexual activity. For those who had become active (15 in the treatment group and 12 in the comparison group), the average age at first intercourse was approximately 11 years. In addition, the researchers found few social or demographic differences between program participants and members of the comparison group. They did note, however, that comparison group teens were more likely to believe that parents opposed sexual intercourse during adolescence, and program participants showed higher levels of self-esteem.

Knowledge Measures

Compared to their peers who received no intervention, at the Time 2 assessment program participants showed greater gains in their understanding of sexual development and STIs ($p < .001$), sexual anatomy and physiology ($p < .001$), and the complications that can result from teen pregnancy ($p < .05$). Moreover, these gains were largely maintained 6 months following the conclusion of the program.

Initiation of Sexual Intercourse

Participation in *Project Taking Charge* may have delayed the initiation of sexual intercourse for teens who had not yet begun having intercourse at the start of the study. The researchers found that 50% of comparison group students who were abstinent at the Time 1 assessment had become sexually active by the final assessment period. In contrast, the figure for program participants was 23%. However, the actual numbers of students in the two groups was small, and the statistical test fell just short of significance ($p = .051$).

On all other measures—including self-esteem, educational aspirations, clarity of sexual values, intentions regarding sexual activity, and communication with parents regarding sexual intercourse and vocational aspirations—the researchers found no difference between the two groups of teens.

Effects on Parents

At the follow-up assessment, parents who participated in *Project Taking Charge* showed significant gains in their knowledge of sexuality and STIs, relative to the comparison group of adults. However, the treatment and comparison groups did not differ on measures of communication about sexual issues with teens.

Summary

Overall, both youth and adult participants in *Project Taking Charge* showed increased knowledge of sexual development, STIs, and sexual anatomy and physiology at the conclusion of the program, and these gains remained strong 6 months following the intervention. There was also an increase in teens' understanding of the complications caused by early pregnancy. In addition, the researchers presented some evidence to suggest that *Project Taking Charge* may have promoted abstinence among teens who had not yet begun having intercourse at the start of the study. They noted, however, that a significance test between participants and their comparison group peers fell just short of significance ($p = .051$).

The researchers had predicted other positive outcomes for program participants, but the intervention appeared to have no effect on participants' self-esteem, educational aspirations, clarity of sexual values, intentions regarding sexual activity, or communication with parents regarding sexual intercourse and vocational aspirations.

PROJECT TAKING CHARGE IN THE COMMUNITY TODAY

In the past 3 years, *Project Taking Charge* has been implemented in communities in five states: Colorado, Connecticut, Ohio, Minnesota, and Texas.

NOTE

1. A full set of program materials, including curriculum manual, resource guide, videotapes, evaluation materials, and more, is available for purchase from Sociometrics at http://www.socio.com/pasha.htm.

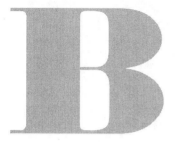

Programs Designed for
Youths in High School

School-Linked Reproductive Health Services (the Self Center): A High School Pregnancy Prevention Program

Kathryn L. Muller, Starr Niego, M. Jane Park, and Janette Mince

Original Program Developers and Evaluators

Laurie Schwab Zabin, PhD
Edward A. Smith, DrPH
Mark R. Emerson
  Johns Hopkins University School of Hygiene and Public Health
  Baltimore, MD

Janet B. Hardy, MDCM
Marilyn B. Hirsch, PhD
  Johns Hopkins University School of Medicine
  Baltimore, MD

School-Linked Reproductive Health Services (the Self Center) was supported by contracts and grants from the Educational Foundation of America, the Ford Foundation, the W.T. Grant Foundation, the Hewlett Foundation, the Charles Stewart Mott Foundation, and the Jessie Smith Noyes Foundation.

Rosalie Streett, MS
Friends and Family Inc.
Baltimore, MD

PROGRAM ABSTRACT

Summary

Originally launched as a partnership between junior and senior high schools and a neighboring clinic, the *Self Center* combines education, counseling, and reproductive services into a comprehensive intervention. Services are provided by a team of nurses and social workers who divide their time between the schools and clinic. School-based components include the following: (a) at least one presentation to each homeroom class per semester to introduce the program and begin discussing values clarification, decision making, and reproductive health; (b) informal discussion groups that arise as students seek advice and information from staff on such themes as pubertal development, drug use, and parenting; and (c) individual counseling sessions, available as needed, with a social worker. At the clinic, reproductive health and extended counseling services are provided, and referrals are given for teens requiring medical care. In addition, clinic staff encourage students to participate in discussion groups and examine educational videos and pamphlets. Although the intervention was launched as a primary prevention effort, secondary prevention might be incorporated as well.

A 3-year field test of the program was conducted in a low-income neighborhood in Baltimore, Maryland, where elevated rates of sexual activity and teen pregnancy had been recorded. Compared to their peers attending comparable schools, students in program schools showed reduced levels of sexual activity and more effective use of contraception; the effects were greatest among younger girls and boys whose use of contraception was minimal at the start of the program. A delay in the onset of sexual activity was also recorded among youths who were abstinent at the start of the program.

Focus

☑ Primary pregnancy prevention   ☐ Secondary pregnancy prevention   ☐ STI/HIV/AIDS prevention

Original Site

☑ School based   ☐ Community based   ☑ Clinic based

Suitable for Use In

This program can be implemented either by school–clinic or community–clinic partnerships. The clinic should be located in close proximity to participating schools or community organizations, or easily accessible to teens.

Approach

- ☑ Abstinence
- ☑ Behavioral skills development
- ☐ Community outreach
- ☑ Contraceptive access
- ☑ Contraceptive education

- ■ ☐ Life option enhancement
- ■ ☐ Self-efficacy/self-esteem
- ■ ☑ Sexuality/HIV/STI education

Original Intervention Sample

Age   The program was intended to serve all students enrolled in two urban schools, one junior high and one senior high (approximately 1,700 students total). Nearly all students regularly attending school were exposed to at least one program component.

Race/ethnicity 100% African American

Program Components

- ■ ☐ Adult involvement
- ■ ☑ Case management
- ■ ☑ Group discussion
- ■ ☑ Lectures
- ■ ☐ Peer counseling/instruction
- ■ ☐ Public service announcements
- ■ ☐ Role play
- ■ ☑ Video
- ■ ☑ Other: Team of student assistants and outreach workers; informal education and games

Program Length

The school-based components of the program operate continuously during the academic year. The program nurse visits each homeroom class at least once each semester, and all program staff are available to students for individual counseling or informal group discussions during lunch/free periods. The clinic services are available to teens year-round—on weekday afternoons and during school vacations.

Staffing Requirements/Training

One social worker (required) and one nurse (if possible) are needed for each participating school or community organization. A program administrator, preferably with training in the field of education or health education, is needed for each clinic site. Other professionals (e.g., physicians) should be on call to provide necessary services and supervision.

BIBLIOGRAPHY

Clark, S. D., Zabin, L. S., & Hardy, J. B. (1984). Sex, contraception, parenthood: Experience and attitudes among urban black young men. *Family Planning Perspectives, 16*(2), 77–82.

Hardy, J. B., King, T., & Repke, J. T. (1987). The Johns Hopkins Adolescent Pregnancy Program: An evaluation. *Obstetrics and Gynecology, 69,* 300–306.

Hardy, J. B., & Zabin, L. S. (1991). *Adolescent pregnancy in an urban environment: Issues, programs and evaluation.* Washington, DC: The Urban Institute Press.

Zabin, L. S. (1991). Adolescent pregnancy and early sexual onset: Problems of evaluation in the school context, and what a school-linked program can do. In J. Brooks-Gunn, R. M. Lerner, & A. C. Peterson (Eds.), *Encyclopedia of adolescence.* New York: Garland.

Zabin, L. S. (1992). School-linked reproductive health services: The Johns Hopkins Program. In B. Miller, J. Card, R. Paikoff, & J. Peterson (Eds.), *Preventing adolescent pregnancy* (pp. 156–184). Newbury Park, CA: Sage Publications.

Zabin, L. S., & Hirsch, M. B. (1984). *Evaluation of pregnancy prevention programs in the school context.* Lexington, MA: Lexington Books.

Zabin, L. S., Hirsch, M. B., Smith, E. A., Smith, M., Emerson, M. R., Smith, M., King, T. M., & Hardy, J. B. (1988). The Baltimore pregnancy prevention program for urban adolescents: II. What did it cost? *Family Planning Perspectives, 20*(4), 188–192.

Zabin, L. S., Hirsch, M. B., Streett, R., Emerson, M. R., Smith, M., Hardy, J. B., et al. (1988). The Baltimore pregnancy prevention program for urban adolescents: I. How did it work? *Family Planning Perspectives, 20*(4), 182–187.

Zabin, L. S., Smith, E. A., Hirsch, M. B., Streett, R. & Hardy, J. B. (1986). Evaluation of a pregnancy prevention program for urban teenagers. *Family Planning Perspectives, 18*(3), 119–126.

Related References by the Developers of the *Self Center*

Weden, M. M., & Zabin, L. S. (2005). Gender and ethnic differences in the co-occurrence of adolescent risk behaviors. *Ethnicity & Health, 10*(3), 213–234.

Zabin, L., Emerson, M. R., Ringers, P. A., & Sedivy, V. (1996). Adolescents with negative pregnancy test results: An accessible risk group. *Journal of the American Medical Association, 275*(2), 113–117.

Zabin, L. S. (1999). Ambivalent feelings about parenthood may lead to inconsistent contraceptive use—and pregnancy. *Family Planning Perspectives, 31*(5), 250–251.

THE PROGRAM

Program Rationale and History

The *Self Center* combined educational, counseling, and reproductive health services in an effort to reduce unintended pregnancy among junior and senior high school students.[1] Services were provided through a collaboration between schools and nearby school-affiliated clinics. The program consisted of both in-school and clinic components, delivered by a shared staff of nurse educators, counselors, and on-call physicians.

The *Self Center* was originally conducted as a demonstration project by the Johns Hopkins School of Medicine and the Baltimore City Departments of Education and Health. The program was implemented and field tested between 1981 and 1984 at a junior and senior high school located in an urban, low-income neighborhood in Baltimore, Maryland. All students at the program schools were African American.

During the original implementation, students had access to program services at both school sites, as well as at a nearby clinic. Education and counseling services were provided by teams of health and social work professionals. In-class presentations, small group discussions, and individual counseling were offered in schools, and peer group discussion as well as group and individual counseling were provided in the clinic. Contraceptive and other reproductive health services (such as pregnancy testing and treatment for sexually transmitted infections [STIs]) were also provided, free of charge, in the clinic.

In addition to enhancing contraceptive access, the *Self Center* helped teens recognize the impact of their behavior on their ability to realize personal, social, and educational goals. For this reason, the program aimed to (a) help teens to understand how sex, unintended pregnancy and premature parenthood could affect their ability to meet personal goals; and (b) empower teens to make responsible decisions. This approach was represented by the program's motto, "Make a life for yourself before you make another life." In the field study, this motto was displayed on program stationery and frequently cited in education and counseling sessions.

The *Self Center* activities and services were not implemented as a stand-alone curriculum, but in addition to the existing state-mandated sex education curriculum provided at Maryland junior and senior high schools at that time.

Because Maryland state law allowed minors to receive reproductive services without parental notification or consent, the *Self Center* was able to provide students with confidential reproductive health services. At the time this study was conducted, there was much debate over whether federal funds for birth control (known as Title X of the Public Health Service Act, enacted in 1970) could be used to provide minors accesses to reproductive health services without parental consent. Several court decisions in the 1970s and 1980s affirmed that no state could require parental consent or notification for providing such services to married or unmarried minors. In recent years, several state legislatures have considered requiring that clinics that receive federal funds involve parents before providing reproductive health services.

As of 2007, 21 states and the District of Columbia explicitly allow minors access to birth control and other reproductive health services without parental consent. Two states, Texas and Utah, require parental consent in clinics or health centers that receive state funding for their family planning programs. Four states (North Dakota, Ohio, Rhode Island, and Wisconsin) have no explicit policy. The remaining states have pending legislation or recognize special circumstances such as the following: (a) minors over the age of 14, (b) minors who are married or have completed high school, (c) minors who are "mature," and (d) minors who already have a child or who have been pregnant. Some states do allow the provider some latitude regarding parental notification (e.g., a clinician may seek consent but is not required to). (See the Alan Guttmacher Institute's September 2007 "State Policies in Brief: Minors' Access to Contraceptive Services.")

Theoretical Framework

This program is rooted in the idea that improving teens' access to reproductive health-related education and medical services will reduce unintended pregnancy. A number of factors, including lack of transportation, difficulty planning ahead for appointments, concerns about confidentiality, and limited financial resources, make negotiating the health care system daunting for many teens. The original program developers saw schools as an ideal place to make first contact with students and to provide a bridge to clinic services. As such, they designed an integrated program linking two schools and a nearby clinic in providing education, guidance, and reproductive health services.

Program Objectives

The overall goal of the *Self Center* was to reduce the incidence of unintended pregnancy among junior and senior high school students. Specifically, the program endeavored to

- increase students' knowledge of physical maturation, human sexuality, contraception, fertility, and awareness of the personal burdens and costs of unintended pregnancy;
- reinforce positive attitudes toward pregnancy prevention and promote realistic attitudes toward premature pregnancy and parenthood;
- postpone first intercourse among adolescents who are not yet sexually active;
- increase the use of professional contraceptive services by adolescents who are sexually active;
- increase the use of effective contraception by adolescents who are sexually active;
- reduce the rates of adolescent pregnancy, abortion, and childbearing.

Since the time of the original implementation of the *Self Center*, overall U.S. teen pregnancy rates have decreased by 36%. Among African American teens, the population served in the original *Self Center* study, the rate has decreased by 40% since the early 1990s. Also since the time of the field test, HIV/AIDS has emerged as a top public health crisis worldwide. Were the *Self Center* to be developed today, there would be a strong emphasis on reducing sexual risk behaviors and promoting consistent and correct condom use.

Program Outline

The *Self Center* consisted of six categories of services—three of which were delivered in school, and three of which were delivered in a nearby clinic. The program staffing, overall educational approach, and basic structure of these components (as implemented in the field study) are described briefly below.

Please note that this information is provided as a model, based on the original study. Particular components may need to be altered to fit the needs of your teens and the values of your schools and community.

Educational Approach

The major thrust of the educational component of the program was to encourage personal responsibility and goal setting so that students would postpone sexual activity until they were more mature. Although abstinence was emphasized as the most effective means of pregnancy prevention, the need for effective contraception for those who chose to be sexually active was also recognized. For this reason, educational activities were designed to help students understand (a) the risks of pregnancy and STIs following unprotected intercourse; (b) the reproductive process, including contraceptive methods and their relative effectiveness and safety; and (c) the potentially adverse consequences of unintended pregnancy for teens' future lives.

Interactive, rather than didactic, presentations were preferable for all but the classroom presentations. In addition, the clinic waiting room provided students with informal educational resources, such as videos, games, posters, and pamphlets on issues regarding sexuality and health. An important tenet of the program was that teens needed to be oriented to their future lives and receive consistent and frequent expressions of expectations for success. In the field study, for example, program staff posted information about community events, local colleges, and training programs, along with other optimistic messages in addition to the more traditional "warnings" about adolescent sexual involvement.

Program Staff

The core service staff for each participating school was a team comprised of a social worker and registered nurse (RN). Each of the social workers was paired with a nurse-midwife or a pediatric nurse practitioner. These teams delivered the bulk of services provided to students. All program staff members were selected for their experience and interest in working with adolescents.

Program teams visited the participating schools each morning and became acquainted with students by giving at least one classroom presentation per semester. Team members were also available in the schools' health offices during students' lunch and free periods for individual consultation or small-group counseling work. The same social worker–nurse teams were available to students in a nearby clinic later in the afternoon. Additional clinic staff included a clinic administrator/educator, a receptionist, a nurse's aide, and a supervising physician.

The original implementation of the *Self Center* also employed a peer resource team of 12 students trained to serve as representatives of and spokespersons for the program. These students wore T-shirts and/or buttons that read, "Ask me about the Self Center," and assisted with tasks such as distributing handouts and talking with drop-in students when staff members were involved in individual counseling sessions.

In-School Services

In-school components of the *Self Center* program were designed to reach junior and senior high school students and to serve four basic functions: (a) to provide instruction in each classroom at least once, and usually more often, during each semester; (b) to serve as a resource for teachers in their routine health and sex education programs; (c) to offer individual and/or small group counseling as needed and/or answer student questions; and (d) to bridge the school and clinic components of the program.

Classroom Presentations

In the field study, staff gave an hour-long presentation to each homeroom class per semester. The presentations introduced students to the program's services and provided information on various topics concerning reproductive health. In addition, program staff were available to offer additional class sessions on related topics by request and to serve as a resource for the school's regular health education program.

Group Discussions

In addition to classroom presentations, the program social worker at each school was available midday during students' lunch or free periods. During these times, students dropped by to ask questions or take advantage of the variety of informal educational materials available in the health offices. The health offices were the site of frequent, spontaneous small-group discussions, ranging from informal "rap sessions" to more focused discussions of problems identified by students or program staff. Staff used the informal discussions to identify students whose emotional needs warranted additional counseling within the program or with outside agencies.

Individual Counseling

Individual counseling services were available to students during the school day. Program social workers publicized the hours they were available for private consultation. Students sought out program staff to discuss personal issues, such as relationships with the opposite sex, problems at home, pregnancy scares, and other confidential matters. Because the academic setting did not allow for prolonged consultations or great privacy, longer-term counseling was provided at the afternoon clinic.

Clinic Services

The *Self Center* clinic services were provided at a storefront clinic located across from one school and four blocks from the other. The clinic operated in the hours after school. In addition to nurse–counselor teams who moved to the clinic in the afternoon, clinic activities were directed by a clinic administrator, a trained health educator. Contraceptive and other reproductive health services (such as pregnancy testing and treatment for STIs) were provided to students at no charge. In addition to reproductive health care, group education and individual counseling were also provided.

Reproductive Health Services

The *Self Center* clinic provided students in program schools with reproductive health and contraceptive services. Students could obtain condoms, spermicide, and oral contraceptives. In addition, students could receive care for a variety of sexuality-related problems, including menstrual irregularity, growth and development problems, STI concerns, pregnancy tests, and birth control concerns. Females seeking oral contraceptives were given a physical exam and counseling in the use of this method. Although the nursing staff served as the primary contacts for students' health concerns, a physician (gynecologist) was also available for consultation and supervision. Clinic staff provided referrals for medical problems other than reproductive health concerns.

Group Education

The clinic waiting room served as a center for informal education through audiovisual resources, games, and small-group encounters. More formal educational sessions were guided by a health educator. Clinic staff were available in the waiting room. Some of the educational sessions were organized around specific topics (proposed by students as well as staff), while others arose from student discussion of personal experiences or concerns. Informal discussions often led to larger group discussions, which then took place in the "Rap Room." Clinic discussion groups and presentations were held on all but 1 day a week, which was reserved for first-time clinic patients. First-time visitors received a special orientation that welcomed them to the clinic and praised them for being sexually responsible.

Individual Counseling

One of the main services provided by the clinic was individual counseling. Although counseling in a school setting is somewhat more accessible to students, clinic counseling is not restricted by rigid schedules, so teens could have longer, regularly scheduled counseling sessions. Students who sought condoms or other birth control methods were required to register for and participate in an initial psychosocial interview. Often the interview revealed areas warranting further exploration through counseling. Staff provided counseling on a broad range of issues, including pubertal development, relationships, and family problems. Few limits were placed on the amount of counseling students could receive.

Program Implementation

There are a number of issues to take into account when preparing to implement the *Self Center* or a similar comprehensive pregnancy prevention program. A brief overview of some of the major issues is provided below.

Confidential Reproductive Health Care for Minors

This program was originally implemented in a state where reproductive-related health care and contraceptives could be provided to teens without parental consent; however, your state laws may limit the ability of your staff to provide confidential care and contraceptive access to minors.

As noted earlier, 21 states and the District of Columbia explicitly allow for minors' access to reproductive health care services without parental consent or notification. Two states, Texas and Utah, require parental consent for such services offered in clinics that receive state funds for family planning. Most other states have restrictions of some kind, but allow for some latitude on the part of the service provider.

An Adjunct Sexuality Curriculum

The *Self Center* program was not a stand-alone sexuality education curriculum. Instead, program services were delivered in addition to the sex education curriculum that was state-mandated at that time. Moreover, *Self Center* program staff members often collaborated with school health educators to assist in delivering the required curriculum.

Staff Skills

Knowledgeable staff members who were capable of communicating well with students were needed to make this program successful. Because informal discussions helped to identify educational and counseling issues, as well as build student trust and rapport, staff needed to be skilled in small-group processes. During the field study, students reported that the *Self Center* staff really cared about them; this perception helped them feel comfortable using program services.

PROGRAM EVALUATION

The Original Evaluation

Design

The original evaluation of the *Self Center* investigated the impact of the intervention on students' fertility-related knowledge, attitudes, and behavior. The researchers followed two analytic strategies. Using a matched-comparison design, they compared teens in participating schools with youths attending schools with similar social and demographic characteristics. Additionally, using a pre-/posttest design, they investigated changes within program school students over the course of the study. Self-administered questionnaires were given to teens at the following points:

- Time 1: fall 1981, prior to the start of the program (all schools)
- Time 2: spring 1982, the end of the first program year (program schools only)
- Time 3: spring 1983, the end of the second program year (program schools only)
- Time 4: spring 1984, the end of the final program year (all schools)

The questionnaires measured students' knowledge regarding sexual health and birth control, attitudes toward teen pregnancy and parenting, sexual history, use of birth control, and any pregnancies experienced. Additionally, the evaluators collected detailed information on program participation through staff-maintained records and student sign-in sheets. An examination of financial records also allowed for an assessment of the relative costs of various program components.

Design Issues

The program was designed, in part, to test the belief that school-linked programs like the *Self Center* could reach young people who otherwise would not be served by professional health facilities. If this assertion proved to be true, program evaluators felt that the impact of the program would be evident among the entire student body in participating schools—not merely among the subset of teens who attended the clinic and, consequently, might be likely to seek similar services in other settings as well. Therefore, the field study of the *Self Center* program was designed to assess changes in the knowledge, attitudes, and behaviors among all students who attended program schools during the time the *Self Center* was in place, rather than only those students who took advantage of various program services.

Moreover, the original evaluators cited and addressed a number of methodological problems that were unique to program evaluations conducted in a school context; these concerns are discussed briefly below and elaborated in the book *Evaluation of Pregnancy Prevention Programs in the School Context.* Should you choose to evaluate your implementation, take care to consider these issues—or seek assistance from an evaluation consultant.

Student mobility. Student mobility into and out of individual schools (due to graduation, moving, or transfer) makes it difficult to identify a fixed population in which behavioral change or the use of particular services can be measured. In statistical terms, it becomes difficult to determine the denominator in calculating the ratio of particular behaviors to a given population, particularly when program effects on the entire student body are used as the key measure of program impact.

Comparability of program and control schools. It is difficult to locate comparable schools to serve as program and comparison/control sites. Schools that appear similar may have important differences that affect the detection of program outcomes. The original evaluators felt that it was more appropriate to use data from the two control schools to establish the presence or absence of change in the absence of the intervention, rather than to compare absolute rates or numbers between the program and control schools at specific points in time.

Attrition among high-risk students. Schools where the need for pregnancy prevention or other special programs is greatest may also have higher than average transience rates and large populations of chronic absentees and/or dropouts. This issue complicates the measurement of program effects, since students who receive program services may not be in attendance when follow-up assessments are administered. In the original field study, data from the comparison schools were used to control for the fact that spring semester dropouts and/or transience might exclude less-motivated or at-risk students from the sample.

Age, grades, and program exposure. Once a program serving multiple grades of students has been in place for several years, older students have had a greater opportunity for longer exposure to the intervention. Data collection and analysis plans must take this factor into consideration. The original field study of *the Self Center* classified students both by their grade level and years of actual exposure to the program. Life table analysis—a statistical method used to determine the probability of an event, such as conception or first intercourse, occurring by a specific age or time—was used to determine specific program effects.

Evaluation Questions

The original field study was designed to address the following questions:

1. Would students at program schools exhibit greater improvement in knowledge of reproductive health, contraception, and the consequences of adolescent parenthood following exposure to the *Self Center*?
2. Would students at program schools show improved attitudes toward pregnancy prevention and more realistic beliefs about premature conception and parenthood following exposure to the *Self Center*?
3. Would nonsexually active students at program schools postpone the initiation of sexual intercourse until a later age following exposure to the *Self Center*?
4. Would students at program schools increase their use of clinic services following exposure to the *Self Center*?
5. Would sexually active students at program schools demonstrate more effective contraceptive use following exposure to the *Self Center*?
6. Would students at program schools exhibit lower rates of pregnancy, abortion, and childbearing following exposure to the *Self Center*?

Data Collection Procedures

A few days before each survey was to be administered, parents were mailed written notification about the study, along with an explanation of the need for students to complete sensitive anonymous questionnaires. Parents were assured that they could withhold consent for their child's participation in the study, and they were provided with a telephone number to call if they had further questions or wished to have their child excused. Only two parents withheld consent, though several called to ask questions or express support for the program. Prior to distributing the questionnaires, homeroom teachers provided students with an additional opportunity to decline to participate; however, very few students refused to complete the surveys.

Questionnaires were distributed to classroom teachers in packets. Teachers were responsible for returning every questionnaire, even those that remained blank. All packets were assigned six-digit classroom identification numbers but were not labeled with individual identifiers.

Because the surveys were completely anonymous, they yielded cross-sectional, rather than longitudinal, data. That is, the analysis considered the entire group of respondents at each assessment period, rather than following the behaviors of individual students over time.

Research Sample

Baseline questionnaires were completed by 667 males and 1,033 females at the two program schools (representing 98% of the junior and senior high students who attended school on the day the Time 1 survey was administered). All students at the program schools were African American. Follow-up surveys were administered each spring over the 3-year period of the study. Lower school enrollment and attendance during the spring yielded smaller research samples. Thus, the Time 2 assessment included 498 male and 793 female students; the Time 3 assessment, 450 male and 764 female students; and the final, Time 4, assessment, 506 males and 695 females. Refusal rates for follow-up at the program schools ranged between 2% and 3%.

The comparison group sample was also drawn from two urban schools. Unlike the program schools, comparison schools were racially mixed. However, only data from the 944 male and 1,002 female African American students who completed the Time 1 survey, and the 860 male and 889 female African American students who completed the Time 4 follow-up, were used for the analysis.

Service Logs

Student contacts with program staff and services were well documented. Staff maintained daily logs of student contacts (both at school and in the clinic). In addition, the clinic had sign-in sheets in the waiting room, and program staff completed registration forms for students seeking individual services, and medical history forms for students receiving care from a nurse or physician. Though they proved quite helpful to program staff, such logs are only required if you choose to evaluate your program.

Evaluation Results

The field study showed that the *Self Center* was particularly effective in changing students' fertility-related knowledge and behaviors. The impact on attitudes was less striking, because participants' attitudes were already quite positive when the program began. These findings are elaborated below.

Knowledge and Attitudes

At the start of the study, students in program and comparison schools scored similarly on the 10-item knowledge test. At the Time 1 assessment, females answered 6.8 questions correctly. After 2 years of program exposure, the average number of correct responses rose to 7.8, and males showed similar significant increases. In contrast, no significant changes were recorded in the scores of students attending comparison schools.

Program evaluators also assessed changes in students' attitudes regarding (a) the acceptability of teenage pregnancy, (b) the ideal ages at which to marry and have children, and (c) the acceptability of intercourse between persons who have just met or who date occasionally. In contrast to the changes in knowledge, the researchers found that these three attitudes were not consistently affected by program exposure. For example, although positive support for adolescent childbearing declined among program females, there was no consistent program effect for males. Similarly, at the start of the study, a large proportion of students reported ideal ages for childbearing that were lower than those considered ideal for marriage. Following the program, these percentages declined for girls but not for boys. Within the comparison schools, no change was found. With respect to attitudes toward "casual sex," evaluators observed no consistent change in program schools and a statistically nonsignificant decline in the comparison schools.

In interpreting these findings, the evaluators noted that the majority of students held rather positive attitudes toward contraception and rather negative attitudes toward adolescent childbearing and casual sex before the program began. Consequently, significant change in these outcomes would be difficult to detect.

Sexual and Contraceptive Behaviors

At the start of the study, the researchers measured high levels of sexual activity in both program and control schools. Over 90% of all junior and senior high males, over 50% of junior high females, and nearly 80% of senior high females reported that they were sexually active. Although large percentages of students (71% of junior high students and 89% of senior high students) reported having used a contraceptive method at some time, far fewer reported using a method at last intercourse. Furthermore, over 10% of sexually active junior high girls and over 22% of senior high girls had already experienced a pregnancy when the Time 1 data were collected.

Onset of sexual activity. The researchers investigated the timing of first coitus among program students only. At the follow-up assessments, they found that students who attended program schools during the entire 3-year study period postponed intercourse for an average of 7 months. Smaller delays were evident for students who had only 1 or 2 years of program exposure. Furthermore, there was a two-thirds reduction in the proportion of girls attending program schools who became sexually active by ages 14 or 15, a time of great risk for unintended pregnancy.

Clinic attendance. Clinic attendance increased dramatically among program school students following exposure to the *Self Center*'s services. When the program began, only 49% of the sexually active female students and 16% of the sexually active male students had visited a clinic for contraceptive assistance. After 1 year of exposure to the program, 63% of sexually active females and 28% of sexually active males had sought professional contraceptive services. After 3 years' exposure, 71% of the females and 48% of the males had used clinic services. No such increase in clinic attendance was observed in the comparison schools.

In addition to increasing the frequency of clinic attendance, the *Self Center* improved the timeliness of clinic visits. Over the course of the study period, significantly more students in program schools attended the clinic within the first

3 months of initiating sexual activity, as compared to their peers attending comparison schools. Furthermore, an increased number of program students sought professional advice on birth control prior to having intercourse for the first time after exposure to the program. In the comparison schools, in contrast, the researchers found no consistent changes in teens' use of reproductive health clinic services.

Contraceptive use. At the Time 1 assessment, nearly 57% of sexually active females and 49% of sexually active males reported using contraception at their last sexual intercourse. After 2 years' exposure to the program, the proportion of students who reported using some method of birth control at their last sexual encounter rose to nearly 77% among sexually active females and almost 56% among sexually active males. In addition, the percentage of females using oral contraceptives increased significantly among all grade levels, particularly among younger girls, following exposure to the program. Unprotected intercourse also dropped to extremely low levels. In all but one subgroup of one grade, fewer than 20% of females who had been exposed to 2 or more years of the program failed to use any contraceptive method at last intercourse. In contrast, in three grades at the comparison schools, 45%–50% of students reported using no method of birth control at all.

Condom use did not change consistently as a result of program exposure. Instead, it appeared to fluctuate with the use of female contraceptive methods. This is not surprising given that condom use as protection against HIV infection or other STIs (as distinct from pregnancy prevention) was not stressed in the original implementation of the *Self Center*.

Note that the original study was conducted between 1981 and 1984. Little was known about HIV/AIDS—its origins or transmission—at that time. When the *Self Center* was developed, AIDS and HIV had not yet entered the lexicon of reproductive health education. Although the word *AIDS* would be used for the first time in 1982 when the first suggestions of sexual transmission arose, the virus that causes AIDS would not be isolated until 1983 by the Institut Pasteur in France. The first cases of AIDS among women were reported in 1983. However, the president of the United States would not publicly use the word until a speech in 1985. Not until 1986, when the cumulative known AIDS-related death toll exceeded 16,000, did the U.S. surgeon general publish a report on AIDS and call for sex education as a means of prevention.

If developed and evaluated today, an intervention like the *Self Center* would have a strong emphasis on risk-reduction behaviors, STI prevention, male condoms, and perhaps female condoms as well.

Pregnancy rates. The evaluators used life table analysis to estimate the cumulative percentage of sexually active students in grades 9–12 who became pregnant at different points during the study period. However, 7th- and 8th-grade students were not included in this analysis due to the small number of pregnancies and less-detailed pregnancy information collected for this group of students.

Program and control schools showed similar pregnancy rates at the Time 1 assessment. However, at 16 months into the program, pregnancy rates at the comparison schools had increased by 50%, reflecting increased rates in the city of Baltimore during this time. At 28 months into the project, the pregnancy rates had increased by 58%. In contrast, after an initial increase of 13%, the pregnancy rates decreased in the program schools. In particular, there was a 22% drop for students exposed to the program for 20 months and a 30% drop for students exposed to the program for the full 28-month program period. Consequently, by the end of the original evaluation, the pregnancy rates in program and controls schools differed by nearly 90%. Using mathematical models, the evaluators concluded that the reductions were due (in equal part) to a decrease in the frequency of intercourse and an increase in the use of effective contraceptives. Additionally, abortion and childbearing rates also dropped in program schools over the course of the field study.

Patterns of Service Utilization

Detailed analyses of the teens' service utilization revealed that 85% of all students enrolled in participating schools were exposed to at least one program component. When adjusted for chronic absenteeism, it still appeared that even chronic absentees were occasionally reached by some aspect of the program. At the same time, the researchers found that nearly all students who regularly attended school had at least one contact with the *Self Center* activities.

Sixty-eight percent of all student contacts with program staff took place in the school setting. Approximately 73% of program school students (96% if estimates are based on those in regular attendance) heard at least one classroom presentation. The popularity of spontaneous in-school discussions, or "rap sessions," is evidenced by the participation of over 50% of all students in these discussions and the fact that they accounted for more than 40% of all student–staff interactions. Fifteen percent of students took part in individual counseling in school, and a slightly higher percentage received such counseling at the clinic. Although over one-quarter of students enrolled at the program schools participated in group education at the clinic, relatively few students attended group sessions unless they also came for some other clinic service.

Finally, nearly 15% of those enrolled in program schools made reproductive health-related medical visits. An examination of students' routes to the clinic supported the hypothesis that the school was a good base from which to encourage clinic attendance. For the vast majority of patients (88%), school contact with program staff preceded their first clinic visit.

The evaluators also considered gender differences in the teens' use of program services. They found that females generally used many more medical, clinic group education, and individual counseling services than did males. However, among junior high school students, males and females used clinic group education and clinic counseling services at comparable rates. The staff also reported that a few students—among the most difficult and needy cases—required inordinate amounts of staff time.

Cost Analyses

The program evaluators examined financial records to determine the costs associated with various of the *Self Center* components. Because the *Self Center* was a comprehensive and multifaceted intervention, the overall costs of the program were high. However, the evaluators concluded that the *Self Center* services could be delivered for less money. The relative costs and effectiveness of program components are outlined below.

Approximately 40% of the total budget was directed toward the school-based components, while 60% went toward the clinic components. The average cost per student served was $122. However, when analyzed by gender, services to females were approximately four times as costly as services provided to males. When analyzed by school level, services for senior high students cost more than double those provided to junior high students. These differences are due in part to the fact that females in general, and senior high females in particular, took part in many medical and counseling services.

One surprising finding was that costs for counseling exceeded those for medical visits. This was attributed to the amount of time social workers spent in individual counseling sessions. Staff members felt it would be difficult to set limits on the amount of counseling provided and still meet student needs. Indeed, they wondered whether this strategy might only increase the number of questions and concerns addressed to physicians and nurses, whose hourly costs were equal to or greater than those of the social workers.

The small-group sessions conducted by social workers in the school attracted large numbers of students, many of whom would not have been reached if services were only offered at the off-campus clinic. This service proved to be extremely cost-effective, with per student costs well below those of classroom presentations. Although classroom presentations involved many more students at a given time, each one required an entire class period to deliver, as well as advance preparation by program staff.

The use of peer resource teams, while gratifying to the students who staffed them, did not appear to contribute to program success. Instead, paid students consumed both staff time and financial resources. Few students at program schools reported that the peer teams influenced their use of program services.

The researchers asserted that cost analyses are primarily useful for estimating maximum program costs and understanding the relative costs of various components. In fact, they conceded that the *Self Center* staffing had been relatively luxurious and that the program could be implemented for less. Specifically, program costs might be reduced with the following modifications:

- Limiting school-based staff to a program social worker (rather than both a nurse and social worker)
- Sharing program staff among participating schools
- Relying on small, in-school discussion groups to disseminate program information and provide a bridge to clinic services

Summary

In summary, the *Self Center* showed multiple positive impacts on students' reproductive health-related knowledge and behaviors. To begin, exposure to the program delayed the onset of sexual activity among teens who were abstinent at the start of the study; it was also associated with a reduction in the frequency of intercourse among sexually active students. Additionally, students who continued to have intercourse used effective methods of birth control following program exposure. Timely clinic attendance also improved among program school students, as reflected in a greater number of clinic visits and earlier clinic attendance following (and in some cases, preceding) the initiation of sexual intercourse. Effective contraceptive use and decreased frequency of intercourse led to a drop in the pregnancy rates among students at program schools, while the rates at comparison schools increased. The field study further demonstrated that abortion and pregnancy rates could be reduced, and sexual onset postponed by the same program. These findings refute the hypothesis that providing teens with contraceptive services or discussing the responsibilities of sexual intercourse will promote increased sexual activity.

The way in which students used the school components as a bridge to the clinic suggests that a visible relationship between the school and the clinic is crucial to program success. In fact, 88% of students who attended the clinic made their first program contact in school. Although the program was costly in terms of staff time, program evaluators felt that the costs were clearly warranted by the savings from unintentional pregnancy, abortions, and births avoided. Nevertheless, program developers and evaluators suggest a number of ways in which program costs might be reduced in the future.

High rates of HIV and other STI infection among teens make it imperative that any future implementation of the *Self Center* address HIV-related risk and prevention behaviors in addition to pregnancy prevention. Promotion of abstinence and safer sex, along with the proper and consistent use of condoms for STI protection, should be emphasized in all program components.

THE *SELF CENTER* IN THE COMMUNITY TODAY

During the past 3 years, the *Self Center* has been implemented in communities in three states. In one state, the program was implemented in five communities.

NOTE

1. A full set of program materials, including program manual, pamphlets, parental notification form, evaluation materials, and more, is available for purchase from Sociometrics at http://www.socio. com/pasha.htm. Although the program originally focused on primary pregnancy prevention, sexual risk reduction and secondary pregnancy prevention activities might easily be incorporated.

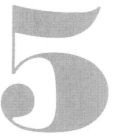

Reducing the Risk: A High School Pregnancy and STI/HIV/AIDS Prevention Program

Kathryn L. Muller, Starr Niego, Margaret S. Kelley, and Janette Mince

Original Program Developers and Evaluators

Richard P. Barth, PhD
   School of Social Welfare
   University of California at Berkeley
   Berkeley, CA

Douglas Kirby, PhD
   ETR Associates
   Scotts Valley, CA

Joyce Fetro, PhD
   San Francisco Unified School District
   San Francisco, CA

Nancy Leland, PhD
   School of Public Health
   University of Minnesota
   Minneapolis, MN

Reducing the Risk was supported by grants from the Stuart Foundation; the William and Flora Hewlett Foundation; and the Division of Research Resources, National Institutes of Health (507-RR07006–22).

PROGRAM ABSTRACT

Summary

Reducing the Risk is a high school–level sexuality education curriculum designed to reduce the frequency of unprotected sexual intercourse through (a) delaying or reducing the frequency of intercourse, or (b) increasing contraceptive and sexually transmitted infection (STI)–protection practice. The 16-session curriculum is intended to serve as one program component, rather than as a comprehensive, stand-alone program. Based on social learning theory, the curriculum aims to change student norms about unprotected sex and perceptions of peer sexual activity, as well as to strengthen parent–child communication concerning abstinence and contraception. The curriculum explicitly emphasizes that students should avoid unprotected intercourse, either by not having sex or by using contraceptives. Lessons are reinforced through role plays, homework activities, quizzes, and skill-building activities.

A field study of the program was conducted in 13 California high schools. Participation in the program significantly increased teens' knowledge and communication with parents regarding abstinence and contraception. In addition, the program significantly reduced the likelihood that students who had not had intercourse at the start of the program would become sexually active by the 18-month follow-up assessment. However, program participation did not affect the frequency of sexual intercourse or the use of contraceptives among teens who were already sexually active at the start of the program.

Focus

☑ Primary pregnancy prevention ☐ Secondary pregnancy prevention ☑ STI/HIV/AIDS prevention

Original Site

☑ School based ☐ Community based ☐ Clinic based

Suitable for Use In

Although the program was originally designed for high schools, it is equally suitable for use in community-based organizations.

Approach

- ☑ Abstinence
- ☑ Behavioral skills development
- ☐ Community outreach
- ☐ Contraceptive access
- ☑ Contraceptive education
- ☐ Life option enhancement
- ☐ Self-efficacy/self-esteem
- ☑ Sexuality/HIV/STI education

Original Intervention Sample

Age, gender   The field study included male and female high school students (average age = 15 years).

Race/ethnicity   61% White, 21% Latino, 9% Asian, 2% African American, 6% Other.

Program Components

- ☑ Adult involvement
- ☐ Case management
- ☑ Group discussion
- ☑ Lectures
- ☐ Peer counseling/instruction
- ☐ Public service announcements
- ☑ Role play
- ☐ Video
- ☑ Other: Clinic and store visits

Program Length

The program consists of 16 lessons, each designed for a 45-minute class period. Most lessons can be expanded to fill two class periods by increasing practice and discussion time.

Staffing Requirements/Training

Regular classroom teachers lead the program. During the original field study, teachers attended a 3-day training session, which focused primarily on practice of the role plays and other class activities. The training also included 3 hours of instruction in reviewing procedures both for obtaining parent and student consent and for collecting program evaluation data.

BIBLIOGRAPHY

Barth, R. P., Leland, N., Kirby, D., & Fetro, J. V. (1992). Enhancing social and cognitive skills. In B. Miller, J. Card, R. Paikoff, & J. Peterson (Eds.), *Preventing adolescent pregnancy* (pp. 53–82). Newbury Park, CA: Sage Publications.

Kirby, D., Barth, R. P., Leland, N., & Fetro, J. V. (1991). *Reducing the Risk:* Impact of a new program on sexual risk-taking. *Family Planning Perspectives, 23*(6), 253–263.

Related References by the Developers of *Reducing the Risk*

Becker, M. G., & Barth, R. P. (2000). Power Through Choices: The development of a sexuality education curriculum for youths in out-of-home care. *Child Welfare, 79*(3), 269–282.

Sangalang, B. B., Barth, R. P., & Painter, J. S. (2006). First-birth outcomes and timing of second births: A statewide case management program for adolescent mothers. *Health & Social Work, 31*(1), 54–63.

THE PROGRAM

Program Rationale and History

Reducing the Risk, a 16-session sexuality education program for high school students, is designed to reduce the frequency of unprotected sexual intercourse through (a) delaying or reducing the frequency of intercourse, or (b) increasing contraceptive practice.[1] The curriculum is intended to be integrated into a broader sexuality education course, rather than as a stand-alone program.

The curriculum aimed to change student norms about unprotected sexual intercourse and perceptions of peer sexual activity, develop effective skills to delay intercourse and/or refuse unprotected sex, and improve parent–child communication concerning abstinence and contraception. The curriculum explicitly emphasized that students should avoid unprotected intercourse, either by not having sex or by using contraceptives. Active student participation was required in role-play situations that simulated those likely to be encountered outside the classroom. Homework assignments provided further reinforcement of class lessons.

A field test of *Reducing the Risk* was conducted during the 1988–1989 school year in 13 California high schools. Funding for the study was provided by the Stuart Foundation, the William and Flora Hewlett Foundation, and the National Institutes of Health.

Theoretical Framework

Reducing the Risk is based on social learning theory (SLT). SLT asserts that the likelihood of engaging in some action, such as using birth control, is determined by four factors:

1. A person's understanding of what must be done to avoid pregnancy
2. The belief that one will be able use the method
3. The belief that the method will be successful at preventing pregnancy
4. The benefit one anticipates from accomplishing the behavior (e.g., preventing pregnancy through effective contraception)

This theory suggests that students need to develop the specific cognitive and social skills that will enable them to resist pressures and successfully negotiate interpersonal encounters. Another important tenet of SLT is that people learn skills by observing others' behavior and then imitating them. In *Reducing the Risk,* teachers and peers first model socially desirable behaviors, such as discussing using birth control with a partner, and then students practice those behaviors in role plays.

Program Objectives

Reducing the Risk provided instruction and practice in using the skills needed to prevent pregnancy and reduce unsafe behavior in high-risk situations. After completing the program, students would be able to

- evaluate the risks and consequences of becoming an adolescent parent or becoming infected with HIV/AIDS or another STI;
- recognize that abstaining from sexual activity or using contraception were the only ways to avoid pregnancy, HIV infection, and other STIs;
- conclude that factual information about conception and protection was essential for avoiding teenage pregnancy, HIV infection, and other STIs; and
- demonstrate effective communication skills for remaining abstinent and for avoiding unprotected sexual intercourse.

Program Content

Reducing the Risk used modeling and repeated practice to enhance teens' skills in resisting unprotected intercourse. Program lessons continually reinforced the message that youths should avoid unprotected intercourse, that the best way to do this was to abstain from sex, and that youths who did not abstain from sex should use contraceptives to guard against pregnancy and STIs. Students also participated in activities that were designed to personalize the consequences of pregnancy and HIV infection. Finally, the curriculum sought to improve parent–child communication about abstinence and contraception.

With its primary emphasis on skill development, *Reducing the Risk* included instruction in the following areas:

- *Refusal statements:* Students learned to say "no" clearly, in a manner that maintained a good relationship but left no ambiguity about the speaker's intent to abstain from sex or unprotected intercourse.

■ *Delay statements and alternative actions:* Students learned ways to avoid a situation or delay acting until they had had sufficient time to decide what to do or say, or until they were prepared to implement a decision.

Program Schedule

The program curriculum spanned 16 classes or lessons. Lessons were designed for 45-minute class periods but could be easily expanded to two periods by increasing practice and discussion time.

Reducing the Risk—Building Skills to Prevent Pregnancy, STI & HIV (also referred to as the *Teacher's Handbook*) provided a comprehensive lesson plan for each class, including a summary of activities and the approximate time required for each, materials needed, detailed steps for leading each activity, student worksheets and handouts, role-play scripts, teacher references, and homework assignments. A brief overview of the lessons is provided below.

Description of Program Sessions

Class 1: Abstinence, Sex, and Protection—Pregnancy Prevention Emphasis. During this introductory class, the teacher demonstrated refusal skills through two versions of a role play. Students participated in a two-part "pregnancy risk" activity to personalize their vulnerability to pregnancy.

Please note that there were two options for Class 1. "Class 1" focused on pregnancy prevention. "Alternate Class 1" focused on HIV/AIDS prevention.

Alternate Class 1: Abstinence, Sex, and Protection—HIV Prevention Emphasis (could be substituted for Class 1 or used in addition to Class 1). The teacher modeled two versions of a role play to demonstrate refusal skills for preventing HIV infection. Students participated in an "HIV Risk" activity to personalize their vulnerability to HIV/AIDS and to symbolically experience modes of transmission.

Class 2: Abstinence—Not Having Sex. Students learned that there are only two ways to avoid pregnancy and HIV: not having sexual intercourse (abstaining) or consistently using protection. This session focused on the advantages of abstinence. Reasons why teens fail to abstain or protect themselves during intercourse were also considered. Students discussed elements of successful male–female communication about abstinence, and they practiced identifying successful communication strategies.

Class 3: Refusals. This class introduced verbal and nonverbal communication skills for refusing sexual activity. Participants watched a demonstration of social skills that were important to abstaining and using protection. Finally, they practiced and studied five characteristics of effective refusals. The homework assignment "Talk to Your Parents" encouraged students and their parents to discuss their sexual attitudes and values.

Class 4: Using Refusal Skills. After students were quizzed on refusal skills, they used role plays to practice applying these skills in difficult situations.

Class 5: Delaying Tactics. After observing a demonstration, students practiced delaying skills in role-play situations. Participants' progress was evaluated with a short quiz.

Class 6: Avoiding High-Risk Situations. Through a class discussion and minilecture, students identified "yellow alert" and "red alert" situations that could lead to unwanted or unprotected sex. Students practiced dealing with the two types of alert situations with the worksheet "Handling Crisis Situations." A second worksheet, "Protection: Myths and Truths," encouraged teens to protect themselves from pregnancy, HIV, AIDS, and other STIs.

Class 7: Getting and Using Protection—I. This class used lectures and demonstrations to provide teens with information on methods for protecting against unplanned pregnancy, HIV/AIDS, and other STIs. For homework, students researched prices and descriptions of nonprescription contraceptive products.

Class 8: Getting and Using Protection—II. The first half of Class 8 included a discussion and visual demonstration of prevention methods, specifically for preventing HIV/AIDS. During the second half of the class, students learned how to locate local clinics for information about protection. They evaluated which methods might be best for them. As an option, this lesson might include a guest speaker from, or a field trip to, a nearby clinic.

Class 9: Knowing and Talking About Protection: Skills Integration—I. This was the first of three lessons in which students applied the communication skills they had learned earlier in the program. A quiz on protection methods was also included. Finally, students watched role plays in which friends talked to each other about issues related to sex and discussed ways to handle similar situations with their own friends.

Class 10: Skills Integration—II. Additional opportunities were provided for teens to practice saying "no" and making decisions about protection. Students also took part in partially scripted role plays involving difficult situations.

Class 11: Skills Integration—III. Students used worksheet and role-play exercises to practice handling situations that might have led to unprotected sex.

Class 12: Preventing HIV/AIDS and Other STIs. Working in small groups, participants explored information about five specific STIs: genital warts (or HPV), gonorrhea, herpes, chlamydia, and HIV. The groups compared forms of transmission, prevention, and treatment for the five infections.

Class 13: HIV/AIDS Risk Behaviors. Class activities were designed to help students apply their knowledge about HIV/AIDS transmission and identify which behaviors would put them at greatest risk for exposure to the virus. Students placed behaviors on a continuum of risk, from no risk to risky, and discussed why certain behaviors were more risky than others.

Class 14: Protecting Oneself From STIs and Pregnancy. This session included several activities to help students develop plans for preventing pregnancy and reducing STI risk through the use of a condom. Participants wrote role-play scripts for scenes involving protection with condoms.

Class 15: Sticking With Abstinence and Protection. Students reported on two homework assignments in which they researched information about protection. The teens discussed and practiced the "self-talk" method designed to help them plan and then follow their plan to avoid sex or unprotected sex.

Class 16: Skills Integration—IV. A discussion about sticking with choices and a final role-play situation provided two opportunities for students to practice avoiding intercourse or unprotected sexual activity.

Program Implementation

Obtaining District and Parent Support

The subject matter of *Reducing the Risk* may provoke controversy, and instructors should make certain that they understand and apply school district policies and state mandates before beginning the program. School board approval and administration support are equally essential. Informed consent from students and their parents is critical when using the *Reducing the Risk* curriculum.

Establishing Classroom Ground Rules

Ground rules for classroom discussion should be established at the start of the program. This creates an atmosphere of trust and comfort in which students feel free to discuss sexuality, birth control, and protection from STIs.

Instructors are advised to follow the principles listed below:

- Students have the "right to remain silent" about any thoughts and actions that they wish to keep private.
- Every question is a good question; every comment is worthy of consideration.
- Teasing, putting others down, or discussing other class members' comments inside or outside the classroom is not tolerated.
- The teacher respects the confidentiality of students' comments (within the constraints permitted by law).
- Students who have, or are aware of, a concern, complaint, or question about the class are encouraged to discuss it with the teacher as soon as possible.
- When discussing issues raised in class with parents, students should provide as accurate a description as possible.
- Nothing said in any role-play exercise should be taken as a sign of interest in having a relationship or having sex (i.e., a "come on"). Because role plays are based on fictional situations, students may say things, as actors, that they would not otherwise say.

Importance of Role Playing

Practicing newly learned skills was a critical piece of the *Reducing the Risk* curriculum. Because situations that could have potentially led to unprotected sex are much more powerful in real life than in the classroom, students needed to "overlearn" refusal and delay skills. Extensive practice increased students' chances of being clear and forceful in real-life romantic situations.

EVALUATING THE PROGRAM

The Original Evaluation

Design

The impact of the *Reducing the Risk* program was measured in a field test conducted with 758 students enrolled in 13 California high schools. A diverse set of measures was used to compare the knowledge, attitudes, and behaviors of two groups of teens: (1) students who took part in the *Reducing the Risk* program (the treatment group) and (2) students who received their school's standard sexuality education curriculum (the comparison group). Questionnaires were administered to all teens at four points in time:

- Time 1: before the *Reducing the Risk* program began
- Time 2: at the conclusion of the program
- Time 3: about 6 months following the program
- Time 4: about 18 months following the program

Recruitment Procedures

To recruit schools for the study, program evaluators sent letters of inquiry to 252 high schools in the 140 California school districts with existing sexuality education programs. To be eligible to participate, schools had to have at least two classes of sexuality education, so that one class could be included in the treatment group, and the second in the comparison group.

Thirty-two high schools expressed strong interest in the study. However, concerns about the subject matter discouraged many from participating, and the final sample included 13 schools. Among the schools that ultimately declined to participate, two reasons were most common: (a) pressure from interest groups concerned about the inclusion of birth control in the curriculum; and (b) reluctance to use the student questionnaire, which was not anonymous and which included questions about sexual intercourse and pregnancy. You and your staff may want to anticipate similar concerns when using *Reducing the Risk* in your own community.

Within the participating schools, teachers volunteered to use the curriculum in their classes. During a 3-day training session held at the start of the study, instructors practiced program exercises and reviewed procedures for obtaining parental and student consent and administering the study survey.

Individual classes were assigned to either the treatment or comparison group; whenever possible, the assignment was random. In schools where classes were unequal in size, the larger classes were assigned to the treatment group to maximize the power of the statistical analysis.

Minimizing Potential "Contamination" Effects

About half of the comparison classes were taught by teachers who also taught one or more treatment classes; this arrangement had implications for the statistical analysis. Although researchers could control for the teachers' general experience and teaching style in their analysis, they could not eliminate possible "contamination" effects. Contamination would result if teachers brought treatment material and techniques into their comparison group classrooms. The researchers tried to address this issue by carefully and repeatedly instructing teachers who taught both treatment and comparison classes not to incorporate any of the *Reducing the Risk* techniques into their comparison classes during the study period.

At the same time, by having some control classes taught by treatment teachers and some by other teachers, the evaluators hoped to reduce potential threats of contamination and differential teaching ability; the researchers reasoned that these biases might cancel, rather than reinforce, each other.

Data Collection Procedures

Participation in the study required "active consent" from students and their parents. Parents were invited to learn more about the curriculum and the evaluation study at an information session that was held in the evening at their child's school. Across all participating schools, fewer than 1% of students were excluded from the program because their parents withheld permission.

The Time 1 and Time 2 assessments were completed by students in their classrooms. The 6-month and 18-month follow-up assessments were conducted in two ways. Some students were recruited by their teachers to complete the survey in school. The remaining students, who received the survey at home, were contacted by telephone to encourage them to return the questionnaire. At the 6-month follow-up, about 25% of students were contacted at home; at the 18-month follow-up, the percentage had increased to more than 50%. Some youths were called more than a dozen times by research staff before responding.

Original Intervention Sample

A total of 46 classes from 13 high schools in 10 school districts participated in the field test. At pretest, 1,033 students completed the assessment (586 in the treatment group and 447 in the comparison group). A total of 758 students, or 73% of the original sample, completed the pretest and 18-month surveys. The researchers found that students who did not complete the 18-month follow-up differed from the other teens in several important ways: At pretest, they were more likely to be older, more likely to be male, more likely to have poor grades, less likely to live with both parents, more likely to have had sex, more likely to have failed to use birth control because sex was not planned, and less likely to have talked to their parents about abstinence.

Evaluation Results

The results indicated that the *Reducing the Risk* curriculum had significant effects in several areas, particularly parent–child communication, knowledge, and the initiation of intercourse.

Effects on Parent–Child Communication

Participation in the program increased teens' communication with their parents about abstinence and birth control. Although comparison group students also showed an increase in communication with their parents over time, the gain among program participants was significantly greater, even 18 months after the intervention. Both parents and students reported that the program made it easier for them to communicate; for many families, this was the first time they had discussed abstinence and birth control at home.

Effects on Knowledge

Many sexuality education programs have produced significant gains in student knowledge. Nevertheless, the gains measured in *Reducing the Risk* were noteworthy for three reasons. First, the curriculum did not focus on knowledge acquisition, but rather on role-playing exercises. Second, comparison group students also received sexuality education, yet the gains recorded for *Reducing the Risk* students were significantly greater. And third, the effects remained significant through the 18-month follow-up assessment.

Effects on Peer Norms

One of the goals of this norm- and skills-based curriculum was to change norms about unprotected sex and to change students' perceptions that "everyone is doing it." Although the curriculum did not seem to diminish students' perceptions about sexual activity among their peers, it apparently prevented those perceptions from worsening over time.

Effects on Initiation and Frequency of Sexual Intercourse

The curriculum apparently reduced the chance that a student would initiate intercourse, possibly by as much as 24%; moreover, it did not increase the frequency of intercourse among students who had already become sexually active, as some of its opponents had feared. In addition, the curriculum appeared to reduce unprotected intercourse among lower-risk students, although no decrease in the overall frequency of sexual activity was recorded.

Effect on Contraceptive Use

Overall, the data indicate that the curriculum did not affect the use of birth control at first intercourse or at most recent intercourse, nor did it affect the frequency of contraceptive use. However, among the subset of teens who became sexually active following the study, program participants were more likely to use contraception.

Summary

The empirical results showed that the 16-session *Reducing the Risk* curriculum, emphasizing the development of skills for resisting unprotected intercourse, was an effective component of a comprehensive sexuality education program. Program participants showed clear gains in knowledge and communication with their parents (at least about the specific issues of abstinence and contraception addressed in homework assignments). The curriculum also delayed intercourse among teens who had not already become sexually active at the start of the intervention.

Among the relatively few students who did initiate intercourse following the study, *Reducing the Risk* participants were more likely than comparison group students to use contraception. However, the curriculum did not significantly affect the frequency of sexual intercourse or the use of birth control among those who had initiated intercourse before the study began.

Overall, the results are particularly impressive in light of the fact that most comparison group students received traditional sex education (rather than no intervention at all). Thus, the field study suggested that *Reducing the Risk* was more effective at producing behavioral changes than the more traditional curricula.

AWARDS AND RECOGNITION

Reducing the Risk has been identified by the Centers for Disease Control and Prevention for inclusion in its Research-to-Classroom Project as a program with credible evidence of reducing sexual risk behaviors. The program is now in its fourth edition.

REDUCING THE RISK IN THE COMMUNITY TODAY

In the past 3 years, *Reducing the Risk* has been implemented in communities in nine states, ranging from Maine to Michigan. It has also been implemented in a community in Canada.

NOTE

1. A full set of program materials, including teacher's handbook, student workbook, pamphlets, evaluation materials, and more, is available for purchase from Sociometrics at http://www.socio.com/pasha.htm.

Reproductive Health Counseling for Young Men: A High School Pregnancy and STI/HIV/AIDS Prevention Program

Ross Danielson, Starr Niego, and Janette Mince

Original Program Developers and Evaluators

Ross Danielson
    Portland State University
    Portland, OR

Anne Plunkett
Merwyn R. Greenlick
    Kaiser Permanente Center for Health Research
    Portland, OR

Shirley Marcy
    Northwest Permanente
    Portland, OR

William Wiest
    Reed College
    Portland, OR

Reproductive Health Counseling for Young Men was supported by grants from the Office of Family Planning, U.S. Department of Health and Human Services.

PROGRAM ABSTRACT

Summary

Originally developed for boys between 15 and 18 years of age, this is a 1-hour, single-session, clinic-based intervention. The program is designed to meet the needs of sexually active and inactive teens, and to promote abstinence as well as contraception. The session begins with a video viewed privately by each teen. The materials address reproductive anatomy, fertility, hernia, testicular self-examination, sexually transmitted infections (STIs) (including HIV/AIDS), contraception (including abstinence), communication skills, and access to health services. A half-hour private consultation with a health care practitioner follows the presentation. Guided by the young men's interests, the consultation may include such topics as sexuality, fertility goals, and reproductive health risks, along with rehearsal and modeling of sexual communication.

A field study of the intervention was conducted with 1,195 high school–aged males visiting health maintenance organizations (HMOs) in two northwestern cities. Compared to a control group of their peers, sexually active program participants were significantly more likely to use effective contraception at the 1-year follow-up assessment, especially if they were not yet sexually active at the time of the intervention. The sexual partners of program participants were also more likely to use effective contraception at the follow-up. Among participants who remained abstinent, the young men reported greater comfort with their decision to delay sexual involvement than did their control group peers.

Focus

☑ Primary pregnancy prevention   ☐ Secondary pregnancy prevention   ☐ STI/HIV/AIDS prevention

Original Site

☑ School based   ☐ Community based   ☑ Clinic based

Suitable for Use In

This program is suitable for use in hospital- or community-based clinics.

Approach

- ☑ Abstinence
- ☑ Behavioral skills development
- ☐ Community outreach
- ☑ Contraceptive access
- ☑ Contraceptive education
- ☐ Life option enhancement
- ☑ Self-efficacy/self-esteem
- ☑ Sexuality/HIV/STI education

Original Intervention Sample

Age, gender   The field study involved 1,195 adolescent males ranging in age from 15 to 18 years.

Race/ethnicity   91% White, 5% African American, 4% Asian, 1% Other.

Program Components

- ■ ☐ Adult involvement
- ■ ☐ Case management
- ■ ☐ Group discussion
- ■ ☐ Lectures
- ■ ☐ Peer counseling/instruction
- ■ ☐ Public service announcements
- ■ ☑ Role play
- ■ ☑ Video
- ■ ☑ Other: Private counseling session

Program Length

The intervention is 1 hour in length, evenly divided between the counseling session and video presentation.

Staffing Requirements/Training

Health care practitioners serve as counselors and provide a brief introduction to the video presentation. In the field study, special training was held to introduce staff to the program's "developmental counseling" strategies, as well as to review the slide and tape presentation. Throughout the study, one of the program leaders was available to answer questions and lead occasional staff meetings.

BIBLIOGRAPHY

Danielson, R., Marcy, S., Plunkett, A., Wiest, W., & Greenlick, M. R. (1990). Reproductive health counseling for young men: What does it do? *Family Planning Perspectives, 22*(3), 115–121.

Related References by the Developers of *Reproductive Health Counseling for Young Men*

Danielson, R., Barbey, A., Cassidy, D., Rosenzweig, J., & Chowdhury, D. (1999). Couple-friendly services in a metropolitan sexually transmitted disease clinic: Views of clients and providers. *Family Planning Perspectives, 31*(4), 195–199.

THE PROGRAM

Program Rationale and History

The *Reproductive Health Counseling for Young Men* program was developed to fill a gap in existing teen pregnancy prevention efforts—notably the involvement of adolescent males.[1] The program was originally targeted toward young men between the ages of 15 and 18, regardless of their previous sexual experience. All intervention activities took place within a single, regularly scheduled medical appointment at participating HMOs in Portland, Oregon, and Vancouver, Washington.

Guided by the belief that health care practitioners could serve as credible sources of sexuality information, the program provided reproductive health information and counseling in a primary health care setting. The two-part, single-session intervention took a broad approach; rather than focusing narrowly on abstinence or (for sexually active young men) contraception, it was also designed to improve participants' knowledge of sexuality and STI prevention, and to promote the practice of testicular self-examination. The intervention further aimed to improve teens' skills and attitudes by encouraging and providing practice in couples communication, as well as promoting greater empathy for female development.

A field study of the intervention was conducted between 1985 and 1987 in Northwest Region Kaiser Permanente, an HMO serving more than 300,000 members in the Portland, Oregon, and Vancouver, Washington, regions. Approximately 1,200 males, ages 15–18, participated in the study.

Theoretical Framework

The *Reproductive Health Counseling for Young Men* program was grounded in previous research demonstrating that teens, parents, and health care professionals believed that HMOs could provide valuable reproductive health information and services to teens. In an earlier project, an HMO had developed a number of innovations, including teen clinics; enhanced access to women's health services and contraception; aggressive attention to women seeking pregnancy testing; newsletters, films, and forums for teens and parents; and extensive community outreach. However, the researchers found that very little attention was ever given to males, despite abundant opportunity, especially in medical visits. Informal research revealed that staff felt less comfortable addressing sexual health topics with young men than they did with women.

The developers of the *Reproductive Health Counseling for Young Men* program recognized the importance of male involvement in contraception. Studies found that "male" methods—condoms and withdrawal—were the most widely used methods of contraception in many teenagers' earliest sexual experiences, and a variety of studies illustrated how the concerns of women's partners were relevant to their use of different contraceptive methods. For these reasons, the program developers hoped to reach and educate adolescent men, especially in their role as partners of young women.

The program is further guided by principles of "developmental counseling." This approach sought to tailor advice and support to the psychosocial and cognitive level of the client, yet provided directive advice for urgent situations. Additionally, counselors strived for discussions that were interactive, concrete, and grounded in the client's personal concerns. In previous research, this method had proved more effective than traditional medically oriented consultations with youths.

Finally, in the intervention, highly explicit information and photography were used to enhance youths' attention and to distinguish this material from other, more general sex education they may have experienced. The original program developers believed that the provision of such "manly" knowledge would be appropriate for the private medical setting in which it was to be viewed. They reasoned that this approach might assuage some of the curiosity of youths with little or no sexual experience. Moreover, they hoped it would reduce virgins' "sexual impatience," boost their sense of manly adequacy, and reduce pressures to begin having intercourse.

Program Objectives

Reproductive Health Counseling for Young Men embraced five educational objectives:

1. To promote abstinence, contraception, and prevention of STI/HIV/AIDS
2. To serve both sexually active and abstinent teens
3. To appeal both to youths and their parents
4. To address the educational and counseling needs of young men without labeling them as sexually active/inactive or as having sexual problems
5. To promote sexual and reproductive health, broadly defined

Program Elements

The 1-hour intervention was divided into two 30-minute components: a video presentation followed by a counseling session. During the original field study, these activities took place within a regular scheduled medical appointment at a health care facility.

Video Presentation

Following a brief introduction and greeting by a health care practitioner, the teen viewed a video program privately, in an examination or conference room. The presentation explicitly addressed reproductive anatomy, fertility, hernia, testicular self-examination, STIs (including HIV/AIDS), sexuality and contraception (including abstinence), communication skills, and access to health services. It was partly adapted from *Young Men's Reproductive Health* and *Young Men's Sexual Responsibility*, both created by researchers at the University of Minnesota School of Public Health.

Counseling Session

Immediately following the video, the health care practitioner returned for a private consultation and counseling session with the teen. Although the session typically focused on abstinence and/or contraception, it was guided by each participant's expressed interests and covered such topics as sexuality, fertility goals, symptoms of STIs, and appropriate use of health care resources. In an effort to enhance teens' familiarity and comfort with contraception, samples of condoms and other products were shown. Finally, staff modeled effective communication with one's partner and then encouraged the youths to practice these skills.

At the time this intervention was being developed, HIV/AIDS was just emerging as a significant public health issue. Until that point, most STIs could be cured by a course of antibiotics. The first year of this study, 1985, was the year that Ryan White (a teen with hemophilia) was denied entry to school because he had HIV—contracted through a blood transfusion. It was also the year Rock Hudson died—the first of many celebrity deaths to follow.

The first case of HIV/AIDS appeared in China during the first year of the study of *Reproductive Health Care Counseling for Young Men*—signaling that the infection was viable in every part of the world. Had *Reproductive Health Care Counseling for Young Men* been developed and evaluated today, condom use, a condom demonstration, and condom use practice would likely have been at the forefront of the activities/discussion points of the counseling segment of this intervention.

Program Implementation

Developmental Counseling

During the field study, program staff aimed to be directive, but not judgmental, during the counseling session and to address any questions or concerns the youths might have. This "developmental" approach—first used with young women—offered highly explicit advice. Moreover, it differed significantly from traditional reproductive counseling, which typically concentrated on the medical history of the teen.

Underlying Principles

The following principles were used by the original program developers to set up and carry out the intervention. They may prove helpful for your own intervention.

- Take a positive view of adolescence and sexuality.
- Acknowledge sexual development as one of the tasks of adolescence.
- Take a broad and positive view of sexuality.
- Tailor the counseling to the cognitive skills of teens.
- Emphasize couples' communication, shared responsibility, and personal responsibility.

- Encourage young men to understand and empathize with their female partners' experiences.
- Recognize the high esteem and trust given to health care professionals regarding health issues.
- Teach teens how and when to access health care services, and invite them to practice discussing reproductive and sexual health issues with health care professionals.

PROGRAM EVALUATION

The Original Evaluation

Design

The effectiveness of *Reproductive Health Counseling for Young Men* was investigated in a field study conducted in two northwestern cities between 1985 and 1987. The study compared two groups of males: adolescent males who took part in the single-session video and counseling intervention (e.g., program participants) and members of a "wait list" control group. Assignment to the two groups was randomly determined.

The researchers investigated the two groups' knowledge of reproductive health, levels of sexual activity, contraceptive use, and for abstinent males only, sexual impatience or feelings about having never engaged in intercourse. Surveys were administered to all teens at two points:

- Time 1: at the youth's recruitment into the study (pretest)
- Time 2: 12 months following the intervention (follow-up)

Evaluation Questions

The researchers hypothesized that program participants would show significant improvement on the following measures, relative to their control group peers:

1. Knowledge of reproductive health
2. Delay in sexual debut
3. Use of contraception if sexually active
4. Acceptance of postponed sexual debut

Recruitment and Data Collection

Young men were recruited by telephone from the population of high school–aged males whose names appeared on active appointment schedules for routine medical services at a large HMO. The plan for participating in the program and completing questionnaires was described to each youth and at least one parent. Consent was then requested, and confidentiality was assured for the information provided on all research instruments. The young men were also promised a $15 travel allowance following completion of the final questionnaire.

With teens who had been randomly assigned to the treatment group, visits were scheduled immediately. For teens assigned to the control group, staff explained that they would call back to arrange an appointment at a later time.

Unless there was a refusal, at least three attempts were made to schedule appointments with each youth. If the client seemed reluctant to schedule a visit, the scheduler asked if the client would prefer to see a male practitioner or a physician instead of a nurse practitioner. In only a few cases did this happen, and these youths were served accordingly. In a few cases, the young man asked to bring a friend or brother along, and this was welcomed.

Staff attempted to reschedule all missed appointments. However, with reminder calls, missed appointments were not a problem, and 81% of teens assigned to the treatment group eventually participated. All youths completed the pretest survey at the time of their recruitment into the study and the follow-up survey 12 months later.

Research Sample

Of the 2,602 potential participants identified by the researchers, 94% were reached by phone, and 56% provided the necessary consent. Scheduling was successfully completed for 1,195 teens, or 46% of the original pool. The final research sample was predominantly middle-class and White, though 5% of participants were African American and 4% Asian. At the pretest assessment, 18% of the youths were high school freshmen, 45% sophomores, 24% juniors, and 24% seniors.

After discarding 23 surveys that could not be matched to baseline instruments, the researchers were left with complete data from 971 teens, or 81% of the initial sample. Overall, the demographic characteristics of the final research sample were similar to those of the HMO population in this age category, except that high school sophomores were overrepresented.

Evaluation Results

Knowledge of Reproductive Health

Analysis of data provided evidence of statistically significant effects on teens' understanding of contraception, STIs, fertility, and transmission and prevention of HIV/AIDS. However, most of these effects were significant only among particular subgroups of participants. For example, program participants were significantly more likely than their control group peers to believe that the birth control pill is very safe ($p < .01$). However, this belief was significant only among those teens who had already become sexually active when the study began. In contrast, on items measuring teens' understanding of fertility, newly sexually active program participants scored significantly higher than their control group peers ($p < .01$). Finally, on a seven-item index of HIV/AIDS-related knowledge, participants showed a modest improvement, relative to the control group. This finding was significant for the entire group of participants ($p < .05$).

Sexual Activity Status

There were few differences in patterns of sexual activity between program participants and members of the control group—at either assessment period. Thus, it appeared that the intervention neither encouraged nor discouraged sexual activity by the teens. Across the two groups, 37% were sexually active during the year prior to the study, and 53% were active during the follow-up period. Among teens who had been abstinent at baseline, 31% were active at the follow-up assessment, while 90% of teens who were sexually active at the pretest remained so through the study period. Although fewer virgins in the intervention group became active in the follow-up year than in the control group, this difference was not statistically significant.

Contraceptive Use

In contrast, the program did appear to have a positive impact on sexually active participants' patterns of contraception, particularly regarding the birth control pill. At the follow-up assessment, among sexually active teens, participants were significantly more likely than control group members to report that their partner was using oral contraception ($p < .05$), especially if they had not yet had intercourse at the time of the intervention ($p < .01$).

Sexual Impatience

Finally, on measures of sexual impatience, program participants reported greater comfort than did their control group peers with postponing sexual involvement.

Summary

Overall, the single-session intervention, combining a video presentation with a private counseling session, showed promise in promoting support for sexual restraint among abstinent males and more effective contraception among sexually active youths. Additionally, the field study data provided no evidence that the onset of sexual activity is affected by young men's participation.

In interpreting the data, the researchers concluded that health care practitioners played an important role in counseling and educating young men about pregnancy prevention. In addition, based on the finding that the intervention had resulted in more consistent use of birth control pills by the young men's partners, the researchers emphasized the importance of working with couples. Indeed, they recommended that providers encourage young men who are engaged in unprotected intercourse to return for a visit *with their partners.*

Finally, the researchers acknowledged that their evaluation tested a well-defined *minimal* intervention; future projects should incorporate individualized strategies or follow-up with youths who appear to be at significant risk for unwanted pregnancy or STI/HIV/AIDS. Such strategies might include referrals for additional services at school, by telephone, or in the community, and visits with one's partner. Providers should also develop strategies for serving youths whose cognitive skills are quite limited.

REPRODUCTIVE HEALTH COUNSELING FOR YOUNG MEN IN THE COMMUNITY TODAY

In the past 3 years, *Reproductive Health Counseling for Young Men* has been implemented in multiple communities in three states.

NOTE

1. A full set of program materials, including program manual, program script, videotape, evaluation materials, and more, is available for purchase from Sociometrics at http://www.socio.com/pasha. htm.

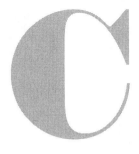

Programs Designed for Youth/Community Collaboration

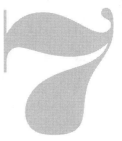

School/Community Program for Sexual Risk Reduction Among Teens: An Adolescent Pregnancy Prevention Program

Starr Niego, William S. Farrell, M. Jane Park, and Janette Mince

Original Program Developer

Murray L. Vincent, EdD
  Department of Health Promotion and Education
  School of Public Health
  University of South Carolina
  Columbia, SC

Original Program Evaluator

Andrew F. Clearie, MSPH
  School of Public Health
  University of South Carolina
  Columbia, SC

School/Community Program for Sexual Risk Reduction Among Teens was supported by grants from U.S. Department of Health and Human Services and South Carolina State Health and Human Services Finance Commission.

PROGRAM ABSTRACT

Summary

The School/Community Program for Sexual Risk Reduction Among Teens (hereafter referred to as the *School/Community Program*) is a community-wide public outreach campaign. It incorporates multiple forms of outreach and public education to engage the entire community in preventing pregnancy among unmarried adolescents. Public schools, universities, church groups and civic organizations are all targeted as sites for training and workshops concerning human physiology, sexual development, self-concept and sexual awareness, values clarification, and communication skills. Abstinence is promoted as the preferred sexual health decision in all activities; for teens who do choose to become sexually active, effective contraception is encouraged. In 1982, the intervention was developed and field tested in a rural, low-income, and predominantly African American community. A significant drop in the pregnancy rate was recorded during the full implementation period of the program.

Focus

☑ Primary pregnancy   ☐ Secondary pregnancy   ☐ STI/HIV/AIDS
   prevention   prevention   prevention

Original Site

☑ School based   ☑ Community based   ☐ Clinic based

Suitable for Use In

This program is suitable for use in any community in collaboration with a variety of organizations, including schools.

Approach

- ☑ Abstinence
- ☑ Behavioral Skills development
- ☑ Community outreach
- ☑ Contraceptive access
- ☑ Contraceptive education
- ☑ Life option enhancement
- ☑ Self-efficacy/self-esteem
- ☑ Sexuality/HIV/STI education

Original Intervention Sample

Age, gender   Rather than targeting a particular group of teens, the program involved an entire community with a population of 18,796 in 1982.

Race/ethnicity The community composition was 58% African American and 42% White.

Program Components

- ☑ Adult involvement
- ☐ Case management

- ■ ☑ Group discussion
- ■ ☑ Lectures
- ■ ☐ Peer counseling/instruction
- ■ ☑ Public service announcements
- ■ ☑ Role play
- ■ ☐ Video
- ■ ☑ Other: Peer education training program

Program Length

The complete program of public service announcements, adult education workshops, and graduate courses for teachers may require a full year to implement.

Staffing/Requirements/Training

The project requires a full-time project director and an on-site coordinator. Both should have a solid knowledge of teen pregnancy and public health strategies.

BIBLIOGRAPHY

Frost, J. J., & Forrest, J. D. (1995). Understanding the impact of effective teenage pregnancy prevention programs. *Family Planning Perspectives, 27*(5), 188–195.

Koo, H. P., Dunteman, G. H., George, C., Green, Y., & Vincent, M. (1994). Reducing adolescent pregnancy through school and community-based education: Denmark, South Carolina revisited. *Family Planning Perspectives, 26*(5), 206–211, 217.

Koo, H. P., Dunteman, G. H., Gogan, H., Johnson, J., Spruyt, A., Cook, T. J., et al. (1990). *Reanalysis of changes in teenage pregnancy rates in Denmark area and comparison counties. Evaluation of the South Carolina School/Community intervention to reduce unintended adolescent pregnancy.* Unpublished manuscript.

Vincent, M. L., Clearie, A. F., & Schluchter, M. D. (1987). Reducing adolescent pregnancy through school and community-based education. *Journal of the American Medical Association, 257*(24), 3382–3386.

Vincent, M. L., Geiger, B. F., Johnson, C., Dills, H. M., & Peebles, K. (1993). *Practical needs assessment and evaluation methods for establishing a successful sexual risk reduction program.* Myrtle Beach, SC: South Carolina Association for the Advancement of Health Education & South Carolina Alliance for Health, Physical Education, Recreation and Dance. Unpublished report.

Vincent, M. L., Lepro, E. G., Baker, S. L., & Garvey, D. G. (1991). Projected public sector savings in a teen pregnancy prevention project. *Journal of Health Education, 22*(4), 208–213.

Related References by the Developers of *School/Community Program*

Lindley, L. L., Reininger, B. M., Vincent, M. L., Richter, D. L., Saunders, R. P., & Shi, L. (1998). Support for school-based sexuality education among South Carolina voters. *Journal of School Health, 68*(5), 205–212.

Paine-Andrews, A., Harris, K. J., Fisher, J. L., Lewis, R. K., Williams, E. L., Fawcett, S. B., et al. (1999). Effects of a replication of a multicomponent model for preventing adolescent pregnancy in three Kansas communities. *Family Planning Perspectives, 31*(4), 182–189.

THE PROGRAM

Program Rationale and History

The *School/Community Program* is a comprehensive, multifaceted approach to public health education.[1] In October 1982, a field study of the program was initiated in a rural, predominantly African American, and low-income community in South Carolina, where the rate of adolescent pregnancy exceeded the state average. Following the program's success in Bamberg County, a second sister project was begun in Hampton County, South Carolina, in March 1992.

Recognizing unintended teenage pregnancy as a major public health concern, the program developers mobilized local residents to participate in a broad-based, community-wide intervention encouraging youths to postpone sexual intercourse. Public schools, universities, church groups, and civic organizations all became sites for training, education, and workshops. Topics included human physiology and reproduction, sexual development, self-concept and sexual awareness, communication skills, and values clarification.

Note: Since the field tests of *School/Community Program* were conducted in 1982 and 1992, the U.S. teen pregnancy rate overall has decreased approximately 36%. Among African American teens, the majority of the population served by this intervention, the teen pregnancy rate has decreased by 40%. During that same time, the U.S. population—indeed, the world—and African Americans in particular, have experienced the spread of the HIV/AIDS epidemic. Had *School/Community Program* been developed today, the emphasis would have been on decreasing sexual risk behaviors and increasing correct and consistent condom use.

Theoretical Framework

The program is guided by three theoretical perspectives. They are viewed as complementary ways of understanding individual and community change. First, the program views sexual risk reduction as an innovation, or a new idea, to be diffused throughout the community. For an innovation to be accepted, it must be perceived as advantageous to the community, consistent with residents' values and needs, easy to understand and carry out, and finally, capable of being tested. Following these principles in their field study, program staff first aimed to increase knowledge, awareness, and commitment among local leaders, who in turn would encourage the larger community to help change adolescents' sexual practices.

Principles of the health belief model suggest that individuals will be likely to engage in health-related behaviors when the following conditions are met:

1. One perceives that the problem (e.g., teen pregnancy or sexually transmitted infections [STIs], including HIV) poses a threat to one's well-being.
2. One understands the benefits and barriers to taking preventive action.
3. One feels able to effectively carry out the recommended actions.

Finally, Bandura's social learning theory elaborates the processes through which intentions can be translated into behavioral change among teens. Bandura asserts that learning occurs through practice and observation of social models; it is mediated by internal beliefs about one's ability to succeed, as well as by others' evaluation of the individual's performance. The *School/Community Program* is designed to expose youths to positive role models, provide opportunities to practice responsible decision making, and enhance teens' sense of efficacy over their life circumstances.

Program Objectives

The overall goal of the original program was to reduce the occurrence of unintended pregnancy among unmarried adolescents. In the process, the program aimed to improve the health and social welfare of the community. Two behavioral objectives were also specified:

1. To postpone adolescents' initial sexual intercourse
2. For teens who choose to be sexually active, to promote effective use of contraception

Hypothesized Outcomes

It was hypothesized that an intensive program of school- and community-based education, accompanied by a continuing stream of pregnancy-prevention messages, would be associated with a decrease in unintended adolescent pregnancy in the target community.

In the original field study, the researchers also outlined subcomponents, such as enhancing self-esteem and increasing decision-making skills. However, no specific hypotheses were stated, and these outcomes were not measured in the study.

The original program developers recognized that the success of the intervention would depend on residents' acceptance of adolescent pregnancy as a public health concern, as well as on their willingness to participate in educational activities. In selecting a target community, the developers sought a location with high need (as reflected in an adolescent pregnancy rate above the state average) and a high level of interest. Because many residents of the mixed-race community came from families in which adolescent pregnancy had occurred, perhaps for several generations, program leaders maintained a nonjudgmental stance. Instead, they highlighted benefits associated with delayed sexual intercourse, including increased opportunities for education and employment.

Education Objectives

In the field study of the program (1982), community residents participated in a continuing program of educational activities. The following objectives, formulated during the original study, were appropriate for participants of all ages:

- To promote the postponement of initial voluntary intercourse as the positive, preferred sexual and health decision for teens
- To help people recognize that early sexual intercourse and pregnancy could create problems that impair one's quality of life
- To understand growth and developmental changes experienced by children, adolescents, and adults
- To develop skills in assertiveness, communication, problem solving, and decision making that were resistant to peer, social, and cultural pressures
- To enhance the self-esteem and future aspirations of all participants
- To understand reproduction and contraception and acquire skills regarding the prevention of pregnancy

Program Activities

The field study of the *School/Community Program* included the following four concurrent and overlapping outreach activities. However, the components of your intervention may vary with the needs and interests of your community.

1. *Public awareness.* At the start of the intervention, program staff saturated the community with messages emphasizing both the consequences of adolescent pregnancy and residents' responsibility to help address the problem. The messages included public service announcements on radio, television, and in the local newspaper; notes sent from school to parents at home; and phone calls from program staff to church representatives.
2. *Community workshops.* Five workshops addressed parenting skills and social relations between children and adults. These sessions were directed toward ministers, clergy, and parents and included sessions on enhancing self-esteem, communication, responsible decision making, and values, as well as reproductive anatomy, physiology, and contraception.

3. *Teacher education.* Public school teachers were invited to participate, at no cost, in 3-credit-hour, graduate-level courses at the local university, where they were introduced to principles of family life and sex education. Enrollment for each course was open on a first-come basis to 25 teachers and guidance counselors. All teachers (grades K through 12) were encouraged to apply the material in their classes. Because no specific sex education program was mandated for the county schools, participants integrated units of the Growth and Development Curriculum within their biology, science, social studies, and other courses.

4. *Peer counselors.* With parental permission, high school students were invited to participate in approximately 70 hours of training. The sessions covered listening, counseling, problem-solving and facilitating skills, along with conflict resolution, understanding human behavior, and teen health issues. Each year, approximately 9–12 students completed the program, which was scheduled before and after the school day, as well as on weekends. Trained peer counselors made presentations to middle and elementary school students.

Finally, in conjunction with the *School/Community Program,* school nurses provided family planning education, referrals to public agencies, and contraceptive services to sexually active youths.

Program Overview

Public Awareness Activities

Efforts to raise community awareness about the importance of delaying sexual intercourse and pregnancy occurred throughout the duration of the program.

Community Workshops and Peer Education Training

Listed below are outlines for the community workshops, which were held on weeknights from 6:30 to 8:00 p.m. A similar curriculum was applied in an expanded format for the peer counselor training sessions.

Session 1: Enhancing Self-Esteem

Learning Objectives

1. Participants assessed their personal levels of self-esteem.
2. Participants identified psychosocial conditions that influenced self-esteem.
3. Participants gained an understanding of basic human needs and wants for a positive self-image.

Content

After a brief introduction, participants reviewed the four conditions of self-esteem (e.g., connectiveness, uniqueness, power, models) and basic needs for a positive self-image. Characteristics of self-accepting individuals were also discussed. The facilitator led a discussion of strategies for increasing self-esteem among adolescents.

Suggested Activities

1. Participants completed the Rosenberg Self-Esteem Scale for self-assessment.
2. Participants wrote brief autobiographies that highlighted their accomplishments and characteristics and shared them with the group.

Session 2: Communication

Learning Objective

This session taught participants how to differentiate between effective and poor communication. They demonstrated the skills of attending, understanding, responding, and taking responsibility.

Content

Combining a lecture/discussion format, the facilitator illustrated communication strategies that enhanced and impeded communication.

Suggested Activities

1. Participants gave examples of roadblocks to communication and their effects on people.
2. Participants were videotaped in role plays, such as parents and teens discussing topics or teens resisting peer pressure in a dating situation. The group critiqued the scenes.

Session 3: Responsible Decision Making

Learning Objectives

1. Participants applied steps in the decision-making process to life situations.
2. Participants described how the decision-making process applied to postponing sexual activity.

Content

After introducing the principles of effective decision making, the facilitator defined each of the steps involved. The importance of careful decision making concerning sexual activity, contraception, and relationships was also discussed.

Suggested Activities

1. Participants identified a problem and carried out the decision-making process, both individually and in a group.
2. The moderator posed questions for reflection and discussion concerning the decision of whether to have sexual intercourse: reasons, consequences, personal values, family and community values, birth control, and partner's feelings.

Session 4: Values

Learning Objectives

1. Participants identified and affirmed their sexual values.
2. Participants applied their values to a life situation.

Content

The facilitator first defined the values-clarification process and then illustrated "the clarifying response," a strategy for encouraging individuals to consider what was most important to them. After considering reasons why teens engaged in early sexual activity, the group considered ways adults might assist youths in incorporating values into sexual decision making.

Suggested Activities

1. Participants chose and ranked the three most and least desirable factors in a sexual relationship. Working with a partner, participants discussed their choices.
2. Participants rank-ordered a list of possible lifetime influences on their values (e.g., family members, friends, records, books, movies, church, school). In small groups, participants discussed their top five influences and considered:
    i. How did these influences affect personal values?
    ii. How did participants feel about the effects of these influences?
    iii. Did participants want to change the influences, or were they satisfied?
    iv. How would participants like their children to develop their personal values?
3. Participants role-played scenarios (e.g., mother/daughter, friend/friend, pastor/parishioner) in which one character sought the other for advice concerning premarital sex. The "counselor" guided the other person through the valuing process.

Session 5: Reproductive Anatomy, Physiology, and Contraception

Learning Objectives

1. Participants described the fertilization process.
2. Participants demonstrated techniques of assertiveness in resisting pressure to have sexual intercourse.
3. Participants described the mechanics and advantages/disadvantages of at least two forms of contraception.
4. Participants identified and refuted common myths regarding the risks of pregnancy and contraception.

Content

The facilitator introduced key concepts of male and female physiology and sexual development. This was followed by a discussion of contraceptive methods, highlighting abstinence as the most effective form of pregnancy prevention.

Suggested Activities

1. Participants discussed the following:
    ▪ What had their parents told them about sex?
    ▪ What are some myths they had heard about sex?
    ▪ What did they wish they had been told about sex?
    ▪ How did they feel about counseling someone about sexuality?
2. Participants role-played effective communication in saying "no" to sex.

Teacher Education

Listed below are sample descriptions and recommended textbooks for the graduate-level courses offered to teachers in conjunction with the *School/Community Program*. Sexuality Education, Curriculum Methods, and Teaching Methods were the three primary courses; seminars on related topics, such as HIV/AIDS Education and Health Promotion in the Elementary School, were taught as well. Each course included at least 45 hours of instruction and a variety of activities: lecture-discussions, small-group discussions, written assignments, demonstrations, and evaluations of curriculum materials.

HEDU 501: Family Life and Sex Education Programs. This course examined problems and questions concerning the inclusion of family life and sex education instruction in health education programs.

Course Objectives

1. To comprehend and internalize the biological, psychological, and sociological bases of human sexuality.
2. To assess the sexual health needs of different populations and construct and coordinate curricula to meet those needs.
3. To understand and describe the negative consequences of immature sexual activity and promote the value and importance of postponing sexual intercourse among teen populations.
4. To understand, describe, and implement teaching methods that facilitate the learning of basic concepts related to human sexuality.
5. To justify the inclusion of the study of human sexuality and family life education in various health education settings.
6. To resolve personal biases and prejudices that may inhibit learning in individual and group interactions.
7. To achieve personal growth toward attaining a comfortable attitude regarding one's sexual potential.

Suggested Text

- Bruess, C. E., & Greenberg, J. S. (2004). *Sexuality education: Theory and practice* (4th ed.). New York: Jones & Bartlett.

HEDU R755: Selected Topics in Health Education—Implementation and Methodologies in Family Life and Sex Education. This course surveyed curriculum options, teaching methods, and community support strategies for improving family life and sex education instruction.

Course Objectives

1. To assess the curricular options for providing educational programs at specific age and maturation levels.
2. To acquire planning skills necessary to sequence learning experiences in individual classes and in extended curriculum plans.
3. To assess the appropriateness of material aids and resources available to supplement instruction.
4. To understand the purpose of, and acquire the ability to function as, a teacher-facilitator in group settings.
5. To acquire the skills required to promote appropriate sexual behavior among teens and to promote abstinence as a positive alternative.

Suggested Texts

- Brindis, C. D. (1991). *Adolescent pregnancy prevention: A guidebook for communities.* Stanford, CA: Health Promotion Resource Center.
- Drolet, J. C., & Clark, K. (Eds.). (1994). *The sexuality education challenge: Promoting healthy sexuality in young people.* Santa Cruz, CA: ETR Associates.
- Farber, N. (2003). *Adolescent pregnancy: Policy and prevention services.* New York: Springer Publishing.

■ Romer, D. (Ed.). (2003). *Reducing adolescent risk: Toward an integrated approach.* Thousand Oaks, CA: Sage Publications.

HEDU R729 Selected Topics in Health Education—Curriculum Planning in Family Life and Sex Education. Participants in this course selected a curriculum design for their school and integrated curricular objectives, content, and learning opportunities into their existing courses.

Course Objectives

1. To review and assess the merits and limitations of family life and sex education curricula currently in use in school districts around the nation.
2. To select and determine appropriate concepts, objectives, content, and learning experiences for one's own school district.
3. To reach group consensus on strategies for integrating the Growth and Development Curriculum into existing courses.

Suggested Texts

■ Fodor, J. T., Dalis, G. T., & Giarratano, S. C. (2002). *Health instruction: Theory and application for community, school, health care and workplace settings* (6th ed.). Dubuque, IA: Kendall/Hunt Publishing Company. (Reprints of periodicals and book chapters related to curriculum development. Display of existing family life and sex education curriculum guides.)
■ Hale, J. A. (2007). *A guide to curriculum mapping: Planning, implementing, sustaining the process.* Thousand Oaks, CA: Corwin Press.
■ Rew, L. (2005). *Adolescent health: A multidisciplinary approach to theory, research and intervention.* Thousand Oaks, CA: Sage Publications.

Student Curriculum

In conjunction with the graduate-level education courses, teachers implemented family life and sex education in their own classrooms. Table 7.1 lists program components from the *School/Community Program's* Growth and Development Curriculum used during the field study. For each topic, the grade level and number of sessions are also noted.

Program Implementation

The *School/Community Program* required support and active participation from community residents, civic leaders, church representatives, teachers, and educational administrators. For this reason, the program director began by reviewing the four steps involved in organizing a community:

■ Gaining acceptance
■ Identifying local needs
■ Entering the community
■ Establishing trust and support

Following these steps enabled the program director to increase community awareness and build the kinds of partnerships that were necessary to implement a comprehensive, multifaceted intervention.

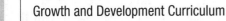

TOPIC	GRADE LEVEL	NUMBER OF SESSIONS
Self-Awareness, Sex Role	K	4
The Changing Self	K–1	7
Family Relationships	1	4
Self-Concept, Awareness of One's Own and Others' Feelings	2	5
Self-Concept, Getting Along With Others	4	4
Socialization, Making Decisions	5	5
Sex Roles in Dating	8–12	4
Saying "No" to Sex	9–10	4
Decision Making and Role Playing	9–12	6
Male and Female Reproductive Anatomy	9–12	6
The Moral Implications of Abortion: Why Not Abortion	9–12	4
Responsible Decision Making, Sexual Development, Family Relationships and Respect for Friends	10	6
Responsible Sexual Decision Making: Alternatives to Sexual Intercourse	10	3
Intelligent Choice of a Sexual Lifestyle	10–11	5
Saying "No" and Meaning It	11–12	4
Individual/Group Counseling	1–12	8

PROGRAM EVALUATION

The Original Evaluation

Initial Design

A matched-area design was used to measure the program's effectiveness. Annual estimated pregnancy rates (EPRs) for adolescent females in the intervention portion of Bamberg County were compared with EPRs in four similar areas. The estimated pregnancy rate is an annual indicator expressing the number of pregnancies that occur per 1,000 females in a population (in this case, per 1,000 females ages 14 through 17 years). The rate is computed as follows:

$$EPR = \frac{\text{Live Births} + \text{Fetal Deaths} + \text{Induced Abortions}}{\text{Number of Females Ages 14–17}} \times 1,000$$

Intervention effectiveness was determined by comparing *average* EPRs within the target population before and after the intervention, and by comparing the difference between preintervention and postintervention pregnancy rates in populations exposed and not exposed to the program.

The first comparison area was the nonintervention portion of the county. Recognizing that the program may have had some spillover effect beyond the target community, three other South Carolina counties were selected for comparison, based on their sociodemographic similarity to Bamberg County in 1982.

Trends in annual, age-specific EPRs for females ages 14 to 17 years were examined. In addition, the average EPR for a given period was calculated as the sum of annual EPRs for the years included, divided by the number of years in the period.

Average EPRs were analyzed across the four comparison areas for the following periods:

- Preintervention period (1981–1982)
- Postintervention period (1984–1985)

Evaluation Question

Program evaluators examined whether the target community showed significantly lower rates of adolescent pregnancy, over time, relative to comparable areas of the state.

Where to Get Data

The estimated pregnancy rate for the original field study was devised using annual data supplied by the Office of Vital Records and Public Health Statistics, South Carolina Department of Health and Environmental Control. This agency provided the number of live births, fetal deaths, and abortions to South Carolina residents by age of resident, by town and county of resident, and by year of occurrence.

The analogous government agencies in your state may be able to provide you with similar data for calculating EPRs in your community for your target population.

Evaluation Results

There was a sharp reduction in the number of adolescent pregnancies in the target community after 1983, when the intervention program had been fully implemented. Among 333 female adolescents in the population, ages 14 to 17 years, there were 18 pregnancies in 1981. In both 1984 and 1985, with 319 girls in the population, 8 pregnancies were recorded. During this period, there was a slight drop in the number of pregnancies in the nonintervention portion of Bamberg County, and an increase in the other three comparison areas. Simultaneously, population levels dropped in all five areas, with the sharpest declines found in the comparison communities located outside Bamberg County. Focusing on EPRs helped adjust for such fluctuations.

After 1983, the EPR in the target community dropped significantly—from 61.7 in 1983 to 25.1 in 1984 and 1985. This meant nearly 37 fewer pregnancies per 1,000 females following the start of the intervention. A less dramatic drop, from 63.1 in 1983 to 58.8 in 1984 and 46.0 in 1985, was measured in the nonintervention portion of the county. In contrast, the pregnancy rates increased somewhat in the three comparison areas outside Bamberg County. For example, in one community, there had been 45.1 pregnancies per 1,000 females in 1983; by 1985 the figure had risen to 54.9. Overall, during the postintervention period (1984–1985), the average EPR for the target community was significantly lower than the average rates in the four comparison groups ($p < .01$ for all comparisons).

Comparing changes in average EPR between the preintervention (1981–1982) and postintervention (1984–1985) periods, there was a significant drop in the rate measured in the target community (estimated decrease between 13.7 and 57.3 pregnancies per 1,000 females, 95% confidence interval). A smaller, nonsignificant decrease was found between the two periods for the nonintervention portion of the county. Outside Bamberg County, the average EPR increased significantly in two of the comparison areas, while no significant change was recorded in the other community.

Comparing the rates of change across counties showed that the drop in EPRs between the intervention and nonintervention portions of Bamberg County was not significant. On the other hand, the increase in EPR among the comparison areas did differ significantly from the decrease measured in the target community ($p < .002$, $p < .001$ and $p < .001$ for the three comparisons).

Secondary Analysis

In 1994 the original program developer joined with a team of researchers to re-analyze the program's effectiveness. Three strategies guided the secondary data analysis:

1. To achieve a closer match between the target and comparison communities, additional sociodemographic data were examined, notably the adolescent pregnancy rate prior to the start of the intervention. A new group of comparison communities was selected for analysis.
2. The pre- and postintervention periods were lengthened to allow for an expanded analysis.
3. EPRs were adjusted to correct for the fact that adolescent females who became pregnant at age 17, but gave birth at age 18, would have been excluded from the original measure.

Across the two evaluation studies, overall trends for the immediate postintervention period (1984–1985) appeared similar, with a steep, significant decline in EPR recorded in the target community. Yet, the secondary analysis also revealed an increase in the pregnancy rate in 1987–1988, to 66 pregnancies per 1,000 females. By 1987–1988, differences in the adjusted EPRs for the target and comparison communities were insignificant.

After examining possible explanations for the upward trend in EPR, program evaluators focused on significant changes in the scope of program activities. Most importantly, in 1987 public opposition led to the termination of the Teen Life Center's contraceptive services for high school students; in 1988 the nurse who had staffed the center resigned. Thus, in 1987–1988 the county health department clinic was the only family planning service available to adolescents, and it was inaccessible by public transportation. The researchers also noted a decline in enrollment for the graduate-level family life and sex education courses. Overall, they linked the lowest rates of adolescent pregnancy to the years of greatest community involvement (1984–1986); once community support and participation declined, adolescent pregnancy returned to preintervention levels. They found additional support for this hypothesis by examining pregnancy prevention activities in the comparison counties. None of these efforts were as comprehensive as the *School/Community Program,* and none of the communities showed a drop in EPR comparable to that measured in the target community during the period of maximum implementation. The secondary analysis confirmed the findings of the original analysis: that the reductions in EPR were due to the intervention.

Summary

There appeared to be a significant decline in the adolescent pregnancy rate in Bamberg County during the full implementation period of the *School/Community Program.* The program encouraged all community members—including parents, teens, teachers, and church representatives—to take responsibility for addressing the problem of unintended pregnancy among unmarried adolescents. In addition to publicizing pregnancy prevention messages in local media, program staff organized workshops for parents and clergy, graduate-level courses for teachers, and peer counseling training for youths. The lessons included human physiology and reproduction, sexual awareness and self-concept, communications skills, and values clarification.

During the immediate postintervention period, the target community showed an average decrease of 35.5 pregnancies per 1,000 adolescent females. As expected, the intervention showed some spillover into the comparison portion of the county. Still, the average EPR for the target community was significantly lower than that of the comparison area of Bamberg County during the full implementation period. Some of the other comparison counties also showed a drop in EPR, but in all cases, the decline in the target community was significantly greater.

However, secondary analysis revealed that in subsequent years, after important elements of the program had been discontinued, the teen pregnancy rate returned to preintervention levels in the target community.

AWARDS AND RECOGNITION

The *School/Community Program* was featured in a Centers for Disease Control video, *Health Education Works*. The program was also selected by the Kansas Health Foundation for replication in three Kansas communities.

SCHOOL/COMMUNITY PROGRAM IN THE COMMUNITY TODAY

During the past 3 years, the *School/Community Program* has been implemented in communities in nine states—ranging from Wisconsin to Texas to North Carolina—as well as in Puerto Rico.

NOTE

1. A full set of program materials, including a resource guide, implementation standards and guidelines, evaluation materials, and more, is available for purchase from Sociometrics at http://www.socio.com/pasha.htm.

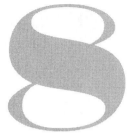

Teen Talk: An Adolescent Pregnancy Prevention Program

Danette M. Schott, Starr Niego, Alisa Mallari, M. Jane Park, and Janette Mince

Original Program Developers and Evaluators

Marvin Eisen, PhD
   Johnson, Bassin & Shaw
   Silver Springs, MD

Alfred L. McAlister, PhD
   Center for Health Promotion
   University of Texas
   Austin, TX

Gail L. Zellman, PhD
   RAND Corporation
   Santa Monica, CA

Teen Talk was supported by contracts and grants from the Family Planning and Genetic Services, Texas Department of Human Resources; the William and Flora Hewlett Foundation; the Hogg Foundation for Mental Health; the National Institute of Child Health & Human Development Grant HD-22982; the Texas Department of Human Services; the University of Texas at Austin Research Institute; and the Lyndon B. Johnson School of Public Affairs, University of Texas at Austin.

PROGRAM ABSTRACT

Summary

Teen Talk is a six-session, collaborative school-based and community health centers–based sex and contraception education intervention intended to reduce adolescent pregnancy. The 12- to 15-hour program begins with two large-group, lecture format presentations covering reproductive physiology, contraception methods, and contraceptive effectiveness. During the remaining four sessions, students participate in small-group discussions that are designed to (a) help teens understand and personalize the risks and consequences of teenage pregnancy, and (b) develop and practice the skills that will make abstinence or obtaining contraception easier decisions to implement. The sessions include games, role plays, and trigger films that encourage group discussion.

A field study of the intervention was conducted in both rural and urban communities in Texas and California. Teens of diverse ethnicities recruited from different agencies and schools participated. Participation in the program was especially beneficial to males, leading to a delay in the onset of sexual activity among male virgins and to the use of more effective contraception among male nonvirgins.

Focus

☑ Primary pregnancy prevention   ☐ Secondary pregnancy prevention   ☐ STI/HIV/AIDS prevention

Original Site

☑ School based   ☑ Community based   ☐ Clinic based

Suitable for Use In

Teen Talk can be implemented in community-based organizations, schools, and school districts, or as a collaboration between community organizations and schools.

Approach

- ■ ☑ Abstinence
- ■ ☑ Behavioral skills development
- ■ ☐ Community outreach
- ■ ☐ Contraceptive access
- ■ ☑ Contraceptive education
- ■ ☐ Life option enhancement
- ■ ☐ Self-efficacy/self-esteem
- ■ ☑ Sexuality/HIV/AIDS/STI education

Original Intervention Sample

Age, gender   The original sample included male and female students between the ages of 13 and 19: 29% were ages 13–14; 67%, ages 15–17; and 4%, ages 18–19.

Race/ethnicity   The original sample population was composed of the following: 15% White, 24% African American, 53% Hispanic, 8% Other.

Program Components

- ■ ☐ Adult involvement
- ■ ☐ Case management
- ■ ☑ Group discussion
- ■ ☑ Lectures
- ■ ☐ Peer counseling/instruction
- ■ ☑ Public service announcements
- ■ ☑ Role play
- ■ ☑ Video
- ■ ☑ Other: Games, audiotape

Program Length

This program is designed to last a total of 12–15 hours. The program schedule is relatively flexible and can be adjusted to suit the particular site. However, it is recommended that the program be given over a span of 2 to 3 weeks: the initial lectures in two 2-hour sessions; and the subsequent group discussions in four 2- to 2.5-hour sessions.

Staffing Requirements/Training

The program requires one lecturer per classroom and one group discussion leader to work with eight students. A 2-day intensive training workshop is recommended to train all group leaders on how to conduct effective group discussion sessions and to familiarize them with the program format and content.

BIBLIOGRAPHY

Eisen, M. (1989). *Testing an intervention model for teen fertility control. Final report to the National Institute of Child Health and Human Development.* Los Altos, CA: Sociometrics Corporation.

Eisen, M., & Zellman, G. (1986). The role of health belief attitudes, sex education, and demographics in predicting adolescents' sexuality knowledge. *Health Education Quarterly, 13,* 9–22.

Eisen, M., & Zellman, G. (1987). Changes in the incidence of sexual intercourse of unmarried teenagers following a community-based sex education program. *Journal of Sex Research, 23,* 527–533.

Eisen, M., & Zellman, G. (1992). A health beliefs field experiment: *Teen Talk.* In B. Miller, J. Card, R. Paikoff, & J. Peterson (Eds.), *Preventing adolescent pregnancy* (pp. 220–264). Newbury Park, CA: Sage Publications.

Eisen, M., Zellman, G., & McAlister, A. (1985). A health belief model approach to adolescents' fertility control: Some pilot findings. *Health Education Quarterly, 12,* 185–210.

Eisen, M., Zellman, G., & McAlister, A. (1990). Evaluating the impact of a theory-based sexuality and contraceptive education program. *Family Planning Perspectives, 22,* 261–271.

Eisen, M., Zellman, G., & McAlister, A. (1992). A health belief model-social learning theory approach to adolescent fertility control: Findings from a controlled field trial. *Health Education Quarterly, 19,* 249–26.

THE PROGRAM

Program Rationale and History

Teen Talk was a theory-based adolescent pregnancy prevention program.[1] This program was developed as a public health approach to sexuality and contraception education and incorporated lectures with group discussions. It was originally field tested in several community-based health centers and schools over a 4-year period

(1984–1988). Given that HIV/AIDS was, at that time, just emerging as a significant public health issue, and that most known sexually transmitted infections (STIs) could be cured with a single treatment of antibiotics, the focus of *Teen Talk* was pregnancy prevention rather than condom use and STI prevention. Within a few years of the completion of the *Teen Talk* field test, teen pregnancy rates would begin to decline, even as STI rates, including HIV, would burgeon worldwide. Communities implementing the program today broaden the original curriculum to include sexual risk prevention.

Teen Talk was implemented in youth groups, health classes, and other community education programs as an alternative to their "usual care" sex and contraception educational outreach curriculum.

Theoretical Framework

The development of *Teen Talk* was guided by two theoretical perspectives, the health belief model (HBM) and social learning theory (SLT). They can be viewed as complementary ways of understanding individual behavior change and are often applied to issues of health behavior modification and primary prevention.

Principles of the HBM suggest that individuals will be likely to engage in health-related behaviors when the following conditions are met:

1. One perceives that the problem (e.g., teen pregnancy or STIs) poses a threat to one's well-being.
2. One understands the benefits of and barriers to taking preventive action.
3. One feels a sense of efficacy in carrying out the recommended actions.

SLT elaborates the processes through which intentions can be translated into behavioral change among teens. SLT asserts that learning occurs through practice and observation of social models; it is mediated by internal beliefs about one's ability to succeed, as well as by others' evaluation of the individual's performance.

Program Objectives

The goal of the program was to research the effectiveness of the theoretical model in affecting health knowledge, attitude, and behavior change. Two behavioral objectives are specified:

- To increase unmarried adolescents' knowledge of and motivation for fertility control (i.e., abstinence or consistent use of effective contraception)
- To determine the impact of *Teen Talk* with respect to participants' subsequent sexual behavior, contraceptive use, and pregnancy status

Hypothesized Outcomes

The research team hypothesized that by applying the principles of the HBM-SLT model and in incorporating both didactic and active learning, *Teen Talk* would result in

- lower incidence of transition to sexual activity status during the 1-year follow-up period;
- higher incidence of effective contraceptive use at first and most recent intercourse among those who became sexually active;
- higher incidence of effective contraceptive use at most recent intercourse among teenagers who were sexually active prior to the intervention;

- more consistent use of effective contraception among those who were sexually active over the 1-year follow-up period;
- older average age at first intercourse for teenagers who became sexually active during the follow-up period.

The researchers assumed that the *Teen Talk* program model would not be equally effective with all age, gender, racial/ethnic, and sexual status groups or in all study sites. Little empirical basis exists, however, for predicting the direction or the magnitude of potential differences.

Educational Objectives

The 12- to 15-hour program was intended to increase teenagers' knowledge and awareness of the following:

- The probability of personally becoming pregnant or causing a partner to become pregnant
- The serious negative personal consequences of teenage maternity and paternity
- The personal and interpersonal benefits of delayed sexual activity and consistent, effective contraceptive use

In addition, the program aimed to decrease

- The psychological, interpersonal, and logistical barriers to abstinence and consistent contraceptive usage.

Program Content

Teen Talk was based on four basic components. These components formed the content of the two lecture sessions and the four discussion sessions.

1. *Presentation of factual information.* This information was presented to the teens in the initial two large-group lectures. The lectures covered topics such as reproductive biology, STIs, and contraception and were intended to provide the teens with factual knowledge about sexuality and contraception.
2. *Group discussion of factual information.* Issues that drew upon the lecture material were discussed in small groups. Discussion emphasized basic concepts of probability and pregnancy risks; social, educational, and economic consequences of premarital pregnancy and parenthood; and pregnancy resolution options, including adoption and abortion.
3. *Group discussion of values, feelings, and emotions.* Further personalization of sexuality issues continued in discussions that emphasized communication in relationships with same-sex peers and opposite-sex partners, as well as for one's own feelings about sexuality.
4. *Making decisions and taking personal responsibility.* In order to solidify these issues in concrete action, this component emphasized actual decision making, making personally and sexually responsible decisions, and learning new skills to implement those decisions.

Program Schedule

Teen Talk was designed to last a total of 12–15 hours. The program schedule was relatively flexible and could be adjusted to suit the particular needs and constraints of the site. However, it is recommended that the program be given over a span of

2 to 3 weeks: the initial lectures in two 2-hour sessions, and the subsequent group discussions in four 2- to 2.5-hour sessions.

Lecture Sessions

Lecture session 1 presented material on Anatomy and Physiology and Sexually Transmitted Infections.

Lecture session 2 presented material on Contraception and Prenatal Development and Care.

This curriculum was a relatively standard sexuality education curriculum. Adapt and/or augment the material, or substitute your own curriculum, provided that the participants learn the same information. This lecture material was important preparation for the heart of the *Teen Talk* program—the four small-group discussion sessions.

Group Discussion Sessions

The small-group discussions (2 to 2.5 hours each) were designed to help group members understand and personalize the risks and consequences of teenage pregnancy, and to develop and practice the skills that would make abstinence or obtaining contraception easier decisions to implement. The four small group discussions are described below.

Group Discussion Session 1: Risks and Consequences

1. Session 1 began with introductions.
2. Group rules were discussed.
3. The first formal exercise ("Communicating in Pairs") was designed to show that without good skills, communication could be very difficult and frustrating. (40 minutes)
4. The "Spinner Game" was designed to help young people grasp the risks and consequences of unprotected intercourse. (20 minutes)
5. The film *Wayne's Decision* was shown in order to help group members comprehend the consequences of an unwanted pregnancy. (15 minutes)
6. The session was brought to a close by asking the group, "How many of you want to be sure that what happened to Wayne and Donna never happens to you?" (10 minutes)

Group Discussion Session 2: How to Avoid Those Risks and Consequences

1. This session began with a warm-up and review of the previous session. This review included a discussion of the consequences of an unwanted pregnancy.
2. Once the consequences were reviewed, a discussion of all the ways to prevent such an unwanted pregnancy followed. (15 minutes)
3. This session then focused on communication skills. *Teen Talk* presented the skills in order of difficulty, so that group members could first practice and receive reinforcement on easier tasks. (20 minutes)
4. Role play provided group members an opportunity to practice these skills.
5. The final exercise showed students how to say "no." This concept was introduced by the film *Mark and Susan*, which portrayed a boy pushing a girl to have sex when she really did not want to.
6. The session ended with a short review and a preview of the next session: addressing communication skills in greater detail.

Group Discussion Session 3: Communication

Focusing on communication skills, this session emphasized the ability to say "no" to intercourse. For those who had decided to say "yes," the session taught group members how to acquire contraceptive devices.

1. This session began with each member sharing what he or she had learned from *Teen Talk* so far. (20 minutes)
2. The film *Mark and Susan*, shown in Session 2, was reviewed. The purpose of this review was to emphasize that Mark and Susan could make just two responsible decisions: They could decide to abstain from sex, or they could mutually decide to have sex.
3. Two sets of role plays followed from the two alternatives discussed above.
4. At the end of the session, each group member committed to returning for the final *Teen Talk* session. (10 minutes)

Group Discussion Session 4: Boy–Girl Communication and Review

1. After a brief warm-up, the session began with a film called *What's to Understand?* This film portrayed communicating in sexual situations.
2. The film set up the two final role plays.
3. The game "Family Feud" was introduced to help group members review what they had learned. It was played in much the same manner as on television.
4. The group ended with an informal party—a chance to socialize and enjoy refreshments together.

You may wish to interview your teen participants prior to the first session, immediately after the last session, and 12 months after the last session to ascertain the program's impact on their knowledge, attitudes, and behavior.

Program Implementation

Training Workshop

In the original field study, a 2-day workshop was held to prepare leaders to implement the program with teens. You may wish to conduct a similar training session for your own staff.

On the first day of training, *Teen Talk* group leaders discussed

- Their role as group leader
- How to present *Teen Talk* activities
- How to run a productive group
- Group development and maintenance

Opportunities for staff to practice facilitating group discussions and role-play exercises were provided in the training. Training participants were encouraged to ask any questions they had about the curriculum.

During the second day of the workshop, participants viewed the following four training video segments:

- *Training Tape 1* introduced *Teen Talk* and the trigger films, guided discussions, role playing, and games that were used to achieve the program's objectives.
- *Training Tape 2* discussed the sequencing of *Teen Talk*. Rules and guidelines were suggested for group leaders, and Group Session 1 was introduced.

- *Training Tape 3* introduced the Group Session 2 curriculum.
- *Training Tape 4* presented information on Group Sessions 3 and 4.

PROGRAM EVALUATION

The Original Evaluation

Design

The original evaluation of *Teen Talk* approximated a randomized field trial. Six family planning service agencies and two grades of one independent school district (representing a total of eight sex and contraceptive education programs) compared their own "usual care" outreach or regular classroom curriculum with the *Teen Talk* program. Each agency recruited its study sample by its usual methods; the school district used its 8th- and 9th-grade population. Across sites, participation was open to all youths between the ages of 13 and 21; no attempt was made to balance the sample by gender, race/ethnicity, or preintervention sexual activity status. At each site, participants were assigned by classroom unit or individually (at some agencies) to the agency's usual program (comparison group) or the *Teen Talk* program (experimental group). Data were collected from individual participants at three points during the study period:

- Time 1: before exposure to the intervention
- Time 2: immediately following the intervention
- Time 3: 12 months after the scheduled program completion date

Evaluation Questions

To assess the outcomes of the field experiment, the program evaluators attempted to answer the following questions.

1. Were teens who were not yet sexually active more likely to remain virgins if they had received the *Teen Talk* intervention? Did significant sex or race/ethnicity differences exist in treatment effects between the *Teen Talk* and comparison programs?
2. Were experimental program teens who became sexually active following the intervention more likely to report initial and consistent contraceptive use than youths in the comparison program? Were there sex or racial/ethnic differences in program effectiveness?
3. Did significant increases occur in contraceptive efficiency from Time 1 to Time 3 among sexually active teenagers? If so, was the *Teen Talk* program more effective than the comparison programs in producing these improvements? Were there sex or race/ethnicity differences in program effectiveness?
4. Were Time 2 health beliefs and sexual knowledge significant predictors of adolescents' fertility control behaviors (i.e., continued abstinence or contraceptive usage) at Time 3? Did the perceptual and knowledge changes (if any) mediate or augment relationships between treatment conditions and fertility control behaviors?

The overall analysis plan involved a four-group approach: (a) Time 1 virgins' abstinence, (b) transition to sexual activity, and (c) initiation of contraceptive use were examined separately for each sex; and (d) Time 1 nonvirgins' contraceptive behavior was examined separately for each sex. Researchers measured abstinence continuation, transition from virginity to sexual activity, and use and changes in use of effective birth control methods at first and most recent post-intervention intercourse. Effective contraceptive methods included pill, condom, diaphragm, foam/jelly, and sponge; ineffective methods were withdrawal, rhythm, and douche.

Data Collection Procedures

Community-based agencies were recruited from two pools: (a) organizations that conducted sexuality education outreach programming with state reimbursement agreements in Texas, and (b) educational groups that received "innovative" information and education (I & E) grants in California. The Texas Department of Human Services Director of Family Planning helped recruit eligible agencies in Texas. In California, the chief of the Office of Family Planning, and the executive director of the California Family Planning Council referred the program evaluators to potential sites in their state. A small independent school district in California's San Francisco Bay area also volunteered to participate in the project as a means of evaluating their curricula for family life and drug/problem behavior education.

The community-based agencies and the school district recruited all participants for the study, organized and coordinated the data collection, and delivered the actual intervention. The agencies were paid up to $5,000 (the exact amount was based on the number of teenagers recruited and retained in the sample) over the study period. The agency sample represented a relatively broad mix of service provider organizations, ranging from an urban Planned Parenthood affiliate to a rural community action program health clinic. The agencies were not representative of all agencies conducting educational outreach nationally, but they did appear typical of agencies and community-based outreach programs operating around the country.

Between June 1986 and August 1987, 1,444 adolescents (ages 13 to 19) completed the baseline (Time 1) interview, and 1,328 (92%) received all or part of the *Teen Talk* or comparison intervention and completed the immediate posttest (Time 2) interview. Agencies attempted to reinterview all adolescents who were exposed to any phase of the project 12 months after the scheduled completion date of their particular intervention program, even if the youths did not actually complete it. Between July 1987 and September 1988, 888 participants (62% of the Time 1 sample and 67% of the Time 2 sample) received the 1-year follow-up (Time 3) interview to assess program impact. Included were 839 participants (58% of the Time 1 sample and 63% of the Time 2 sample) from the seven sites who completed all three data collection cycles (i.e., baseline, immediate posttest, and 1-year follow-up).

Evaluation Results

The intervention results were encouraging, but mixed. Sexual experience (Time 1 virginity/nonvirginity) and gender were important mediators of the effects of the *Teen Talk* and comparison programs on key pregnancy avoidance measures.

Time 1 Virgins' Abstinence

For those who had not had intercourse prior to the intervention, more males in the *Teen Talk* program maintained their abstinence over the follow-up year ($p < .05$). For females, no difference was found between the *Teen Talk* and comparison programs.

Transition to Sexual Activity and Initiation of Contraceptive Use

Female Time 1 virgins who attended the comparison programs were more likely to use an effective contraceptive method at their most recent intercourse and more likely to use contraception than those who attended the *Teen Talk* program ($p < .01$).

The *Teen Talk* program and comparison programs were equally effective for sexually inexperienced males. Both programs significantly increased contraceptive use.

Time 1 Nonvirgin Contraceptive Behavior

Sexually active teens in both programs increased their contraceptive use. For males, *Teen Talk* led to significantly greater follow-up contraceptive use than did the comparison programs ($p < .05$); for females, the interventions produced equivalent improvement.

Positive Time 2 perceptions of the benefits of effective birth control use predicted contraceptive efficiency for two of the four analytic groupings and predicted transitions to sexual activity in the follow-up year for males. Finally, exposure to sexuality education prior to the study was associated with greater Time 3 contraceptive use, regardless of the program attended, for two of the four groups.

Summary

In summary, the *Teen Talk* intervention, with its emphasis on refusal skills, role-playing, and guided practice, was more effective for high-risk males in the sample experimental group than in the comparison groups, but it appeared to have less salience for females in general and for females who were just making the transition to sexual intercourse in particular. Even so, this field experiment was the first published, prospectively designed outcome evaluation to demonstrate a significant increase in sexually experienced teenagers' use of effective contraceptive methods over at least a 1-year follow-up period. It was also the first published evaluation featuring random assignment of participants to intervention programs to show significant impact in delaying first intercourse over at least a 12-month period for either males or females.

TEEN TALK IN THE COMMUNITY TODAY

In the past 3 years, *Teen Talk* has been implemented in communities in nine states ranging from Tennessee to Montana to Hawaii. It has also been implemented in Puerto Rico.

NOTE

1. A full set of program materials, including curriculum, training manual, training videotapes, handouts, evaluation materials, and more, is available for purchase from Sociometrics at http://www.socio.com/pasha.htm.

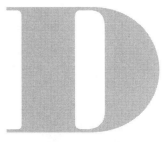

Programs Designed for Youths of All Ages

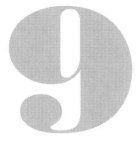

Tailoring Family Planning Services to the Special Needs of Adolescents: New Adolescent Approach Protocols

Kathryn L. Muller, Starr Niego, and Janette Mince

Original Program Developer

Lynn Cooper Breckenmaker
   Family Health Council of Central Pennsylvania
   Camp Hill, PA

Original Program Evaluator

Laraine Winter, PhD
   Family Health Council of Central Pennsylvania
   Camp Hill, PA

PROGRAM ABSTRACT

Summary

This family planning clinic–based intervention was originally developed for teens younger than 18 years of age. It is based on the premise that regular contraceptive

---

Tailoring Family Planning Services to the Special Needs of Adolescents was supported by a grant from the Ford Foundation.

use by teens can be increased by offering information, social support, and counseling, in addition to health and medical services. Accordingly, the program aims to provide family planning services in a manner that will increase teens' sense of comfort, increase their self-confidence, and reduce any fears that may discourage regular and effective contraception.

A key component of the intervention was the Personal Information Form, a one-page questionnaire designed to aid staff in understanding teens' concerns, providing counsel, and identifying patients who may be at greatest risk for early pregnancy. To ease teens' anxiety, the first appointment is divided into two visits, with education and counseling provided in the first session, and the medical examination (and contraceptive prescription) deferred until the second. The intervention also includes: (a) counseling and education in a one-on-one rather than a group setting; (b) use of visual aids; (c) a follow-up visit scheduled 6 weeks after the initial appointment; and (d) encouragement of participation by family members, partners, and friends, while respecting the patient's right to confidential services.

A field study was conducted with 1,261 teens attending six family planning clinics. Compared to their peers receiving standard services, program participants showed significantly greater gains in knowledge and contraceptive use at the 6- and 12-month follow-up assessments. Participants also experienced significantly fewer pregnancies over the following year than their comparison group peers.

Focus

☑ Primary pregnancy prevention   ☐ Secondary pregnancy prevention   ☑ STI/HIV/AIDS prevention

Original Site

☐ School based   ☑ Community based   ☑ Clinic based

Suitable for Use In

This program is suitable for use in community-, hospital- or school-based family planning clinics.

Approach

- ☐ Abstinence
- ☑ Behavioral skills development
- ☐ Community outreach
- ☑ Contraceptive access
- ☑ Contraceptive education
- ☐ Life option enhancement
- ☐ Self-efficacy/self-esteem
- ☑ Sexuality/HIV/STI education

Original Intervention Sample

Age, gender   The field study involved 1,261 adolescent females, of whom 40% were age 17; 34%, age 16; and 16%, age 15.

Race/ethnicity   95% White, 1% African American, 4% Other (mostly Hispanic).

Program Components

- ☑ Adult involvement
- ☐ Case management
- ☐ Group discussion

- ■ ☐ Lectures
- ■ ☐ Peer counseling/instruction
- ■ ☐ Public service announcements
- ■ ☐ Role Play
- ■ ☐ Video
- ■ ☑ Other: Visual instructional aids (e.g., posters, pelvic model)

Program Length

A 6-week period is required for the initial two-part visit and a follow-up appointment. Additional visits are scheduled as necessary.

Staffing Requirements/Training

In addition to the regular clinic staff (e.g., gynecologist, nurse practitioner, receptionist), a counselor-educator is needed to review the Personal Information Form and lead the educational segment of each patient's first visit. All program staff should receive training in adolescent cognitive and sexual development.

BIBLIOGRAPHY

Breckenmaker, L. C., & Winter, L. (1989). *Tailoring family planning services to the special needs of adolescents (final report)*. Camp Hill, PA: Family Health Council of Central Pennsylvania.

Winter, L., & Breckenmaker, L. C. (1991). Tailoring family planning services to the special needs of adolescents. *Family Planning Perspectives, 23*(1), 24–30.

Related References by the Developers of *Tailoring Family Planning*

Winter, L., & Goldy, A. S. (1993). Effects of prebehavioral cognitive work on adolescents' acceptance of condoms. *Health Psychology, 12*(4), 308–312.

THE PROGRAM

Program Rationale and History

At the time of this study, adolescent family planning clinic patients in central Pennsylvania were at high risk for noncompliance with contraceptive methods, discontinuation of clinic services, and unintended pregnancy.[1] According to earlier research, the average teen waited nearly a year after becoming sexually active to make her first clinic visit; furthermore, one-third of all teens made their first clinic visit for the purpose of obtaining pregnancy tests. Concerns that led teenagers to avoid family planning clinics included fear of parental disclosure, fear of the pelvic examination, and fear of contraceptive methods. Family planning clinics did not typically address such concerns. In contrast, the *Tailoring Family Planning* program was based on the premise that family planning clinics could increase regular contraceptive use by offering teens information, social support, and counseling, in addition to health and medical services.

A basic consideration guiding development of the program was teenagers' minimal medical needs in comparison to their need for information, social support, and counseling. Among the special requirements considered during program development were the need for age-appropriate education, reassurance of confidentiality, information, and reassurance about the pelvic examination, as well as counseling regarding such concerns as patients' apprehensions about contraception.

A field study of the program was conducted with 1,261 teens attending six family planning clinics in central Pennsylvania. When this study was conducted, during the mid-1980s, teen pregnancy rates were still on the rise in the United States. Unwanted teen pregnancy was a significant public health issue that needed to be addressed. At the same time, researchers had not yet settled on a final name for the virus that was sweeping the world or the virus-related syndrome that was killing people across the globe. Hence, the focus was contraception. If developed today, an intervention such as *Tailoring Family Planning* would have included a strong emphasis on consistent, correct condom use and on preventing risky sexual behaviors.

Program Objectives

The program was designed to alter relevant features of family planning clinic service delivery to address young clients' fears and to increase their sense of comfort. Specifically, *Tailoring Family Planning* sought to

1. Increase the amount of contraceptive counseling and education provided to teen clients
2. Identify client fears or concerns likely to interfere with effective contraception
3. Provide teens with reassurance and social support
4. Encourage the participation of teens' parents, friends, and sexual partners, while respecting teens' right to confidential services
5. Increase teens' comfort with the medical examination
6. Increase the opportunity for patient follow-up, allowing clinic staff to identify problems early on and provide additional counseling to high-risk teens

Hypothesized Outcomes

By providing in-depth counseling and education, addressing young clients' fears, and increasing their comfort with clinic procedures such as the pelvic examination, *Tailoring Family Planning* aimed to increase effective contraception and decrease unintended pregnancy. Specifically, researchers predicted that program participation would be associated with

- Increased comfort/satisfaction with the clinic
- Increased knowledge about effective contraceptive methods
- Increased confidence regarding contraception
- More effective contraceptive use
- Reduced pregnancy rates

Educational Objectives

The intervention also included the following educational objectives:

- To provide teens with basic information about anatomy, reproduction, contraception, and sexually transmitted infections
- To address misconceptions and fears regarding clinic procedures and contraceptive methods
- To provide descriptions of contraceptive alternatives, including abstinence
- To explain what clients should expect from the medical and pelvic examinations
- To provide detailed instructions for the client's chosen method of contraception

Program Elements

Tailoring Family Planning encompassed a total family planning service delivery system for adolescents. Written protocols provided clinic staff with guidance on all aspects of agency activities, ranging from suggestions for making the environment "teen-friendly" to detailed guidelines for conducting the medical examination and patient follow-up. The major differences between the new protocols introduced in *Tailoring Family Planning* and traditional family planning services were (a) in-depth, individualized counseling and education; (b) more frequent clinic visits; and (c) special staff training regarding adolescent sexual and cognitive development. Critical components of the intervention are highlighted below.

Agency Environment

The majority of agency environment guidelines were standard practice for all family planning agencies serving teens. The most significant change was the posting of additional instructional signs to help direct the teens at every step of their visit. For example, one program recommendation was to post a sign in the waiting room that read, "Let the receptionist know you are here." Suggested posted instructions in the examination room told patients, "How to prepare for your exam."

Staff Training

One of the cornerstones of the program was the fact that all clinic staff received training in adolescent psychological and sexual development, as well as protocol administration.

First Contact With Patient

Very specific telephone protocols were developed for the clinic receptionist. Additions to standard agency protocols included offering the teen directions to the agency, assuring confidentiality to every teen, providing specific information about what her visit would entail, and asking if she needed a temporary birth control method for the interim period. Guidelines for dealing with clients who were only interested in pregnancy testing are also specified.

The program provided general guidelines for the receptionist's interaction with teens at their first clinic visit. Examples included personalizing the interaction by using the teen's first name, making sure to act in a sensitive manner, and providing the teen with condoms and foam as a temporary method of contraception.

Personal Information Form

A key component of the intervention was the Personal Information Form, a one-page questionnaire designed to help clinic staff understand teens' concerns, tailor the counseling and education session to their needs and developmental level, and identify patients at highest risk for unintended pregnancy. Teens who were very young, were developmentally slow, lacked future plans, lacked parental support, thought that pregnancy would be okay, had infrequent intercourse, had short-term sexual relationships, and/or had not initiated the family planning visit themselves were considered to be at especially high risk for unintended pregnancy.

Among the questions asked on the Personal Information Form were the reason for the patient's visit, how she felt about visiting the clinic, whether she was currently having sexual intercourse, whether she was using a contraceptive method (and if so, which one), whether her parents knew about her visit, whether her partner knew about and approved of her visit, whether she had fears about or anticipated any problems with using a method of birth control, what her future plans were, and how she would feel about becoming pregnant. The form was primarily intended to be used as a counseling tool to identify potential problems and initiate discussion with the teenager. Once identified, specific fears about the effects of oral contraceptives or about the pelvic examination, for example, could be discussed at greater length.

The Personal Information Form also served as a tool for counseling and educating teens in a family planning clinic. Questionnaire items prompted the teen to think about important issues, including plans for the future, misconceptions about birth control, and the ways in which pregnancy might affect her life. After the teen completed the form, it was reviewed by the counselor/educator, who then discussed the responses with her. Specific protocol guidelines assisted the counselor during this discussion.

Two-Part Initial Clinic Visit

Tailoring Family Planning split the traditional "initial visit" into two parts for teen clients. The two appointments were generally scheduled no more than 2 weeks apart. At the first visit, the teen received counseling/education regarding anatomy and physiology, sexuality, pregnancy, contraception, and sexually transmitted infections (STIs). The counselor reviewed the Personal Information Form with the teen, corrected any misperceptions, and provided general information regarding contraceptive alternatives, including abstinence. The purpose, procedures, and what to expect from the medical and pelvic examinations were also explained at this visit. Finally, the teen was given temporary birth control (condoms and foam) before she left the clinic.

At the second visit, teens underwent the medical and pelvic examinations, received a prescription contraceptive, and were provided with specific instructions regarding the contraceptive method they had chosen. A 6-week follow-up appointment was scheduled at this time.

The two-visit system accomplished several objectives. First, it enabled the teenager to absorb more information during the counseling and education session by reducing anxiety about the pending pelvic examination. Second, it allowed the counselor to take more time with the client without disrupting clinic scheduling. Third, it put the teenager in more frequent contact with the clinic.

Counseling and Education Sessions

Clinic staff were provided with a list of general points to address during the counseling and education sessions. Included were specific guidelines for reviewing the Personal Information Form with patients; brief instructions for discussions of physiology and anatomy, contraceptive alternatives, and STIs; and detailed instructions to be provided once teens had chosen a contraceptive method. Counselors were reminded to individualize their sessions and to employ visual aids to make information more concrete.

Involvement of Others in the Family Planning Visit

The program strongly advocated that teens' parents, friends, or sexual partners participate in family planning visits. Because the need for assurance of confidentiality was especially important to teens, a special subprotocol was designed to assist the counselor/educator in the event that a parent, boyfriend, or friend accompanied the teen. In addition to providing reassurance about her right to confidential services, counselors were encouraged to spend time alone with the teen to determine what, if any, information she did not wish to disclose to the accompanying person(s).

Medical Examination

A summary of recommendations was provided for the medical examination, most of which were standard protocol for family planning clinics serving teens. Guidelines primarily focused on steps that staff could take to ensure that the teenager felt as comfortable as possible during the examination.

Exit Counseling Session

The program also provided guidelines for counseling patients after they received the medical examination, contraceptive prescription, and specific instructions for the method they had selected. Although most of the guidelines were standard family planning clinic practice, the importance of providing teens with support and encouragement before they left the clinic was underscored.

Patient Follow-Up

Teens were required to make a follow-up visit approximately 6 weeks after their initial visit. The purpose of this visit was to assess whether they were experiencing any problems with their contraceptive method and to provide additional counseling for high-risk teens. Additional visits were scheduled as needed, depending upon the contraceptive method chosen and the individual needs of the teen.

Program Schedule

A 6-week period was required to implement the initial two-part clinic visit and the mandatory follow-up appointment. Additional visits were scheduled as needed, depending upon the teen's choice of contraceptive method and her individual needs.

It is important to note that *Tailoring Family Planning* required about 45 additional minutes per client to administer, compared to the shorter traditional family planning service protocols. Table 9.1 indicates the additional time required for each protocol, and the visit during which it was used.

Program Implementation

One of the key aspects of this program was the fact that all project staff receive training in (a) protocol administration and (b) teen sexual and cognitive development. In the original field study of the program, clinic staff attended a special 2-day training session prior to administering any of the protocols. Day 1 was devoted to lectures on adolescent psychosocial and cognitive development and adolescent sexuality. Day 2 was devoted to instruction on implementing the protocols and the various evaluation measures. You may want to organize a similar session for your staff.

9.1 | Protocol Time Requirements

CLINIC VISIT	PROTOCOL(S)	ADDITIONAL TIME
General	*Agency environment*	*N/A*
Visit 1:	First contact	5 min.
Part 1	Counseling & education[1]	15 min.
Visit 1:	Medical exam	
Part 2	Counseling & education[2]/exit counseling	10 min.
6-Week follow-up	Follow-up	15 min.

1. Includes following the subprotocols General Points, Personal Information Form, Other Person Involvement, and Brief Contraceptive Instructions.
2. Includes following subprotocol Specific Method Instructions.

Staffing

During the original field study, a project coordinator was designated at each participating clinic site; this individual was responsible for supervising program implementation and collection of the evaluation data. Additionally, the project coordinator was responsible for (a) training staff hired after the initial training session, (b) supervising staff who were involved in implementing the protocols, and (c) examining all forms to ensure correct completion.

Protocol Problems

Overall, in the field study, staff reported few problems in using the new protocols. However, clinic schedules needed to be altered significantly to allow for the additional time required to follow the protocols. Additional staff time was also required to train personnel who had been hired after the study began.

EVALUATING THE PROGRAM

The Original Evaluation

Design

The effectiveness of *Tailoring Family Planning* was investigated in a field study involving 1,261 teenage girls attending six nonmetropolitan family planning clinics. Three sites agreed to use the new family planning protocols, and three others continued with their usual service delivery practices. The study compared contraceptive use and pregnancy outcomes between teens receiving the two types of services.

To examine the effect of the program over time, measures were taken at three points:

- Time 1: the patient's first clinic visit during the field study period (index visit)
- Time 2: 6 months following the first visit (6-month follow-up)
- Time 3: 1 year following the initial visit (12-month follow-up)

In addition, a group of 251 teens completed two surveys during a preliminary phase of the study.

Evaluation Questions

The field study addressed the following questions:

1. Did *Tailoring Family Planning* increase teens' sense of comfort with the clinic?
2. Did *Tailoring Family Planning* help young clients use contraception more effectively?
3. Did *Tailoring Family Planning* help young clients avoid pregnancy?
4. Did the increased frequency of clinic visits required by *Tailoring Family Planning* lead to greater attrition among teenage patients?

Site Selection

Six family planning sites were contracted to participate in the project. Of this group, three clinics agreed to use *Tailoring Family Planning* (Lock Haven Family Planning, Adams County Family Planning and Health Center, and Mifflin/Juniata/Huntingdon

Women's Health Services), and the remaining three, serving as comparison sites, continued with their regular program of service delivery (Family Health Services of South Central Pennsylvania, Altoona Hospital Family Planning, and Family Health Services Inc.).

The evaluators' choice of clinics was guided by several criteria. First, all sites participating in the study showed comparable demographic characteristics, including racial and age distribution, per capita income of municipalities, and percentages of families below poverty. Second, the clinics employed the same staffing pattern—a modified form of primary nursing in which the client interacts with a receptionist and only one or two other staff members during her visit. And, importantly, patient continuation rates during the year prior to the study were higher in the comparison sites than in those using *Tailoring Family Planning.* This was a safeguard to ensure that program clinics showed no advantage in patient retention prior to the study.

Random assignment of clinics to treatment condition was not possible, because some of the clinic directors were unwilling to make the changes in patient scheduling that would be required to implement the new program.

Staff Training

Two special training sessions were held for agency project coordinators—one for sites implementing *Tailoring Family Planning* and one for the comparison sites. Topics covered included project coordinator responsibilities, evaluation tools, timelines, and scheduling considerations.

Data Collection Procedures

During the 2-month preliminary phase of the study, measures of patient knowledge and satisfaction were collected from 251 teenagers who made initial or annual visits to the six participating clinics. Because random assignment of patients to condition was not possible, it was especially important that study sites be equivalent prior to the intervention. Comparisons of these preliminary data revealed that although there were no differences in knowledge scores between the participants at the program and comparison group sites (indicating that the sites were similar in terms of the information they were providing to clients), satisfaction scores were higher in the program sites ($p < .05$). One possible explanation for this difference was that program staff planning to use the new protocols might have shown increased enthusiasm in their work (a phenomenon also referred to as the "Hawthorne effect"). It is also important to note that some staff members at program sites had participated in the development of the intervention and may have begun implementing parts of the program before the study officially started.

Data Collection Schedule

The data collection schedule for the study is shown in Table 9.2.

Research Sample

A total of 1,261 patients took part in the study. The majority of this group (62%) were making initial clinic visits; 39% were making annual/return visits. Although participants ranged between 11 and 18 years of age, nearly three-fourths of the teens were either 16 or 17. The few participating 18-year-olds—all considered to be at high risk for early pregnancy—were enrolled at the discretion of clinic staff.

The sample was almost exclusively White (nearly 98%), with a few African American and Hispanic participants. The single largest religious group in the sample was Roman Catholic (22%), followed by Methodist (18%) and Lutheran (10%).

| Data Collection Schedule

	PRELIMINARY MEASURES	INDEX VISIT	6-MONTH FOLLOW-UP	12-MONTH FOLLOW-UP
Knowledge Quiz	X	X	X	X
Client Satisfaction Survey	X	X		
No Show/Continuation Report		X	X	X
Method Use Questionnaire		X	X	X

Preliminary knowledge and satisfaction data were collected from 251 patients. During the 6-month treatment phase of the study, data were collected on an additional 1,010 patients (425 at program sites, 585 at comparison sites).

Evaluation Results

Evaluation measures assessed (a) the knowledge patients acquired during the course of the program; (b) patient satisfaction with clinic services; and (c) contraceptive-related behaviors and outcomes, including pregnancy. The effect of *Tailoring Family Planning* on each of these outcomes is discussed separately below.

Patient Knowledge

In general, clients at all sites scored quite high on the Knowledge Quiz. In fact, all but 5 of the 11 items were answered correctly by at least 95% of the clients. Nevertheless, in both administrations of the quiz, clients at program clinics scored significantly higher than their comparison group peers ($p < .0001$ for both). Since the sites did not differ on this measure during the preliminary phase of the study, differences in the teens' scores can only be attributed to the intervention.

Client Satisfaction

Program evaluators found no evidence that the program sites produced significantly greater patient satisfaction than the comparison sites. In general, patients in both sites reported very high levels of satisfaction with clinic services, with mean scores for most clients falling between 9 and 10 (10 representing the highest possible score).

Continuation Rates

Continuation rates during the year following patients' index visits were equivalent for the two groups of teens, with 39% of program participants and 38% of their comparison group peers returning for their 12-month visits. In addition, the division of the first appointment into two visits did not seem to be a problem for program participants, as nearly all attended their second visit. In sum, teens who took part in *Tailoring Family Planning* did not drop out at a higher rate than those who received standard services.

Contraceptive Method Use

The Method Use Questionnaire, which was completed by a clinic staff member at the 6- and 12-month follow-up assessments, measured clients' contraceptive experiences, including method problems, side effects, and whether the client had continued using the same method or had changed to a different method (and if so, which method). The questionnaire also assessed whether a pregnancy had occurred since the Time 1 assessment.

- *Use of original contraceptive method:* In general, the large majority of clients in both groups of clinics who returned for follow-up visits continued to use the method they were initially prescribed. However, significantly more program clients than comparison group clients stayed with their original method at both the 6-month (92% and 85%, respectively, $p < .001$) and 12-month assessments (90% and 81%, respectively, $p < .05$).
- *Use of any contraceptive method:* The percentage of program participants who continued to use any method (their original method or any other, including condoms) consistently exceeded that of their comparison group peers. However, the difference was statistically significant only at the 6-month follow-up assessment ($p < .001$).
- *Difficulty dealing with method problems:* Clients were asked to rate their experience coping with method problems. At 6 months, program participants reported significantly greater ease in coping ($p < .01$) than did their comparison group peers. At 12 months, this pattern held only for those teens whose index visit was their initial clinic visit, and the difference in coping was only marginally significant ($p < .10$).
- *Continued use of method despite problems:* Investigators explored whether teens continued to use their contraceptive method after experiencing a problem (either a side effect or other problem, such as cost or partner objections). At the 6-month follow-up, 79% of program participants, but only 56% of comparison group members, continued to use their method despite experiencing one or more problems ($p < .001$). This difference was even larger at the 12-month follow-up ($p < .001$), with over 70% of program participants (vs. 40% of comparison group members) continuing to use their method despite problems.
- *Pregnancy rates:* There were a total of 45 known pregnancies during the year following the preliminary assessment—13 in program sites and 32 in comparison sites. This difference was marginally significant ($p = .06$).

Summary

Compared to their peers receiving standard family planning services, teenage clients participating in the *Tailoring Family Planning* program (a) learned more during the educational session; (b) were more likely to be using their original contraceptive method (or any method); (c) experienced less difficulty in dealing with method problems; and (d) were more likely to continue using their prescribed method, despite problems, at the 6-month follow-up assessment. Furthermore, teenage patients who attended program clinics were somewhat less likely to become pregnant over the following year than those who received standard family planning services.

The evaluators also found that the new protocols introduced in *Tailoring Family Planning* were not associated with a greater dropout rate by family planning patients. Yet, contrary to expectations, patients who received the new protocols did not report significantly greater satisfaction with clinic services. Program participants and their comparison group peers reported equivalent, high levels of satisfaction with the family planning services they received.

Overall, the findings lent support to the idea that teenage family planning patients benefited from specialized services. The tailored protocols helped teen patients use their methods successfully, continue to use them despite problems, deal with problems more easily, and use another method after switching from their original method. Moreover, the protocols seemed to have helped patients avoid pregnancy.

The cost of the intervention was primarily due to the extra personnel time needed to counsel and instruct patients. Still, the researchers concluded that the time and effort required to meet teens' special needs were justified by the youths' improved knowledge, increased contraceptive use, and lower pregnancy rates.

Future Evaluators of This Program

The researchers felt that their evaluation was hampered by the inability to determine what happened to clients who dropped out of the study. They also had to exclude follow-up data for many clients who returned late for their annual visit. A proportion of "dropouts" may have simply been tardy in scheduling their 12-month visit and would have provided data had the follow-up period been longer.

Furthermore, the researchers expressed some concerns regarding the evaluation measures, particularly the Knowledge Quiz. While the quiz did yield interpretable data, the overall scores were very high, and the reliability low. It was recommended that future studies use a longer and more difficult quiz. In addition, the evaluators found an overwhelmingly positive bias in Client Satisfaction Survey ratings. Finally, clinic staff had difficulty maintaining the No Show/Continuation Report that recorded clients' compliance with appointments. As a result, program evaluators used the number of clients who completed the Method Use Questionnaire at the 6- and 12-month follow-ups to calculate patient continuation rates.

The evaluators recommended that future studies employ a more vigorous follow-up system, fewer measures (a more challenging quiz, administered once, and the Method Use Questionnaire), and a longer treatment phase and follow-up period to track patients and obtain outcome data. This design would be easier for clinics to implement, require less data management, and yield a larger sample size with greater information on dropouts.

TAILORING FAMILY PLANNING IN THE COMMUNITY TODAY

In the past 3 years, 10 communities in five states, from South Carolina to Michigan to Colorado, have implemented *Tailoring Family Planning*.

NOTE

1. A full set of program materials, including a program manual, forms, brochures, evaluation materials, and more, is available for purchase from Sociometrics at http://www.socio.com/pasha.htm.

Secondary Pregnancy

Prevention

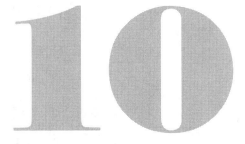

A Health Care Program for First-Time Adolescent Mothers and Their Infants: A Second Pregnancy Prevention Program for Teen Mothers

J. Barry Gurdin, Starr Niego, and Janette Mince

Original Program Developer

Ann L. O'Sullivan, PhD, FAAN
　School of Nursing
　University of Pennsylvania
　Philadelphia, PA

Original Program Evaluator

Barbara S. Jacobsen, MS
　School of Nursing
　University of Pennsylvania
　Philadelphia, PA

A Health Care Program for First-Time Adolescent Mothers and Their Infants was supported by a grant from the Robert Wood Johnson Foundation (Grant #07689).

PROGRAM ABSTRACT

Summary

Originally designed for low-income, unwed teens, this program combines secondary and tertiary pregnancy prevention goals. It aims to help first-time mothers prevent repeat pregnancies, return to school, improve immunization rates for their infants, and reduce their use of hospital emergency room services for routine infant care. A variety of services are offered in the context of a teen baby clinic, including (a) well-baby care at 2 weeks, and when the baby is 2, 4, 6, 9, 12, 15, and 18 months of age; (b) family planning discussions and referral, as appropriate, to a birth control clinic; (c) instruction in parenting skills; and (d) informal parenting education through videos, slides, and discussions with nurse practitioners or trained volunteers.

The effectiveness of the program was assessed in a study in which 243 African American teen mothers at an urban teaching hospital were randomly assigned to either the intervention (n = 120) or control group (n = 132). Compared to members of the control group, who received traditional well-baby services only, intervention participants experienced significantly fewer repeat pregnancies and were more likely to obtain full immunization for their newborns. Mothers who continued attending the clinic for the duration of the program also reduced their use of the emergency room for routine infant medical care.

Focus

☐ Primary pregnancy prevention   ☑ Secondary pregnancy prevention   ☐ STI/HIV/AIDS prevention

Original Site

☐ School based   ☐ Community based   ☑ Clinic based

Suitable for Use In

This program is suitable for use in hospital- or community-based pediatrics clinics, providing that medical and counseling services are available.

Approach

- ■ ☐ Abstinence
- ■ ☑ Behavioral skills development
- ■ ☐ Community outreach
- ■ ☐ Contraceptive access
- ■ ☑ Contraceptive education
- ■ ☑ Life option enhancement
- ■ ☐ Self-efficacy/self-esteem
- ■ ☑ Sexuality/HIV/STI education

Original Intervention Sample

Age, gender   The field study involved 243 first-time mothers less than 18 years of age (average age = 16.5 years).

Race/ethnicity   100% African American.

Program Components

- ■ ☐ Adult involvement
- ■ ☑ Case management
- ■ ☑ Group discussion (in waiting room)
- ■ ☐ Lectures
- ■ ☐ Peer counseling/instruction
- ■ ☐ Public service announcements
- ■ ☐ Role play
- ■ ☑ Video
- ■ ☑ Other: Informal parenting education through one-on-one discussions and educational materials

Program Length

In the field study, participants received services from delivery until their children reached 18 months of age.

Staffing Requirements/Training

In the field study, the clinic was staffed by a pediatrician, a master's level nurse practitioner, and a social worker, who all worked part-time. A half-time master's level nurse practitioner served as program director. Trained volunteers were recruited to serve as informal parent educators in the clinic waiting room.

BIBLIOGRAPHY

O'Sullivan, A., & Jacobsen, B. (1992). A randomized trial of a health care program for first-time adolescent mothers and their infants. *Nursing Research, 41,* 210–215.

Related References by the Developers of the *Health Care Program for First-Time Adolescent Mothers and Their Infants*

O'Sullivan, A. L., & Apriceno-Tesoro, T. (1993). Prevention: Adolescent health. *American Nurses Association Publications, CH-27 5M,* 53–61.

Rew, L., Koniak-Griffin, D., Lewis, M. A., Miles, M., & O'Sullivan, A. L. (2000). Secondary data analysis: New perspective for adolescent research. *Nursing Outlook, 48*(5), 223–229.

THE PROGRAM

Program Rationale and History

This intervention was designed both to meet the multiple, interrelated needs of teenage mothers and their infants, who were at risk for long-term physical, psychological, and socioeconomic difficulties, and to prevent repeat pregnancies.[1] Located within a teen baby clinic, the program combined regular well-baby checkups with reproductive health counseling; referrals for contraception; and parenting education, modeling, and support. In addition, staff members encouraged the young mothers to return to school and reduce their use of hospital emergency services for routine infant care. Services were delivered by a team of medical and social service providers.

A field study and evaluation of the program were conducted in the mid-1980s with 243 unwed teenage African American mothers receiving Medicaid. Program services were provided in a well-baby clinic located in a teaching hospital in Philadelphia, Pennsylvania.

Rationale for the Program

This program was developed in recognition of the complex challenges and everyday needs of unmarried teenage mothers and their infants. In particular, babies born to teenage mothers frequently have low birth weights and are at increased risk for developmental delays, mental retardation, and other neurological disorders. In addition, young mothers frequently drop out of school and have few financial resources with which to support their children. With low levels of educational and vocational achievement, the mothers' opportunities may be severely limited over time.

The program developers also found that teenage mothers often did not understand the importance of regular health care. They tended to miss appointments for routine well-baby checkups but visit the emergency room when their infants displayed only minor symptoms.

A review of services provided to teenage mothers in other countries suggested to researchers that counseling, health care, and education programs could improve the well-being of teenage mothers and their infants. For this reason, the program developers created a comprehensive program combining traditional well-baby care with special counseling and educational services tailored to the needs of teenage mothers (e.g., reproductive health counseling, parenting education). Regular clinic visits were used as an opportunity to reinforce program messages about health care, educational achievement, and parenting skills. Preventing repeat pregnancy was also emphasized as an explicit goal of the intervention.

Program Objectives

The multiple components of the *Health Care Program for First-Time Adolescent Mothers and Their Infants* were designed to meet the following objectives:

1. To reduce the repeat pregnancy rate among adolescent mothers
2. To increase mothers' attendance in school after giving birth
3. To increase the proportion of mothers who obtained full immunization for their infants
4. To reduce teenage mothers' use of the emergency room for routine infant care

Program Overview

The *Health Care Program for First-Time Adolescent Mothers and Their Infants* provided a wide range of basic information on topics essential for the well-being of new mothers and their infants. To accommodate the needs and lifestyles of participants, the program was designed to be flexible, and numerous opportunities were provided for informal education and discussion. Critical features of the intervention are highlighted below; examples are provided from the original field study of the intervention.

Setting

The program was designed to be implemented in a hospital clinic. During the field study, all activities took place in the teen baby clinic to which the participating mothers had agreed to bring their newborn for well-infant care.

Staffing

The team of staff members included a pediatrician, a social worker, and a nurse practitioner, all of whom were knowledgeable about adolescent development and comfortable working with teen mothers. For the field study, in which 120 mothers participated, one pediatrician, one social worker, and one master's level nurse practitioner were all employed on a part-time basis. One additional nurse practitioner staffed the program half-time; in addition to providing nursing care, she served as director and oversaw all administrative tasks. In the waiting room, trained volunteers were also available to discuss and model parenting skills with the young mothers.

To minimize the costs of services, the pediatrician and nurse practitioners alternated in providing care. The social worker spoke with all participants during their first well-baby check visit to the clinic, when the baby was 2-weeks old, and thereafter, by referral from other staff members. Relying on trained volunteers—rather than nurse practitioners—to provide informal educational activities in the waiting room also helped to reduce personnel costs.

Regular Well-Baby Visits

Well-baby care was provided in accordance with guidelines issued by the American Academy of Pediatrics. That is, mothers and their infants were scheduled for routine checkups at the clinic, first at 2 weeks postpartum, and then when the baby reached 2, 4, 6, 9, 12, 15, and 18 months of age.

Special Care

In addition to routine well-baby care, the following services were delivered to each participating teen. During the field study, these services were incorporated into the mothers' regular clinic visits.

Repeat Pregnancy Prevention. At the 2-week clinic visit (the first well-baby check), the social worker interviewed each mother to determine her understanding of contraception and family planning. When appropriate, the social worker counseled and educated the young woman and referred her to a nearby birth control clinic. During subsequent clinic visits, the pediatrician and nurse practitioners continued to inquire about the mother's use of family planning. When appropriate, they suggested that she speak again with the social worker or visit a reproductive health clinic.

Parenting Education. Parenting education began at the 2-week clinic visit (the first well-baby check) and continued for the duration of the program. During the first visit, the social worker discussed and modeled good parenting skills by demonstrating how to properly hold and feed a baby. The mother was encouraged to ask any questions she had about health care, growth and development, and parenting.

Additional, informal education took place in the waiting room. During the field study, for example, trained volunteers and nurse practitioners were available to discuss health care and parenting skills on a one-to-one basis with mothers in the clinic waiting room. They answered questions and concerns, modeled skills, and provided counseling and support. Also available were numerous educational brochures providing information on a variety of parenting issues, including proper nutrition for mother and baby, choosing a contraceptive method, selecting a car seat, installing a smoke detector, and taking an infant's temperature. For your implementation of the program, you may wish to use similar commercially available materials or obtain comparable ones from appropriate agencies in your local community (e.g., Planned Parenthood, County Health Department).

As part of the parenting education component, staff members discouraged teen mothers from visiting the emergency room when their infants showed only minor symptoms. They also showed the women how to take care of minor health problems, such as diaper rash and runny noses.

Encouragement for School Reenrollment. Along with pregnancy prevention, support for school participation began during the first clinic visit and continued for the duration of the program. All staff members—including the pediatrician, nurse practitioner, and social worker—asked about the young woman's educational plans and encouraged her to return to school. They assisted her in making the necessary arrangements and researching options for child care.

Full Infant Immunization. During clinic visits, staff members reminded teen mothers about the importance of obtaining full immunization for their infants. In the field study, participants were provided with copies of their infants' immunization records, free of charge, no matter how many times they lost these papers. Staff explained that the records would be required when enrolling a child in day care, Head Start, preschool, or kindergarten.

Additional Supports

Program staff anticipated that the teen mothers would have difficulty keeping their scheduled appointments. To encourage continued participation in the program, staff members contacted mothers who missed a scheduled appointment, either by calling or sending a letter. Reminders were sent each week for a 6-week period following the first clinic visit; for subsequent appointments, the reminders continued for 8 weeks. In addition, reminder calls for all visits were attempted the day before each scheduled visit.

Program Implementation

Before the program began, staff took part in a training session that was designed to (a) introduce the framework for the intervention and the services that would be provided; (b) provide basic information about adolescent psychosocial and cognitive development, adolescent sexuality, and the challenges faced by teen mothers; and (c) convey basic strategies for communicating with, and providing support to, adolescent mothers.

Time was allotted to recruit and train a group of volunteer parent educators who would be comfortable working with teenage mothers. Training covered the same material as described above; it also provided opportunities for the volunteer educators to practice modeling parenting skills and supporting and communicating with teens. In your setting, you may want to invite a psychologist, health educator, or social worker who can share his/her expertise and experience working with adolescent mothers.

EVALUATING THE PROGRAM

The Original Evaluation

Design

The effectiveness of the *Health Care Program for First-Time Adolescent Mothers and Their Infants* was investigated in an 18-month study conducted with 243 mothers attending a hospital clinic in Philadelphia, Pennsylvania. The young women were randomly assigned either to (a) the treatment/intervention group, who took part in a comprehensive program providing well-baby care, parenting education, family planning counseling and referrals, as well as support for continuing their education; or (b) the control group, who received traditional well-baby care only, without any additional services. To compare the two groups, a variety of measures were recorded for the mothers and their babies, from the time of enrollment in the study, through the young women's regular visits to the clinic, and until the infant reached 18 months of age. Using medical records, these measures were recorded regardless of whether the mother and her child continued attending the clinic for the duration of the study.

Evaluation Questions

The researchers hypothesized that members of the treatment/intervention group would show the following outcomes, compared to their control group peers receiving traditional well-baby services only:

1. A higher rate of clinic attendance
2. A higher rate of school enrollment
3. A higher immunization rate for their babies
4. Less-frequent use of the emergency room for routine infant care
5. A lower repeat pregnancy rate

Data Collection Procedures

Teenage mothers were recruited for the study during their postpartum stay in a participating hospital. The researchers invited young women who (a) were 17 years of age or under, (b) had decided to keep their child, and (c) could provide consent as emancipated minors. Those who agreed to participate and met the eligibility criteria were randomly assigned to either the intervention (n = 120) or control group (n = 123).

At recruitment, the researchers measured a number of demographic variables, both by reviewing patient charts and by asking participants directly. Subsequently, they relied on chart reviews to measure the mothers' clinic attendance and infant immunization rates. At a final 18-month interview, participants were asked whether they had experienced a repeat pregnancy or returned to school; the latter measure was verified using school records, and immunization data were verified using infant charts.

Research Sample

Of the 300 teens recruited for the study, 58 (18%) refused to participate, and 29 (9%) were lost due to administrative reasons at the hospital. Thus, the final sample included 243 mothers, all of whom were African American and receiving Medicaid. Additionally, most of the teens had not been pregnant previously, had experienced no complications during delivery, and had received about 5 months of prenatal care. Although many teens dropped out of the two groups over the duration of the study, through the 18-month follow-up interview the researchers were able to gather complete data for 91% of the original research sample.

Evaluation Results

Clinic Attendance

Beginning with the first scheduled clinic visit 2 weeks postpartum, and continuing for the duration of the study, program participants showed a significantly higher clinic attendance rate than their control group peers. At the 2-week visit, for example, 92% of the treatment group, versus 76% of the control group, kept their appointments ($p = .002$). By the final appointment, 18 months postpartum, 40% of program participants continued to attend the clinic; in contrast, only 18% of their control group peers did so. Although the dropout rate was high for both groups, it was nearly twice as great within the control group.

School Enrollment

At the conclusion of the study, the researchers found no significant difference between the two groups' rate of school enrollment. Regardless of whether school records or self-reports were used, the researchers found that approximately 50% of the mothers in both groups had reenrolled in school following the birth of their child.

Infant Immunization Status

Mothers in the treatment group were significantly more likely than their control group peers to have obtained full immunization for their infants ($p < .02$). Within the treatment group, 33% of the infants (37 of the 113 infants for whom data were available) had received full immunization; in contrast, within the control group, full immunization was recorded for 18% of infants (20 of the 111 for whom data were available). The researchers found no differences in the immunization rates recorded among infants whose mothers had dropped out from either intervention; however, when they focused on "continued attenders," the difference approached significance ($p = .058$). That is, 60% of treatment group infants whose mothers continued attending the clinic for the duration of the study, versus 36% of this subset of control group infants, had received full immunization.

Emergency Room Use

The researchers noted that both groups of mothers used the emergency room to a high degree. They found that 76% of program participants (85 of the 110 mothers for whom data were available) visited the emergency room at least once during the course of the study. Among control group mothers, 85% (96 of 113 mothers for whom data were available) did so. In a χ^2 test, this difference was not significant at the $p = .05$ level. However, the two groups of continued attenders did differ significantly on this measure ($p < .03$), with 81% of intervention participants (39 of 48 mothers) and 100% of the control group (22 of 22 mothers) making at least one visit to the emergency room during the course of the study.

Repeat Pregnancy

Teens who took part in the *Health Care Program for First-Time Adolescent Mothers and Their Infants* were significantly less likely to have experienced a repeat pregnancy by the conclusion of the study ($p < .003$). In particular, at the 18-month interview, repeat pregnancies were reported by 13 of the 108 intervention participants (12%) for whom complete data were available. Within the comparison group, in contrast, the repeat pregnancy rate was 28% (32 of the 113 mothers for whom complete data were available). In subsequent analyses, the researchers determined that the repeat pregnancy rates did not differ significantly for teens who remained in their respective programs, but did differ between those teens who had dropped out ($p = .02$). That is, 15% of mothers who dropped out of the treatment group experienced a repeat pregnancy (9 pregnancies, n = 60), while 32% of dropouts from the control group did so (29 pregnancies, n = 91).

Across the sample, the researchers found that teens who remained in the study for only the 2-week or 2-month visits had a higher repeat pregnancy rate than those who continued attending the clinic for at least 6 months. Moreover, within the treatment group, both continued attenders and dropouts who were followed through the 18-month assessment were half as likely to experience a repeat pregnancy rate as their corresponding control group peers.

Summary

At the conclusion of the 18-month study of the *Health Care Program for First-Time Adolescent Mothers and Their Infants,* program participants showed a number of positive outcomes, relative to their control group peers. Overall, participation in the program's comprehensive set of education, counseling, and support services for teen mothers was associated with significantly higher clinic attendance and higher rates of full infant immunization, as compared to participation only in routine well-baby care. On measures of emergency room use, significantly fewer visits were made by program participants, but only within the subset of teens who continued attending the clinic for the duration of the study. The program appeared to have no impact on school enrollment, with more than half of the mothers in both the treatment and control groups returning to school.

The researchers found that program participants were significantly less likely to have experienced a repeat pregnancy at the 18-month follow-up than were their control group peers. Assuming that the average annual cost to taxpayers (federal, state, and local) of each birth to a teenage parent through the age of 19 cost the public $21,667 (as calculated in 2004), and the intervention prevented 19 pregnancies (as calculated by the researchers), the program saved $411,673 in public funds [see Hoffman, S. D. (2006). *By the numbers: The public costs of childbearing.* Washington, DC: National Campaign to Prevent Teen Pregnancy]. It should also be noted that mothers who attended *either* the treatment or control clinic for at least 6 months were more likely than dropouts to avoid a repeat pregnancy. Thus, it appeared that involvement in a special well-baby program was itself helpful in preventing a repeat pregnancy during adolescence.

Within both the treatment and control groups, large numbers of mothers dropped out of the study. Yet, the researchers noted that it is not uncommon for teenage mothers who are poor to drop out of special education and service programs. They suggested that future interventions might aim to involve the teen's entire family, to improve knowledge about family planning, and to change the young women's attitudes about the future.

NOTE

1. A full set of program materials, including sample educational pamphlets, appointment reminder notices, evaluation materials, and more, is available for purchase from Sociometrics at http://www.socio.com/pasha.htm.

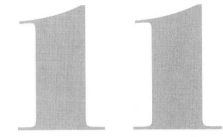

Queens Hospital Center's Teenage Program: A Second Pregnancy Prevention Program for Young Men and Women

J. Barry Gurdin, Alisa Mallari, M. Jane Park, and Janette Mince

Original Program Developers

Jill M. Rabin, MD

Vicki Seltzer, MD

Department of Obstetrics & Gynecology

The Queens Hospital Center Affiliation of the Long Island Jewish Medical Center

Long Island Campus for the Albert Einstein College of Medicine

New Hyde Park, NY

Original Program Evaluator

Simcha Pollack, PhD

Department of Quantitative Analysis

Queens Hospital Center's Teenage Program was supported by grants from the New York State Department of Health Offices of Adolescent Pregnancy and Planning, and New York City Health and Hospital Corporations Division to Reduce Low Birth Weight Infants.

131

St. John's University
Jamaica, NY

PROGRAM ABSTRACT

Summary

Based upon the premise that a teen's first pregnancy may stem from underlying unmet needs, the *Queens Hospital Center's Teenage Program* provides a comprehensive set of services including medical care, psychosocial support, and education to the adolescent, her partner, and her family. This approach emphasizes early intervention, beginning at pregnancy. For the duration of the intervention, each patient and her infant remain with a team of providers: an ob-gyn, pediatrician, social worker, and health educator. The program also has a physician/practitioner "on call" 24 hours a day. Reproductive health and family life education classes are offered to the patient, her partner, and her family. In an effort to prevent repeat pregnancies and sexually transmitted infections (STIs), the program encourages the teen's partner to participate in education, support, and counseling activities. Access to other services is enhanced by the program's location in a multiservice center which houses many social service agencies.

A field study of the intervention was conducted in Queens, New York, with 498 adolescents and their infants. Program participants were more likely to attend clinics regularly, use contraception more frequently and attend and graduate from high school than were teen mothers in a comparison group. Both the participating teen mothers and their infants experienced better health outcomes than those in the comparison group. The investigators also found a significantly reduced repeat pregnancy rate among participating mothers. Only 9% of the adolescent mothers in the program had a repeat pregnancy, as compared to 70% of the comparison group. Moreover, the teenage mothers' repeat pregnancy rate declined with each successive year of program participation.

Focus

☐ Primary pregnancy prevention   ☑ Secondary pregnancy prevention   ☐ STI/HIV/AIDS prevention

Original Site

☐ School based   ☑ Community based   ☑ Clinic based

Suitable for Use In

This program is suitable for use in hospital- or community-based clinics, providing that comprehensive medical and counseling services are available.

Approach

- ☑ Abstinence
- ☑ Behavioral skills development
- ☑ Community outreach
- ☑ Contraceptive access
- ☑ Contraceptive education
- ☑ Life option enhancement
- ☐ Efficacy/self-esteem
- ☑ Sexuality/HIV/STI education

Original Intervention Sample

Age   The field study included 498 first-time mothers, who were all under age 20 when their child was born (average age at delivery was 17 years).

Race/ethnicity   The ethnic makeup of the program clients was 90% African American, 6% Hispanic, and 4% Other (including Asian, Native American, East Indian, and White).

Program Components

- ☑ Adult involvement
- ☑ Case management
- ☑ Group discussion
- ☐ Lectures
- ☑ Peer counseling/instruction
- ☐ Public service announcements
- ☐ Role play
- ☐ Video
- ☑ Other: Partner and family involvement

Program Length

During the field study, participants were eligible to receive services from pregnancy until they reached their 20th birthday. Family life education classes were held on a biweekly basis for the duration of the program.

Staffing Requirements/Training

Your team of providers should include physicians, nurses, social workers, health educators, and additional staff as needed. In the field study, which served 498 mothers, the staff consisted of a team of physicians—drawn from a rotating pool of two pediatricians and one or two obstetrician-gynecologists (ob-gyns)—three registered nurses and six nurses' aides, six social workers, two male counselors, two health educators, one coordinating manager, and six to eight clerical assistants. Clergy were also available as needed. In 1984, the program also began recruiting peer counselors to offer presentations in the waiting room.

During the field study, the coordinating manager held regular weekly meetings to train the staff. Additionally, each group of service providers (e.g., physicians, social workers, health educators) held their own meetings to discuss training issues particular to their specialty.

BIBLIOGRAPHY

Rabin, J. M., Seltzer, V., & Pollack, S. (1991). The long-term benefits of a comprehensive teenage pregnancy program. *Clinical Pediatrics, 30*(5), 305–309.

Rabin, J. M., Seltzer, V., & Pollack, S. (1992). The benefits of a comprehensive teenage pregnancy program. *The American Journal of Gynecologic Health, 4*(3), 66–74.

Seltzer, V. L., Rabin, J., & Benjamin, F. (1989). Teenagers' awareness of the Acquired Immunodeficiency Syndrome and the impact on their sexual behavior. *Obstetrics & Gynecology, 74*(1), 55–59.

THE PROGRAM

Program Rationale and History

The *Queens Hospital Center's Teenage Program* was developed in 1982 to respond to the high adolescent pregnancy rates in the South Jamaica community in Queens,

New York.[1] Recognizing that many of the causes and adverse consequences of teenage pregnancy are functions of socioeconomic, rather than medical or age factors, the program attempted to address underlying social and economic problems faced by adolescent mothers and their families.

The program adopted a team approach to respond to the many needs of pregnant and parenting teens. Upon enrollment in the program, the pregnant adolescent was assigned a team of professionals for the duration of her care. Each team— drawn from the program's interdisciplinary staff of ob-gyns, pediatricians, social workers, and health educators—tailored the broad array of program services to the specific needs of each adolescent. In addition to medical services for the mother and her child, the program provided contraceptive and STI (including HIV/AIDS) counseling, contraception, and HIV testing, as well as ongoing education in reproductive health and family life for the patient, her partner, and family. Vocational and educational assistance, supportive counseling, and social work services were also provided to the mother and her partner. Indeed, the program actively involved the teen's partner in education, support, and counseling, particularly with respect to prevention of repeat pregnancy and STIs.

A field study of the program was conducted between 1982 and 1989 with a diverse group of 498 adolescent mothers (and their infants) who were enrolled in Queens Hospital Center's mother–baby family planning clinic. The program was established by Queens Hospital Center's affiliation of the Long Island Jewish Medical Center's Departments of Obstetrics & Gynecology and Community Medicine and Ambulatory Care. Funding was provided by New York State's Department of Health Offices of Adolescent Pregnancy and Family Planning, as well as by New York City's Health and Hospital Corporations Division to Reduce Low Birth Weight Infants.

Theoretical Framework

The development of *Queens Hospital Center's Teenage Program* was based upon the premise that the causes and many of the adverse consequences of teenage pregnancy reflect an ongoing cycle of unmet needs, including the need for parenting education and economic, psychological, and emotional support.

The developers postulated that a teen's first pregnancy may be a "red flag" signifying the underlying problem: an upbringing marked by unmet basic needs. If not addressed, a teen mother risks experiencing a repeat pregnancy with more serious consequences than those of the first pregnancy (e.g., prematurity, low birth weight, and intrauterine growth retardation). Therefore, to successfully prevent repeat adolescent pregnancy and its negative consequences, it is essential to fully address the needs of adolescent mothers.

Program Goals

The overall aims of the program were to

1. reduce the teenage pregnancy rate (including repeat pregnancies, whether ending in live birth or termination; see "An Update on the Population" later in this program section);
2. improve maternal and infant health outcomes;
3. assist participants in making positive choices for their reproductive health and for their adult lives.

Program Objectives

The *Queens Hospital Center's Teenage Program* sought to

1. provide adolescent mothers and their partners with health care information regarding prevention of unwanted pregnancies, STIs, and HIV/AIDS;

2. treat and counsel adolescents for pregnancy, STIs, and HIV/AIDS;
3. enable teens to become more responsible and self-sufficient by staying in school and learning marketable skills;
4. increase adolescent mothers' return to school;
5. increase the participation of pregnant teenagers in preparing for the birth of their children and in obtaining care for their infants;
6. involve the partners and families of the teenage mothers in the complete care of teenage mothers and their children;
7. discuss with teenage mothers such options as a foster home or adoption;
8. encourage abstinence.

Program Components

Recruitment

Between 1982 and 1986, pregnant adolescents were automatically referred to the program when they visited the clinic for prenatal care. In addition, program staff and other hospital personnel recruited patients through brochure dissemination and other activities. In the original implementation, referrals were provided by family and friends of the pregnant teens, as well as by local clergy. One of the program developers also visited local high schools to familiarize teachers, administrators, and students with the services available through the *Queens Hospital Center's Teenage Program*.

Community of Care

Upon entry into the program, each teen is seen by a social worker for an intake interview and then assigned a health care provider. To ensure continuity of care, this same provider met with the teen at all subsequent visits. A team consisting of an ob-gyn, a pediatrician, a social worker, and a health educator oversaw and directed the care of each patient from the prenatal period throughout the mother's participation in the program.

Accessibility

In the field study of the program, several features enhanced participants' access to services. The program's location in a multiservice center put teens in close proximity to many agencies offering a range of services in areas such as housing, nutrition, and day care. In addition, the center itself was convenient to bus lines. In 1986, the program began offering evening clinic hours (4:00 to 8:00 P.M.) 2 days a week, allowing teens to visit after school using their bus passes. A physician/practitioner 24-hour "on call" system provided access to services at any time. Day care was also available during the teens' visits to the center.

Staffing

Providing the constellation of services offered by the *Queens Hospital Center's Teenage Program* required an interdisciplinary staff committed to a team approach in serving adolescent mothers and their children. In the original implementation, which served 498 mothers and their children, the staff included a team of physicians (drawn from a rotating pool of two pediatricians and one or two ob-gyns), three registered nurses and six nurses' aides, six social workers, two male counselors, two health educators, and one coordinating manager. Clergy were also available as needed. In 1984, the program also began recruiting peer counselors to offer presentations in the waiting room. Finally, the program was served by approximately six to eight clerical staff.

Services

The Queens Hospital Center's Teenage Program. The program provided adolescent mothers, their children, their partners, and their families with a comprehensive set of services, as explained below. All services were provided in the program's multi-service center. However, a number of participants continued attending regular high school programs during pregnancy and postpartum.

Sex, Birth Control, and Parenting Education. The main educational component of the program provided all male and female participants with sex and birth control education. Reproductive and family life education were taught in ongoing biweekly meetings, led by a registered nurse, physician, or health educator, and involving the patient, her partner, and her family. During pregnancy, teens participated in childbirth preparation and Lamaze classes led by registered nurses or other hospital staff.

Parenting education was offered as well. Social workers conducted workshops designed to educate male partners of adolescent mothers on questions of paternity and responsibility. They also discussed with each participant options such as foster home placement and adoption.

Complete Medical and Follow-Up Care for Mother and Child. Obstetrical and postpartum care was offered by a staff of physicians, nurse practitioners, physician's assistants, social workers, and a program administrator. Attending obstetricians supervised prenatal and postpartum care. In the original implementation, pregnant teens delivered at the Queens Hospital Center's labor and delivery unit. Intrapartum care was provided by resident physicians with attending supervision. All services were provided at the Queens Hospital Center's facilities. Over the duration of the field study, these services included well-woman care, internal medicine, family planning, and a range of specialized services.

Infant care was provided in accordance with the American Academy of Pediatrics protocols. The program followed standard protocols for every aspect of medical care, including intake, preeclampsia, amniocentesis, and referrals. These protocols did not specify how much time should be spent on any services—providers devoted as much time as needed to complete the service.

HIV Counseling, Testing, and Education. HIV-related services were integrated into the regular biweekly family life education classes. Additional services were provided on an individual basis, as needed, by the physicians and/or social workers. When appropriate, the young women's partners were also included.

Vocational and Educational Assistance. Program staff—primarily the social workers—worked closely with local organizations providing vocational services to ensure that each of the participants had the opportunity to receive vocational training, job training, and job placement services. Program participants also received educational assistance to complete high school or to receive their graduate equivalency degree (GED). The male counselors provided educational and vocational assistance to partners.

Supportive Counseling and Social Work Services. Psychological and social service counseling and guidance began during the teen's first visit and were provided thereafter as needed. Each teen was assigned to a team so that she could establish close relationships with her service providers. In the event that the teen needed specialized assistance that went beyond the team's expertise, the staff referred the adolescent to appropriate community agencies and served as a liaison and facilitator to ensure that the required services were provided.

Presentations by Peer Counselors

Peer counselors were selected from teenagers in the community and from among program clients. They received training to ensure that they interacted with the participants in a supportive and knowledgeable manner. Peer counselors provided waiting room presentations in the form of plays they had written. Their role was to provide adolescents with information on abstinence, birth control, relationships, HIV/AIDS, and other adolescent issues. They also conducted workshops in schools, churches, and health fairs in the community. For their work, the peer counselors received stipends.

Training

Regular weekly meetings provided opportunities to educate staff about discussing family planning and contraception, HIV prevention, and adolescent sexuality with program participants. Over the course of the program, training focused on additional issues that emerged in teens' lives, including domestic violence, postpartum depression, and educational development.

In addition, each group of professionals (e.g., social workers, physicians) held their own staff meetings to discuss service or training issues particular to their specialty. The social workers met on a biweekly basis, and the physicians convened once each month. Peer counselors also received training from program staff to develop skills in communicating family life information and ideas to adolescent mothers.

Coordination

The coordinating manager used the weekly staff meetings to ensure smooth program functioning and to resolve any conflicts among staff. In addition, the meetings provided an opportunity to discuss findings from quality assurance visits (see below) along with strategies to address deficiencies, inconsistencies, and other concerns about service.

Protocols

Program staff followed all of the standard American College of Gynecologists and American Academy of Pediatrics protocols (e.g., for prenatal and well-baby care and immunization schedules). No special protocols were developed for the program. Although no specialized charts or forms were developed, staff kept extensive notes documenting the services provided to teens over the duration of the program. These notes were included in the medical records for each participant.

Strict quality assurance protocols were put in place for the duration of the program. Official site visits were conducted regularly by the Queens Health Center, Department of Health, and all granting agencies. Selected files were inspected for accuracy and completeness. Files were also monitored more frequently by program administrators.

Financing Medical Care

Although the programs continued after the completion of the field study, changes in public and private financing and delivery of health care services posed challenges to many programs providing comprehensive medical care such as *Queens Hospital Center's Teenage Program*. For example, teens needed to be enrolled in the managed care plan of which the Queens Hospital Center was a member in order to have the program services covered by Medicaid. If a teen who was enrolled in another plan wished to receive program services, program staff would provide instructions on how to switch plans. As another example, males seeking treatment for STIs needed to be referred to other agencies. This disrupted patients' relationships with program staff and made patient follow-up more difficult. Restrictions in your setting may be more, or less, stringent.

Program Implementation

Community Outreach

The success of a multifaceted program such as *Queens Hospital Center's Teenage Program* depends in large part on the ability to integrate the program into the community. It is essential to identify community resources and enlist community support. Residents, leaders in hospital medicine, church representatives, social workers, teachers, educational administrators, and local media can all be involved in this effort. For this reason, the program director should begin by outlining how the program can best gain local acceptance, what the local needs are, how to enter the community, and how to establish trust and support in the community. A good strategy will enable the program director to build the kinds of partnerships that are necessary to implement a comprehensive, multifaceted intervention such as the *Queens Hospital Center's Teenage Program.*

In the field study, health fairs, workshops, seminars, and lectures to churches, schools, and community agencies all proved to be successful venues for contacting the target population. The following provides a brief overview of community outreach activities used in the original implementation. These activities can serve as starting points for your own implementation.

Raising Public Awareness

It is important to focus some effort on public awareness of the program in order to establish credibility and acceptance. Increase the visibility of the program in your milieu through newspaper articles. Report on the program's location and its accessibility to public transportation, and help inform young people who need the medical, social, vocational, housing, and educational services your program will be providing. Public announcements on the radio and television, in church and community bulletins, at commercial cinemas, and the local sites of the World Wide Web may be good resources for "getting out the word" about the program.

Community Workshops

Another way to get the whole community involved is to offer informative workshops on the services provided in the program, and how issues of adolescent pregnancy are affecting the community, what residents can do to help, and so forth. The health educators and social workers on your staff can help to educate and inform your community about the benefits and services the program provides. For your own intervention, these workshops may also provide the opportunity to identify existing community resources that provide some of the services you plan to offer.

An Update on the Population

At the time this study was conducted in the early and mid-1980s, the teen pregnancy rate in the United States was still on the rise. The overall teen birth rate in the United States hit its peak in 1990 and has been declining ever since. According to a report published by the Alan Guttmacher Institute, fewer than 747,000 young women between the ages of 15 and 19 became pregnant in 2002, and approximately 425,500 births resulted from those pregnancies. This represents an overall decline of about 36% since 1989 when more than 1,015,000 young women became pregnant (their births were reflected in the high number of teen births, nearly

522,000, in 1990). Some ethnic subpopulations have experienced a greater decline. Teens are waiting longer before engaging in sexual intercourse. The condom has become the most popular form of contraception at first intercourse. [See *U.S. Teenage Pregnancy Statistics: National and State Trends by Race and Ethnicity.* (2006). Alan Guttmacher Institute: New York.]

Despite this progress in reducing teen pregnancies and increasing condom use, one in five teens under the age of 18 whose parents do not know that they obtain contraceptive services would continue to have sex, but would either rely on withdrawal or not use any contraceptives if the law required that their parents be notified of their clinic visit.

PROGRAM EVALUATION

The Original Evaluation

Design

The effectiveness of the *Queens Hospital Center's Teenage Program* was investigated in a study of adolescent mothers and their newborns attending the mother–baby family planning clinic from 1982 to 1989. The study compared a group of teen mothers enrolled in the *Queens Hospital Center's Teenage Program* housed at the multiservice center with a comparison group of pregnant and parenting adolescents who received care at the Queens Hospital Center's Adult Obstetric Clinic from 1980–1981 (before the program's inception) and who continued to receive care with their newborns at the hospital's adult family planning and pediatrics clinics through 1989 or until they reached age 20.

Evaluation Questions

The evaluation of the *Queens Hospital Center's Teenage Program* examined the following questions:

1. Did participation in the *Queens Hospital Center's Teenage Program* increase utilization of health care services by teen mothers and their children?
2. Did participation in the *Queens Hospital Center's Teenage Program* improve maternal and infant health?
3. Did participation in the *Queens Hospital Center's Teenage Program* improve teens' educational and vocational status?
4. Did participation in the *Queens Hospital Center's Teenage Program* increase teen mothers' use of contraceptives?
5. Did participation in the *Queens Hospital Center's Teenage Program* decrease the rate of repeat pregnancy among teen mothers?
6. Did any of these outcomes change with prolonged exposure to the program?

Recruitment Procedures

A Department of Health Office at the intervention and comparison sites assisted in tracking pregnant patients. From 1980 to 1981, all patients who were seen for prenatal care were examined at the Queens Hospital Center's Adult Obstetrics and Gynecology Clinic. Between 1982 and 1986, all pregnant teenagers were automatically referred to the adolescent program. In addition, program staff and other hospital personnel recruited patients through brochure dissemination and other activities. Young women were eligible if they were under the age of 20 at delivery. Criteria for exclusion from the study included any preexisting hypertension; diabetes; cardiac, renal, endocrinologic, or neurologic disease; multiple gestation; or known drug abuse.

Quality Control

There was no significant difference in the quality of medical care received by teens in the intervention and comparison groups. Medical and nursing protocols were uniform for each clinic and compiled by Queens Hospital Center's Departments of Obstetrics and Gynecology, Community Medicine, and Ambulatory Care and Nursing. A Quality Assurance Committee was responsible for each site's records. The Queens Hospital Center's personnel department's standards for hiring qualified health care professionals remained consistent from 1980 to 1986. Intrapartum care was provided to both groups by resident physicians with attending supervision at the Queens Hospital Center's labor and delivery unit.

Data Collection Procedures

The data were retrospectively abstracted from outpatient and inpatient medical charts prior to July 1985 and prospectively collected from July 1985 onward.

To assess questions relating to maternal and fetal health outcomes, researchers examined numerous prenatal, intrapartum, and postpartum factors, including services received and behavioral influences, as well as clinical outcome variables. These data were recorded by clinicians in the medical charts of the teens and their infants.

From the social workers' charts, the researchers obtained data regarding the student and occupational status of the patient, contraceptive use, and subsequent pregnancy, including pregnancy resolution during the patient's adolescence.

Sample

Adolescents in the sample were defined as those under 20 years of age. The age of teens in both the intervention and comparison groups ranged from 13 and 19 years. The intervention group consisted of 498 adolescents who were enrolled for prenatal care at Queens Hospital Center's adolescent pregnancy program between 1982 and 1986. They received care with their newborns until their 20th birthday.

The comparison group consisted of 91 adolescents who received care at the Queens Hospital Center's adult prenatal clinic from 1980 to 1981, before the *Queens Hospital Center's Teenage Program* began. Individuals in the comparison group continued to receive care with their newborns at the hospital's adult family planning and pediatrics clinics through 1989, or until they reached age 20. The mean age for both groups at delivery was 17. Less than 5% of individuals in both the intervention and comparison groups were lost by the time of follow-up.

There was no difference between adolescents in the intervention and comparison groups with respect to age, socioeconomic status, completed years of school, prior poor obstetrical outcome, or employment status of head of household. The facilities used by the intervention and comparison teens are about 3 miles apart, both located in neighborhoods characterized by high drug use and crime, as well as a high incidence of adverse health outcomes such as low birth weight and neonatal death.

As in virtually every clinical study, there were missing observations for a small number of participants. In this study, 85% of the comparison group and 91% of the intervention group had a complete set of data. However, there were large differences between the two groups on the variances calculated for many outcome measures. The evaluator corrected for this result by employing a formula that decreased the degrees of freedom to produce meaningful results.

Evaluation Results

The results of the study indicate that the *Queens Hospital Center's Teenage Program* had significant positive effects on teen mothers and their children. Moreover, many of the outcomes improved with each successive year of program participation.

Utilization of Health Care Services

Patients in the program entered care earlier and averaged more prenatal visits per trimester of care than comparison patients. Over 75% of the intervention group regularly attended the program's mother–baby clinic, compared to 18% of the comparison group attending the hospital's regular adult gynecology and pediatrics clinics ($p < .0001$). Furthermore, with each subsequent year of the program, a greater proportion of the intervention group attended the program. By 1989, 87% of this group did so.

Maternal and Infant Health Outcomes

There were many positive effects measured for the health of both the mother and the child. Compared to their peers in the comparison group, program participants showed lower indices of maternal morbidity ($p < .0001$), including lower incidence of premature labor and deliveries closer to term, as well as less infection and anemia during labor. Babies born to program patients displayed significantly less distress and weighed more than the newborns of the comparison patients ($p < .001$). Subsequent maternal morbidity was lower among the intervention group (18% vs. 36%, $p < .0001$), as was subsequent infant morbidity ($p < .001$). Mothers in the intervention group were also more likely to breast-feed their infants for at least 3 months than were members of the comparison group (21% vs. 1%, $p < .0001$).

Educational and Occupational Status

Participation in the *Queens Hospital Center's Teenage Program* also had positive effects on the adolescent mothers' educational and occupational status. More teens in the intervention group attended school on a regular basis than did their comparison group peers (77% vs. 38%, $p < .0001$). Not only did school attendance increase with each year of the program, but by 1989, over 95% of the teens in the intervention group who had regularly attended school had graduated from high school, earned a high school GED, or were within 6 months of graduation from one of these programs. Those in the intervention group sought and maintained employment more often and more consistently than did teens in the comparison group (48% vs. 22%, $p < .0001$).

Contraceptive Use

Contraceptive use was more frequent among program participants (85% vs. 22%, $p < .0001$). By 1989, over 96% of program patients used some form of contraception on a regular basis. This also improved for each year of program participation.

Repeat Pregnancy

The repeat pregnancy rate was lower in the intervention group, with 9% becoming pregnant versus 70% in the comparison group. Pregnancy resolution differed between the groups as well. Among the teens who experienced a repeat pregnancy, 6% of the intervention group and 34% in the comparison group chose to terminate their pregnancies ($p < .0001$). For all years of the program, repeat pregnancy, whether ending in live birth or termination, declined significantly with each successive year ($p < .0001$).

Summary

The results of the evaluation indicate that a comprehensive service program can effectively increase contraceptive use and prevent repeat pregnancy among a group of adolescents considered to be at very high risk—teen mothers from urban, low-income neighborhoods. Teen mothers who participated in the *Queens Hospital Center's Teenage Program* also showed other positive outcomes compared to a group of teen mothers who received routine care. Among program participants, the researchers measured an increased use of recommended health care services by both the mothers and their children, from the prenatal period through the first few years of the child's life. Similarly, mothers and children demonstrated better health outcomes for the duration of the study. In addition, program participation had a positive effect on educational and vocational achievement, with participating teen mothers significantly more likely to attend high school and to seek and maintain employment.

Researchers attribute the success of the program to the concerted efforts to maintain contact with the patient for the duration of the program. The evidence that scores improved over the duration of the program indicates that over time, the program gained acceptance by teenagers in the targeted area.

NOTE

1. A full set of program materials, including pamphlets, service provider handbook, evaluation materials, and more, is available for purchase from Sociometrics at http://www.socio.com/pasha.htm.

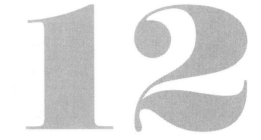

Family Growth Center: A Community-Based Social Support Program for Teen Mothers and Their Families

Diana Dull Akers and Janette Mince

Original Program Developers

Richard Solomon, MD
Department of Pediatrics and Communicable Diseases
University of Michigan
Ann Arbor, MI

Linda Solomon, MEd
Ann Arbor, MI

PROGRAM ABSTRACT

Summary

The *Family Growth Center* (*FGC*) is a comprehensive, community-based family support program designed to reduce repeat pregnancy and school dropout rates among adolescent mothers. The program was originally developed in the early

Family Growth Center was supported by contracts and grants from the Allegheny General Hospital, the Maternal and Child Health Bureau, the American Academy of Pediatrics, the Children's Trust Fund, the Heinz Endowment, the Commonwealth of Pennsylvania, and Gateway Health Plan.

143

1990s to address the escalating problem of adolescent pregnancy in several of Pittsburgh's urban neighborhoods, where approximately 20% of babies were born to adolescents. Teen mothers in the original study faced multiple socioeconomic risk factors in communities where resources to serve them were either lacking or inaccessible.

The goal of the *FGC* pilot project was to promote the health and development of teen mothers and their children using the family support center approach. This approach argues that family support programs promote the flow of resources and support to the new mother and her family so that she and her parents have the time, knowledge, and skills to carry out parenting responsibilities competently. The *FGC* program aims to provide teen mothers in high-risk neighborhoods (i.e., low socioeconomic status, high infant mortality, low educational status) with a comprehensive set of educational and support services, *offered within family and neighborhood contexts.* An informal philosophy of *FGC* is to meet families where they're at and lead them where they want to go.

FGC objectives included providing teen mothers with social support, teaching and helping them with parenting tasks, fostering the health and development of both teens and their babies, and promoting maternal education accomplishments, all through a network of support services that involves both family and neighborhood organizations. Young women are recruited for the program (by *FGC* perinatal counselors/coaches) when they arrive at participating hospital clinics for perinatal visits. Thereafter, they are offered the following intervention components, coordinated by *FGC* case managers:

1. *Perinatal coaching.* During the mother's stay in the hospital, staff help enhance her appreciation of the sensory and interactional abilities of her newborn, while collecting baseline clinical information for the program's contracted social workers (case managers).
2. *Home visits.* After the birth of the baby, social workers offer general social support, parenting advice, and crisis intervention to the new mother in her own home on a weekly or every-other-week basis. The case manager-to-adolescent family ratio is about 1:15 to 1:20, depending on demands/needs and staffing resources.
3. *Center-based services.* Once the baby reaches 6 months of age, the mother is offered services at a designated *FGC* location (a dwelling centrally located within the targeted high-risk neighborhood). Specific activities and services offered at the *FGC* included: bimonthly parenting classes, supervised day care, counseling, transportation and recreation, and advocacy and referral services (e.g., information on medical, educational, and housing options, etc.).

In the evaluated field study of the *FGC* pilot program, 88 adolescent mothers were consecutively recruited over 18 months from the perinatal clinic or newborn nursery at the project's university-affiliated hospital. Adolescents who were first-time mothers and lived in one of the high-risk neighborhoods served by the *FGC* were recruited into the intervention group. Young women who lived in other neighborhoods were recruited into a no-intervention control group. Of those who agreed to participate, 49 were assigned to the intervention condition, and 39 to the control; an attrition group was formed to follow the 25 young women (15 intervention, 10 control) who dropped out during the first 12 months.

Protocol assessment measures were diverse and included interview and questionnaire data (e.g., Adult-Adolescent Parenting Inventory, Beck Depression Inventory, Interpersonal Support Evaluation List, and the Family APGAR), videotaped interactional data between mother and child, and psychosocial and behavioral outcomes of mothers and their children.

Results

No significant demographic differences were found among the intervention, control, or attrition groups in terms of maternal age or socioeconomic status. Similarly, few differences existed between the groups on baseline psychosocial measures. However, the researchers did find that the attrition group reported significantly less depression and more family support, which may account for their dropping out of the study. The results of an evaluation of the program's impact from 1991–1994 emphasized a variety of outcomes; two will be emphasized here: (a) school dropout rates and (b) repeat pregnancy rates.

School Dropout Rates

Researchers found that the proportion of intervention group mothers who dropped out of school (3/34) was significantly less than the proportion of the control group (12/29) at the Time 1 analysis ($p = .002$), which was approximately 2 years following recruitment into the project. The same pattern held 1 year later (Time 2), when 2 out of the remaining 31 intervention group mothers and 8 out of the remaining 17 control group mothers had dropped out of school ($p = .019$).

Repeat Pregnancy Rates

Significant differences in the frequency of repeat pregnancies were observed between mothers in the intervention and control groups. At Time 1, 3 repeat pregnancies occurred in the intervention group (less than 10%) versus 11 repeat pregnancies (38%) in the control group ($p = .006$).

The Time 2 pattern was the same, with a total of 7 repeat pregnancies among intervention group mothers and 21 within the control group ($p = .020$). Moreover, during the 3-year follow-up period, several adolescent mothers in the control group experienced more than one subsequent pregnancy after the birth of their first child.

In sum, teen mothers participating in *FGC* had marked decreases in repeat pregnancy and school dropout rates compared to a control population.

Focus

☐ Primary pregnancy prevention ☑ Secondary pregnancy prevention ☐ STI/HIV/AIDS prevention

Original Site

☐ School based ☑ Community based ☐ Clinic based

Suitable for Use In

FGC recognizes the family and neighborhood as two of the most important contexts of a teenager's life. As such, implementation of the *FGC* program takes place across multiple locations, including the teen mother's home, the *FGC*, and the participating local hospital(s) in the geographic region. (The location of your *FGC* will need to be jointly determined by your staff and community.) Depending on the resources and community networking strategies of any given *FGC* program, additional program-related sites may be involved in *FGC* service offerings (e.g., neighborhood family preservation service centers, nutrition services centers, off-site day-care facilities, etc.).

Approach

- ■ ☐ Abstinence
- ■ ☑ Behavioral skills development

- ☑ Community outreach
- ☑ Contraceptive access
- ☑ Contraceptive education
- ☑ Life option enhancement
- ☑ Self-efficacy/self-esteem
- ☑ Sexuality/HIV/AIDS/STI education

Original Intervention Sample

Age, gender   The original sample included 34 intervention and 29 control first-time pregnant teen mothers and their infants.

Race/ethnicity   The original intervention sample population was 97% African American and 3% White. The original control sample population was 48% African American and 52% White.

Program Components

- ☑ Adult involvement
- ☑ Case management
- ☑ Group discussion
- ☑ Lectures (parenting education)
- ☑ Peer counseling/instruction
- ☐ Public service announcements
- ☑ Role play
- ☐ Video
- ☑ Other: Games, audiotape, recreational activities

Program Length

This is an intensive, multiyear intervention designed to begin when teens enter the prenatal units (or newborn nursery units) of their community hospital. Teens, infants, and families are visited by case managers in the teen's homes for the first 6-month "nesting period" and then introduced to the *FGC* array of services. Use of these services may continue for at least 2 years after teens' entry into the program; continuation of services beyond this period will be up to the discretion of your program.

Staffing Requirements/Training

Program director. The program director is a senior-level position responsible for the overall design, implementation, and administration of the *FGC* program. Considerable experience and advanced degrees in education, social work, child development, or other relevant fields are required. Your program may choose to have both a program director and program coordinator in your *FGC* program, or strictly a program director who performs both sets of responsibilities.

Program coordinator. The program coordinator is also a senior-level position in charge of administration, staffing, and daily implementation of the program. Considerable experience and advanced degrees in education, social work, and/or child development are preferred.

Case managers (also called "home visitors"). Case managers serve a critical role as the main point of contact between teens, their families, and the *FGC.* They are responsible for conducting in-home visits with teens and their infants. This position requires advanced credentials in social work (i.e., MSW or LCSW) or family and child development. Bilingual reading, writing, and speaking skills may be required for this position by your program.

Parent support coordinators. Parent support coordinators collaborate with senior staff to deliver services to teens and their families. Responsibilities include record keeping of service utilization, training and supervision of volunteer staff, parenting workshop design and delivery, and so forth. They also work with *FGC* advocates and case managers to coordinate services to clients. An MEd or MSW degree is preferred, as is experience working with teens, families, and/or young children. Bilingual reading, writing, and speaking skills are highly desirable.

Advocate(s). Advocates work at the *FGC* site and provide a variety of information and referral services (e.g., information on area housing, medical options, nutrition services, etc.). Staff training should be provided for this position by the *FGC*. A BA or BS in a related field and/or relevant experience working with teens, families, and/or young children is preferred for this position. Bilingual reading, writing, and speaking skills may also be desirable, depending on your milieu.

Transportation staff. One or more drivers should be hired to drive an *FGC* van or other vehicle that serves teen clients and their families, providing them transportation to the *FGC* site and select other community locations. Transportation staff should have a clean driving record and appropriate state class licenses for this position.

Recommended staff, depending on your program resources, include the following:

- *Short-term day-care assistants/social and recreational activity assistants:* College students seeking internship opportunities or early childhood education credits would be a good fit for these positions. Your program will determine the appropriate amount of training (e.g., number of ECE units, day-care experience, etc.) for these positions.
- *Child development specialist:* Depending on your program resources, you may opt to employ a child development specialist who could offer support and training services to program staff, as well as run the pilot program's developmental day-care program (a valuable but optional component of the *FGC* program).
- *Volunteer staff:* Like most community service programs, volunteers may be a highly desirable addition to your *FGC* staff. In addition to seeking volunteers from your general community (including local high schools and/or college students seeking internships), the *FGC* program is greatly aided by the volunteer role of *FGC* grandparents who help contact pregnant teens as they arrive at area hospitals' perinatal units.

We recommend an ongoing series of staff development and training workshops, educational seminars, and orientation meetings for all communities implementing an *FGC* program. The replication kit contains materials for one such staff development offering (an example of an infant mental health series), but most programs should offer a wider range of training and support services to staff.

BIBLIOGRAPHY

Dunst, C. J., & Trivette, C. M. (1994). Aims and principles of family support programs. In C. J. Dunst, C. M. Trivette, & A. G. Deal (Eds.), *Supporting and strengthening families: Vol. 1. Methods, strategies and practices.* Cambridge, MA: Brookline Books.

Dunst, C. J., Trivette, C. M., Starnes, A. L., Hamby, D. W., & Gordon, N. J. (1993). *Building and evaluating family support initiatives: A national study of programs for persons with developmental disabilities.* Baltimore, MD: Paul H. Brooks.

Helfer, R., Bristor, M., Cullen, B., & Wilson, A. (1987). The perinatal period: A window of opportunity for enhancing parent-infant communication: An approach to prevention. *Child Abuse & Neglect, 11,* 565–579.

Solomon, R., & Liefeld, C. P. (1998). Effectiveness of a family support center approach to adolescent mothers: Repeat pregnancy and school drop-out rates. *Family Relations, 47,* 139–144.

THE PROGRAM

Program Rationale and History

FGC was developed by Dr. Richard Solomon, a pediatrician and clinical associate professor of pediatrics, to address the escalating problem of teen pregnancy in several of Pittsburgh's North Side neighborhoods.[1] At the time of the program's inception in the early 1990s, approximately 20% of all babies born on Pittsburgh's North Side were born to teenagers. The average infant mortality rate in these neighborhoods ranged from 23 per thousand to 32 per thousand. The urban neighborhoods served by the *FGC* were—and remain—quite poor.

Since the development of this program, overall rates of teen pregnancy have declined by approximately 36% from the time of the peak in the early 1990s. However, there remains room for improvement.

Despite many socioeconomic risk factors, resources for teen mothers were either lacking or inaccessible before the establishment of the *FGC*. The goal of the *FGC* pilot program was to promote the health and development of first-time pregnant teenagers and their child(ren) using the family support center approach. The project aimed to provide teen mothers with a comprehensive set of services, including perinatal coaching, home visits, and an array of *FGC* center-based services, all within a family and neighborhood context. The core elements of these services were

1. early contact with the teen mothers, both perinatally and in the newborn nursery;
2. involvement of the nuclear and extended family;
3. issues-oriented parenting groups;
4. community involvement.

An extensive, 3-year longitudinal evaluation component was implemented to assess the effectiveness of the *FGC* pilot program (see below). Solomon's *FGC* pilot program was funded as a SPRANS grant (Special Projects of Regional and National Significance) from the Maternal and Child Health Bureau and the American Academy of Pediatrics. The pilot program also enjoyed significant local partnering from Pittsburgh foundations, businesses, and community social service agencies and associations.

Theoretical Framework

The *FGC* program utilized two models, or theoretical frameworks, for screening and serving at-risk children and their families.

Ecological Model. According to this model, family-system function and child factors mediate both macroscopic and microscopic influences that ultimately affect the child's self-esteem. The macroscopic domains include high-risk status (i.e., risk factors associated with poor outcomes), social support, life stress, and parenting skills. The more microscopic domains include the child's temperament, attachment (level of security), home stimulation, and the degree to which parents help the child accomplish his/her developmental tasks.

According to this model, the child's chances for an improved sense of self-esteem are increased to the extent that more of these domains are positively mediated by the family's function. Applying these principles, the original developers of the *FGC* attempted to address the ecological domains/factors affecting Pittsburgh teens and their families through a secondary prevention, community-based approach.

Family Support Model. *FGC* also drew heavily on the family support model. Other researchers have defined the family support model as efforts to empower families by focusing on building skills within the family to support overall family functioning, and enhance parenting in particular.

Pilot Project Goals

The overarching goals of *FGC* included lowering the rates of repeat pregnancy and lowering school dropout rates. Specific objectives of the project included

- providing teen mothers with an array of social support services;
- providing teen mothers and their children with access/transportation to needed services;
- enhancing parenting abilities for young parents;
- fostering the health and development of both teens and their babies;
- promoting maternal educational accomplishments and the general educational status of families.

Program Implementation

FGC was designed to begin when first-time pregnant teenagers entered their participating local hospital's prenatal unit and were contacted by *FGC* program staff (often a trained *FGC* grandmother or other trained volunteer). However, some teens made initial contact with the *FGC* program in their community later in their child's life (e.g., in the newborn nursery or during their child's first year, as the mother became aware of the program through various recruitment efforts). Thereafter, they were offered the following intervention components for a time period determined by the *FGC* site.

Perinatal Coaching

Parenting support began in the perinatal unit and continued in the newborn nursery, as *FGC* trained staff (and/or hospital staff) offered perinatal coaching to the new mothers. During the mother's stay in the hospital, *FGC* staff helped enhance her appreciation of the sensory and interactional abilities of her newborn while collecting baseline clinical information for the project case managers or other social work staff.

Case Management Through Home Visits

The case manager was the main point of contact between *FGC* and the teen mother in need of services. Case managers (trained social workers) offered general social support, parenting advice, and crisis intervention to the new mother in her own home on a weekly or biweekly visit schedule. Special efforts were made to establish trust and rapport with not only the teen mother and her child, but also the family support network that may have been involved in the teen parent's life. Case managers helped teens establish family goals (staying in school, being an effective parent, delaying second pregnancy, etc.) that guided the intervention. Case managers also helped introduce teen mothers and their families to the array of services offered through *FGC*, including parenting classes, workshops, grandmothers' groups, advocacy/referral services, and transportation services. Case managers managed 15–20 cases at any given time.

FGC Parenting Classes

The *FGC* parenting curriculum was designed to help teenagers enhance their abilities to care for themselves and their children. These classes helped teenagers meet not only the needs of their children, but also their own needs as adolescents. *FGC* parenting classes were provided in a nonjudgmental atmosphere, where trust, intimacy, and openness were encouraged. Goals included promoting the parent's understanding of bonding and attachment; increasing empathy in teenagers; increasing self-esteem and self-concept to enhance the quality of the parent–child relationship; helping parents learn alternatives to physical and verbal violence; and increasing teen parents' awareness of the developmental needs of their children.

FGC Advocacy Services

FGC advocates worked at the *FGC* centers to provide program clients and their families with a variety of information and referral services. Advocates worked both directly with clients (walk-ins, by phone) and indirectly on clients' behalf (e.g., seeking information from other social service agencies, etc.). Advocates also provided program monitoring support to *FGC* administration by tracking the attendance of teen parents and their families in *FGC* parenting classes, grandmothers' groups, and other social/recreational activities.

Transportation Services

Transportation was provided so that clients could attend *FGC* sponsored classes, workshops, and related events (in some cases, these services also extended to transportation to area hospitals, medical professionals, and social service agency appointments). Free transportation increased the utilization of services among *FGC* teen mothers and their children.

Grandmothers' Support Groups

Grandparents, particularly grandmothers, played a significant role in the life of teen parents and their children. In order to support grandmothers in the challenges of supporting their children and grandchildren, *FGC* offered a variety of Grandmothers' Support Group sessions. These were loosely structured discussions around general themes such as caregiver stress, grandparent's roles, setting boundaries, and so forth.

Social and Recreational Activities

FGC maintained a strong social/recreational component. The primary focus was on parent/child activities, but family and community members were involved as much as possible. Recreational activities included trips to parks, museums, educational centers, amusement parks, cultural events, and so forth.

Developmental Day Camps

FGC offered developmental day camps composed of small groups of children ranging in age from birth to 4 years. These camps focused on the developmental domains of language skills, fine and gross motor skills, cognitive growth, emotional support, and social interaction. Developmental day camps were designed to meet each child's needs and skills levels. (Whether your *FGC* program offers developmental day camps will be highly contingent on the funding and resources your program has to provide this therapeutic service.)

Optional Additional Program Components

Beyond the core program components noted above, your program may choose to offer one or more of the following optional program components: car seat programs, literacy programs, buddy projects, clothing distribution projects, playground/development projects, and so forth.

Staff Development Series

FGC recognized the importance of fostering personal and professional growth through staff development by offering a series of training workshops and support activities to program staff. These were individually tailored to each *FGC* setting, but included services that assisted staff in working closely with at-risk families, avoiding burnout, enhancing team-building strategies, and the like.

PROGRAM EVALUATION

The Original Evaluation

Design

Between 1992 and 1995, an extensive, longitudinal evaluation was conducted to assess the effectiveness of the original *FGC* pilot program in Pittsburgh, Pennsylvania. Eighty-eight teen mothers were recruited from the perinatal clinics and newborn nursery of Allegheny General Hospital in Pittsburgh (25 teens dropped out of the study in the first year, for a final sample size of 63). Subjects were assigned to either an intervention or control group, based upon neighborhood of residence.

A broad range of variables was measured in the evaluation, including social support, parenting attitudes, maternal depression, mother–infant attachment, parenting knowledge, life stresses, and personality types. Protocol assessment measures were diverse and included interview and questionnaire data, and psychosocial and behavioral outcomes of mothers and their children.

Specifically, the 3-year evaluation design[2] included data from baseline and repeated questionnaire measures collected from each teen mother at the time of delivery, in her home during the first 6 months of the infant's life, and at 12- and 18-month postnatal university lab visits.

Outcome Evaluation Questions

In conducting the evaluation of the *FGC* pilot program, evaluators attempted to answer a broad range of questions about the effects of the program on teen parents' mother–infant interaction and quality of attachment, and teen parents' knowledge of parenting concepts and principles. However, the two central questions for the evaluation were as follows:

1. Did teen parents who took part in the program show significantly lower repeat pregnancy rates—defined as the total number of subsequent second or third pregnancies of the initially first-time pregnant teenagers—than those in the control group?
2. Did teen parents who took part in the *FGC* program show significantly lower school dropout rates than those in the control group?

In addition, the *FGC* planners and funders investigated the broader process of setting up, managing, and maintaining a comprehensive, multiyear program serving teen parents and their children living in high-risk neighborhoods. The research design included mechanisms for monitoring satisfaction with *FGC* services, as well as intensity and types of services used.

Participant Recruitment

Eighty-eight adolescent mothers were consecutively recruited, over 18 months, from the perinatal clinic or newborn nursery at Allegheny General Hospital. First-time pregnant teenagers whose zip codes indicated residence in one of the high-risk neighborhoods served by *FGC* were assigned to the intervention group. Teen mothers living outside those identified zip codes, in other high-risk neighborhoods, were assigned to the control group.

Final Sample Composition

Of the adolescent mothers who were eligible and consented to participate in the study, 49 teens and babies were assigned to the intervention group and 39 teens and babies were assigned to the control group. In this original sample, there were 16 early adolescents (ages 13 to 15 years), 29 middle adolescents (ages 16 to 17 years), and 41 older adolescents (ages 18 to 19 years). Twenty-five teen mothers (28%), referred to as the attrition group, dropped out of the project in the first 12 months. Of the remaining 63 pairs of subjects, 34 were in the intervention group, and 29 were in the control group. Study groups were comparable at enrollment by age, marital status, socioeconomic status, social support, parenting attitudes, maternal depression, and life stresses.

Data Collection Procedures

Upon enrollment, baseline and repeated measures were obtained from the intervention and control groups. These included measures of parenting knowledge, family support, life stresses, depression, and other measures of importance to the *FGC* pilot project. Baseline measures were obtained by perinatal coaches in the newborn nursery and/or perinatal unit, and in the home by the program's parent support coordinator. Newborn nursery measures included the Maternal Social Support Index, the Family APGAR, and the Adolescent-Adult Parenting Index. Home-based measures included the Beck Depression Inventory and the Family Stress Checklist.

Parenting knowledge and parenting beliefs were also assessed at this time using the Adult Adolescent Parenting Index (AAPI).

Evaluation Results

Results of the evaluation demonstrated that *FGC* had a significant impact on two key criteria: repeat pregnancy rates and school dropout rates.

Repeat Pregnancy Rates

Significant differences in repeat pregnancy rates were observed between mothers in the intervention group and those in the control group. Four repeat pregnancies (nearly 12%) occurred in the intervention group, whereas 12 repeat pregnancies (41%) were reported in the control group at Time 1 ($t = 2.34$, $p = .02$). Time 2 analyses also demonstrated significant differences between groups, as a total of 7 repeat pregnancies occurred in the intervention group, compared to 21 repeat pregnancies in the control group ($t = 2.84$, $p = .02$).

School Dropout Rates

Similar successes were found in the area of school dropout rates. Results of a chi-square test revealed that the school dropout rate in the intervention group (<10%) was significantly less than the control group's dropout rate (nearly 42%) at the Time 1 analysis. The same test performed at Time 2 revealed that the intervention group had significantly fewer school dropouts (6%) compared to school dropouts in the control group (28%). Put another way, only 3 of 34 of the intervention group versus 12 of 29 in the control group dropped out of school; moreover, 4 mothers in the intervention group enrolled in community college, compared to 0 in the control group.

Summary

The evaluators reached the following conclusions about *FGC:*

- *The program appears to have been effective in reaching two of its central goals.* The pilot program helped teens delay second pregnancies and stay in school when compared to a control group of demographically similar adolescent mothers. Tracking of birth control status and assisting adolescents in obtaining birth control (e.g., Depo-Provera) were critical to success.

- *Early contact with adolescent mothers is critical.* The program established early contact with adolescent mothers in both the newborn nursery and perinatal lab. This contact enhanced trust and facilitated *FGC*'s transition into the family; it took an average of 6 months, and as long as 15 months, to establish a relationship.
- *Families appreciate and benefit from issue-oriented parenting groups/classes.* While much of the intervention, education, and social support was conducted on an individual basis through the efforts of case managers, parenting groups catalyzed change in a way that individual work could not. Parenting groups, defined by the age of the children, participated in classes covering issues such as development, feeding, sleeping, behavior, and so forth. These groups allowed teens to bond as a group through age-related interests and the needs of their child or infant.
- *Community involvement and networking are key components of a successful family support program.* Family support approaches promote a community-based orientation and emphasize the importance and value of diverse, comprehensive forms of social support for strengthening family functioning. *FGC* became a hub of activity, focused on recreational events, picnics, "kiddy camps," and museum visits, all of which brought people together, promoting a sense of "community" and diminishing isolation. Moreover, the assistance and collaborations with existing community service programs and agencies were critical to the sustainability of the program.
- *Teen parent support programs need to involve both the nuclear and extended family, particularly grandmothers.* Extended family can play a critical role in the lives of teen parents. Family support programs need to acknowledge the contributions and concerns of extended family. Initially, many grandmothers of the newborns in this study were highly suspicious of *FGC* staff's efforts to intervene and provide social support. *FGC* gradually earned the grandmothers' support and respect as staff worked to promote the teen mothers' and infants' development.
- *When needed services, advocacy, and counseling are offered in a comprehensive program, they are utilized by teen parents.* *FGC* staff in the pilot study focused much of their efforts on teaching teen mothers about family planning options and on keeping the mothers in school. Services were offered and used to help teen parents meet these goals. For example, *FGC* mothers and infants utilized the van services consistently, which contributed to their improved compliance with doctors' appointments and increased attendance at *FGC* parenting classes and functions. Self-reported satisfaction surveys revealed that teen mothers listed their case workers' care and availability, help with getting services, day care, and recreational programming as the most important aspects of their *FGC* experiences.

AWARDS AND RECOGNITION

FGC has been honored in the following ways:

- 1992: Site visit from Senator Jay Rockefeller's Commission on Families: Model Programs
- 1993: "Medical Program of the Year" 1993, Health Education Center Award, Pittsburgh

- 1994: "Citation for Commendable Service: Family Growth Center Pilot Project," Healthy Tomorrows Partnership for Children, Maternal and Child Health Bureau
- 1995: University of Pittsburgh/Allegheny County Department of Health and Human Services, "Progress Toward Change" award

FGC IN THE COMMUNITY TODAY

In the past 3 years, *FGC* has been implemented in Los Angeles, California, and in Taos, New Mexico.

NOTES

1. A full set of program materials, including facilitator's manual, curricular guidelines, staff orientation manual, case manager log, evaluation materials, and more, is available for purchase from Sociometrics at http://www.socio.com/pasha.htm.
2. Questionnaire, survey, and videotaped data were compiled at 0, 12, 18, and 24 months postnatally for mother and child. Data reflecting repeat pregnancy and school status (i.e., attendance, completion, or dropout) was compiled three times during the course of the project: Time 0 (time of entry), Time 1 (approximately 2 years after initial recruitment began), and Time 2 (approximately 3 years after initial recruitment began).

PART III

STI/HIV/AIDS

Prevention

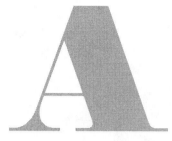

Programs Designed for Youths in Middle School or Junior High School

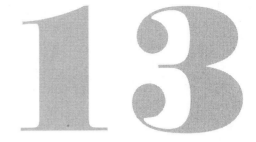

Aban Aya Youth Project: Preventing High-Risk Behaviors Among African American Youths in Grades 5–8

Tabitha A. Benner

Original Program Developers and Evaluators

Brian R. Flay, DPhil

Sally Graumlich, EdD, CHES

The Aban Aya Team
    Institute for Health Research and Policy
    University of Illinois
    Chicago, IL

PROGRAM ABSTRACT

Summary

The *Aban Aya Youth Project (Aban Aya)* is an Afrocentric social development curriculum taught over a 4-year period, beginning in the 5th grade. The number of lessons varies each year. This curriculum encourages abstinence, protection from unsafe sex, and avoidance of drugs and alcohol. The name of the intervention is drawn from two words in the Akan (Ghanaian) language: *Aban* (fence) signifies double/social protection; *Aya* (the unfurling fern) signifies self-determination. The purpose of this intervention is to promote abstinence from sex and to teach students how to avoid drugs and alcohol, and how to resolve conflicts nonviolently.

The *Aban Aya Youth Project* was supported by grants from the National Institute on Drug Abuse (R01DA11019) and the National Institute for Child Health and Development (U01HD30078).

Aban Aya was developed to address multiple "problem behaviors," such as violence, substance abuse, delinquency, and sexual activity, simultaneously in a long-term intervention specifically for African American youths in grades 5–8. The longitudinal evaluation of the program involved 12 schools in the metropolitan Chicago area between 1994 and 1998.

At baseline, 1,153 5th graders participated in the pencil-and-paper assessment. Of the group that completed the baseline survey, 668 were still in attendance in the participating schools at the conclusion of the program.

The group was fairly evenly divided between males and females; the average age was 10.8 years. All participants were African American. Follow-up assessments were conducted at the conclusion of grades 5 through 8 for all students in the test schools with parental consent at the time of assessment. Students who transferred out of the test schools were not followed for the purposes of the study.

Participating schools were assigned to one of three conditions using a randomized block design. The first experimental condition, the social development curriculum (SDC) included 16–21 classroom-based lessons each year. The second experimental condition, the school/community intervention (SCI), included SDC plus a parent/community element. The control condition, health enhancement curriculum (HEC), was equal to SDC in intensity, and focused on general health, nutrition, and physical activity.

At study conclusion, there were no significant intervention effects for girls. For boys, however, the SDC significantly reduced the rate of increase in violent behavior (by 35% compared with HEC), provoking behavior (41%), school delinquency (31%), drug use (32%), and recent sexual intercourse (44%). SDC also improved the rate of increase in condom use (95%) as compared to HEC.

Focus

☑ Primary pregnancy prevention   ☐ Secondary pregnancy prevention   ☑ STI/HIV/AIDS prevention

Original Site

☑ School based   ☐ Community based   ☐ Clinic based

Suitable for Use in

Aban Aya is suitable for use in middle schools, grades 5–8. Owing to the number of sessions and the cumulative nature of the learning, the intervention is not recommended for use outside the classroom.

Approach

- ☑ Abstinence
- ☑ Behavioral skills development
- ☐ Community outreach
- ☐ Contraceptive access
- ☑ Contraceptive education
- ☐ Life option enhancement
- ☑ Self-efficacy/self-esteem
- ☑ Sexuality/HIV/AIDS/STI education

Original Intervention Sample

Age, gender   The baseline sample was 49.5% male and averaged 10.8 years at the beginning of 5th grade.

Race/ethnicity   All participants were African American.

Program Components

- ☑ Adult involvement
- ☐ Case management
- ☑ Group discussion
- ☑ Lectures
- ☐ Peer counseling/instruction
- ☑ Public service announcements
- ☑ Role play
- ☑ Video
- ☑ Other: Homework, some with parental participation

Program Length

The SDC, discussed later in the chapter, is classroom based and involves 16–21 lessons each year in grades 5–8. The lessons are designed to be taught in a typical classroom period and last approximately 40–45 minutes each. The learning is cumulative.

Staffing Requirements/Training

In the original implementation, health educators delivered the curriculum in social studies class. In order to ensure fidelity of implementation, two training sessions were held before each lesson during which health educators role-played the activities and senior project staff provided feedback. In addition, each year, the regular classroom teachers received a 4-hour workshop to provide an overview of program content and philosophy.

There is no formal training program required for implementing *Aban Aya*. However, training is an essential component in prevention programs. Often, instructors find prevention methods differ from teaching methods they normally use. Hence, training can improve the instructors' understanding of concepts that drive prevention programs and increase their competence in prevention strategies. Also, training helps to increase the fidelity of implementation of your program and increase the likelihood that the program will become sustained in your school or agency as the instructors become more comfortable and supportive of the program.

BIBLIOGRAPHY

Flay, B. R., Graumlich, S., Segawa, E., Burns, J. L., & Holliday, M. Y. (2004). Effects of 2 prevention programs on high-risk behaviors among African American youth. *Archives of Pediatric & Adolescent Medicine, 158*(4), 377–384.

Related References by the Developers of *Aban Aya*

Fagen, M. C., & Flay, B. R. (2006). Sustaining a school-based prevention program: Results from the Aban Aya sustainability project. *Health Education & Behavior,* doi:10.1177/1090198106291376.
Ngwe, J. E., Liu, L. C., Flay, B. R., Segawa, E., & Aban Aya Team. (2004). Violence prevention among African American adolescent males. *American Journal of Health Behavior, 28*(Suppl. 1), 24–37.
Segawa, E., Ngwe, J. E., Li, Y., & Flay, B. R. (2005). Evaluation of the effects of the Aban Aya Youth Project in reducing violence among African American adolescent males using latent class growth mixture modeling techniques. *Evaluation Review, 29*(2), 128–148.

THE PROGRAM

Program Rationale and History

Unsafe sex, substance abuse, and violence have been, and continue to be, significant challenges facing urban African American youths.[1] Compared to youths of other ethnicities at the time of this study, African American youths were more likely to initiate sexual intercourse at an earlier age and had higher lifetime rates of sexual intercourse and more sexual partners in their lifetimes, with resulting higher rates of pregnancy and HIV infection. Urban youths also had unrealistic ideas about what "everybody is doing," in addition to getting mixed messages about how to solve their problems.

Aban Aya was designed to teach skills in a developmentally appropriate environment and in a culturally sensitive manner to lessen behavioral risks. The purpose of this intervention was to promote abstinence from sexual intercourse and to teach students how to prevent sexually transmitted infections (STIs), avoid drugs and alcohol, and resolve conflicts in a nonviolent manner. *Aban Aya* also taught knowledge, skills, and information needed to promote African American pride, a positive sense of self, and how to set positive goals.

Aban Aya was taught over a 4-year period, beginning in 5th grade. The number of lessons varied from year to year until the program's conclusion in 8th grade. The intervention was classroom based and designed to teach cognitive-behavioral skills to strengthen a broad range of protective behaviors, including self-esteem, problem solving, assertive communication, decision making, conflict resolution, violence prevention, peer-pressure resistance, and safe sex. It also addressed delinquency, substance abuse, interpersonal relationships, and provocative behaviors.

In the original implementation, *Aban Aya* was taught during the period normally reserved for social studies in an effort to ensure maximum attendance. Each lesson was designed to be taught in 40–45 minutes.

Theoretical Framework

The conceptual framework of *Aban Aya* was derived from theories of behavior change to focus the intervention on risk and on protective factors and skills related to the target behaviors.

The intervention also incorporated Nguzo Saba principles, which promoted African American cultural values, such as unity, self-determination, and responsibility; culturally-based teaching methods (storytelling and proverbs); and African and African American history and literature.

Program Overview

Over the course of the 4-year program, the curriculum provided accurate information about risky behaviors (unsafe sex, violence, alcohol, and drug use), changed student perceptions of acceptable behavior, and altered dangerous norms (weapon carrying, drug trafficking, sexual activity, fighting, etc.). The curriculum emphasized spiral learning, with review and reinforcements following the end of the lessons. These reviews took place once or twice a month for the duration of the school year. The curriculum also included such social skills as decision making, conflict resolution, and negotiation and refusal skills. Major concepts of the curriculum were integrated using the "Check Yourself" problem-solving model:

Stop

Calm down.

Understand the situation.

Think

What are my choices?

What are the consequences of each choice?

Act

Try the best choice.

Review.

Target Behaviors and Content

From grade 5 onward, the curriculum addressed violence, school delinquency, and substance abuse. In grade 6, the curriculum expanded to include provoking behaviors, condom use, and recent sexual intercourse.

The content in *Aban Aya* was broken down into three primary categories, as delineated in Table 13.1. These concepts and skills were presented and revisited throughout the 4 years of the intervention in varying levels of intensity, and with attention to the increasing levels of intellectual and social development of the students.

13.1 | Three Primary Categories of Aban Aya

Skills
- Anger management
- Communication
- Negotiation
- Conflict resolution
- Social networking
- Decision making
- Problem solving
- Goal setting
- Refusal skills
- Stress management

Sense of self and purpose
- Empathy
- Career planning
- Feelings
- Personal strengths
- Cultural pride
- Mentors
- Communalism

Culture, values, and history
- Influence of racism and stereotypes on self and community
- African American heritage
- Ethnic values (Nguzo Saba)
- Normative beliefs
- Environmental influences
- Role models

In all four grades, the *Aban Aya* curriculum utilized a variety of teaching strategies and tools. They included those listed below.

Cooperative Learning Strategies. *Aban Aya* used small learning groups to encourage support, cooperation, and respect among the students. These groups, called Ujima learning groups, were built around the African proverb, "A single bracelet does not jingle." (*Ujima* is the Swahili term for "collective work.") Ujima learning groups taught young people the importance of "working together to get things done." Ujima groups also provided students with an opportunity to practice being more supportive of one another.

Special Assignments. Special assignments (completed outside the classroom) were designed to reinforce information and skills students learned in class, and to provide an opportunity for students and parents to discuss topics openly.

Parent Special Assignments. Several special assignments were identified in the curriculum as parent interactive assignments. The assignments were designed to encourage parent–child interaction. Parents signed these assignments as evidence of their participation.

Small-Group Discussions. Students expressed their thoughts and ideas in large- and small-group discussions. The use of group discussions enabled students to feel that their opinions and thoughts were valuable.

Proverbs. *Aban Aya* used African proverbs and African American quotes to introduce each lesson. Students were encouraged to explain or give examples of the quotes or proverbs in their own words. Each proverb was related to the lesson in which it was introduced.

Role Playing. Role playing was used to reinforce skills taught in *Aban Aya*. Role-play situations were included in many of the lessons. By role playing, each student was encouraged to experience situations and/or give feedback on skills taught in *Aban Aya*.

Storytelling. Storytelling was used to model skills taught in the curriculum. It also allowed students to use their imagination to come up with alternatives to decisions that were made in the story.

Games and Other Activities. *Aban Aya* developed several age-appropriate learning games specifically designed to increase retention or review and reinforce skills and information learned previously.

Anonymous Question Box. *Aban Aya* gave students the opportunity to ask questions about African American history, violence, AIDS, sexuality, and other related topics without fear of being identified. Students were instructed to write down their questions and place them in a box in the classroom.

Program Implementation

Some activities required a small amount of preparation in advance (for example when the educator displayed his/her goal shield to the class). Other activities required coordination with school officials (such as the presentation of student-created public service announcements over the school's public address system).

There was no formal training program for *Aban Aya* educators. However, college-trained health educators were engaged to deliver the intervention in the original implementation, often with the help of the classroom teacher.

EVALUATING THE PROGRAM

The Original Evaluation

Study Design

Aban Aya was implemented in a sample of 12 high-risk, poor, predominantly African American schools in the Chicago area between 1994 and 1998. Inclusion criteria for the participating schools included enrollment of 80% African American and fewer than 10% Hispanic students; grades K–8 (or through 6 if all students progressed to a single middle school or junior high); enrollment greater than 500, not a magnet or charter school; and not on academic probation.

Eligible schools (n = 155 inner-city and near-suburban schools) were stratified into quartiles of risk, based on a combined risk proxy score. The proxies of risk included attendance and truancy, mobility, family income, standardized test scores, and report card data. Using a randomized block design, researchers then assigned to each of the three conditions (health education control, social development curriculum, and school/community; this discussion focuses on the comparison of the first two conditions) two inner-city schools from the middle of the highest risk quartile, one inner-city school from the middle of the second risk quartile, and one suburban school. Schools signed an agreement to participate in the 4-year study and agreed not to participate in any other prevention initiative. Schools were paid $250 for each participating classroom, for up to four per year.

Students (n = 1,153) completed surveys in classrooms at the beginning and end of 5th grade, and at the end of each subsequent year. Survey questions were modified for a 4th grade reading level and cultural sensitivity through feedback from focus groups and pilot testing. To ensure the completion of the surveys, *Aban Aya* staff (rather than classroom teachers or the health educators assigned to that class) administered the instrument, reading the questions aloud. Researchers used identification numbers rather than names for tracking; all responses were confidential.

Study Population

Participants (n = 1,153) were 5th graders in 12 Chicago area schools in the 1994–1995 school year, including students who transferred in, but excluding those who transferred out. Owing to an annual turnover rate of approximately 20%, only 668 of the 1,153 students who completed a baseline survey at the beginning of grade 5 remained at the end of grade 8. The final sample was 49.5% male, with an average age of 10.8 years (SD = 0.6) at the beginning of 5th grade. Approximately 77% were receiving federally subsidized school lunches, and 47% lived in two-parent households.

Parents were informed of the study and given the option to deny consent for their child to participate. Fewer than 1% of parents denied consent during grades 5–7, and 1.7% did so in grade 8. At baseline, 93.2% of students with parental consent completed the survey. Noncompletions were due primarily to absenteeism.

The Evaluation

Starting in the spring of grade 5, three versions of the survey were randomly assigned to classrooms at each wave of data collection. The core section, answered by all students, included items assessing demographics and all of the behavioral outcomes except school delinquency. Measures were based on instruments previously used with inner-city populations. Pilot testing and feedback from focus groups ensured the cultural sensitivity of the surveys.

13.2 | Program Effects for Boys

MEASURE	RELATIVE REDUCTION*	P	EFFECT SIZE
Violence	35%	.05	0.31
Provoking behavior	41%	.10	0.29
School delinquency	31%	.06	0.29
Substance use	32%	.05	0.42
Recent sexual intercourse	44%	.08	0.44
Condom use	95%*	.28	0.38
Combined model	51%	.002	0.052

* Improvement rather than reduction, for condom use.

Outcomes were defined as an increase in safer sex and abstinence, as well as decreases in violence, provoking behavior (added in 6th grade), and substance use. Violence, school delinquency, and substance use were measured from grade 5 onward. Provoking behaviors, recent sexual intercourse, and condom use were added to the survey starting in grade 6.

Evaluation Results

Overall, there were no significant program effects for girls. When compared to their control-group counterparts, boys reported movement in the desired direction on all outcome measures.

At baseline, boys engaged in higher levels of behaviors than girls for all behaviors ($p < .001$) except provoking ($p = 0.17$). The prevalence of all behaviors increased over time across gender and condition. The increase in negative behaviors from 5th grade to 8th grade was less for boys in the intervention versus boys in the control groups (violence by 35%, provoking behavior by 41%, school delinquency by 31%, drug use by 32%, and recent sexual intercourse by 44%). The relative improvement rate for condom use was 95%.

Table 13.2 highlights relative reductions, p values, and effect sizes for boys in the intervention as compared to boys in the control group.

Summary

The *Aban Aya* team developed a culturally sensitive intervention for delivery in the classroom for inner-city African American youths in grades 5–8. The intervention targeted multiple risky behaviors. Results of the randomized controlled trial demonstrated that a single curriculum or intervention could have large effects on multiple behaviors, at least for boys.

According to the research team, the evaluation of *Aban Aya* supported evidence that the dominant prevention strategies worked better for boys than for girls, suggesting an area for future research.

NOTE

1. A full set of program materials, including facilitator's manual, student handbook, poster, evaluation materials, and more, is available for purchase from Sociometrics at http://www.socio.com/pasha.htm.

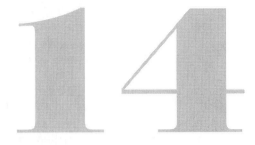

Youth AIDS Prevention Project (YAPP): An Adolescent STI/HIV/AIDS Prevention Program for Junior High School Youths

J. Barry Gurdin, Starr Niego, and Janette Mince

Original Program Developers and Evaluators

Susan R. Levy, PhD
Brian R. Flay, DPhil
Arden Handler, DrPH
Jamila Rashid, MPH
Kyle Weeks, MA
  Prevention Research Center
  University of Illinois at Chicago
  Chicago, IL

PROGRAM ABSTRACT

Summary

Originally designed for high-risk youths, including African Americans, the *Youth AIDS Prevention Project (YAPP)* aims to prevent sexually transmitted infections

_____

Youth AIDS Prevention Project was supported by a grant from the National Institute of Mental Health (MH 45470).

(STIs), HIV/AIDS, and substance abuse among junior high school students. Guiding the program is social cognitive theory, which targets teens' knowledge, attitudes, self-efficacy, intentions, and behaviors regarding high-risk activities. The intervention includes 10 sessions for 7th-grade students, delivered in regularly scheduled health or science classes, and a five-part booster session offered 1 year later, when the teens have entered 8th grade. Classes cover transmission and prevention of STIs and HIV/AIDS, the importance of using condoms for those who choose to have sex, and the development of decision-making and resistance/negotiation skills. In addition to lectures and class discussions, active learning is emphasized, with opportunities for students to participate in small-group exercises and role plays. There are also homework activities and opportunities for parental involvement.

A field study of the intervention was conducted in 15 high-risk school districts in Chicago. Research focused on the group of students who first became sexually active during the study period. Following the booster session, these students reported less-frequent sexual intercourse and greater use of condoms with spermicidal foam or lubricant in the past 30 days; they also expressed greater intention to use condoms with foam in the future.

Focus

☐ Primary pregnancy prevention   ☐ Secondary pregnancy prevention   ☑ STI/HIV/AIDS prevention

Original Site

☑ School based   ☐ Community based   ☐ Clinic based

Suitable for Use In

This intervention is most suitable for 7th-grade classrooms, with the 5-lesson booster program offered in 8th-grade classrooms 1 year later. The intervention could also be used in community-based organizations serving teens between the ages of 12 and 14 years.

Approach

- ☑ Abstinence
- ☑ Behavioral skills development
- ☐ Community outreach
- ☐ Contraceptive access
- ☑ Contraceptive education
- ☐ Life option enhancement
- ☑ Self-efficacy/self-esteem
- ☑ Sexuality/HIV/STI education

Original Intervention Sample

Age, gender   The original group of program participants included 1,459 7th-grade students, of whom 48% were male. The booster program for 8th-grade students involved 1,001 teens.

Race/ethnicity   Approximately 58% African American, 21% White, 16% Hispanic, 5% Other.

Program Components

- ☑ Adult involvement
- ☐ Case management

- ☑ Group discussion
- ☑ Lectures
- ☐ Peer counseling/instruction
- ☐ Public service announcements
- ☑ Role play
- ☑ Video
- ☐ Other

Program Length

During the first year of the program, 10 class sessions are offered, one per day over a 2-week period. A 1-week, 5-session booster program should be held 1 year later. The lessons are designed to last approximately 40–45 minutes.

Staffing Requirements/Training

Ideally, a professional, master's-level health educator who has received special training in HIV/AIDS leads the program; one instructor is required per class session. However, *YAPP* was designed for regular classroom teachers (with modest training) to deliver *YAPP* to their classes. The additional training is recommended to familiarize teachers with the *YAPP* curriculum.

BIBLIOGRAPHY

Levy, S. R., Handler, A., Weeks, K., Lampman, C., Flay, B. R., & Rashid, J. (1994). Adolescent risk for HIV as viewed by youth and their parents. *Family and Community Health, 17*(1), 30–41.

Levy, S. R., Perhats, C., Weeks, K., Handler, A. S., Zhu, C., & Flay, B. R. (1995). Impact of a school-based AIDS prevention program on risk and protective behavior for newly sexually active students. *Journal of School Health, 65*(4), 145–151.

Levy, S. R., Weeks, K., Handler, A., Perhats, C., Franck, J. A., Hedeker, D., et al. (1995). A longitudinal comparison of the AIDS-related attitudes and knowledge of parents and their children. *Family Planning Perspectives, 27*(1), 4–10, 17.

Weeks, K., Levy, S. R., Gordon, A. K., Handler, A., Perhats, C., & Flay, B. R. (1997). Does parental involvement make a difference? The impact of parent-interactive activities on students in a school-based AIDS prevention program. *AIDS Education and Prevention, 9*(Suppl. 1), 90–106.

Weeks, K., Levy, S. R., Zhu, C., Perhats, C., Handler, A., & Flay, B. R. (1995). Impact of a school-based AIDS prevention program on young adolescents' self-efficacy skills. *Health Education Research, 10*(3), 329–344.

Related References by the Developers of *YAPP*

Levy, S. R., Anderson, E. E., Issel, L. M., Willis, M. A., Dancy, B. L., Jacobson, K.M., et al. (2004). Using multilevel, multisource needs assessment data for planning community interventions. *Health Promotion Practice, 5*(1), 59–68.

Levy, S. R., Baldyga, W., & Jurkowski, J. M. (2003). Developing community health promotion interventions: Selecting partners and fostering collaboration. *Health Promotion Practice, 4*(3), 314–322.

THE PROGRAM

Program Rationale and History

YAPP integrated human sexuality, drug, STI/HIV/AIDS, and risk reduction education for junior high school students.[1] Based on social cognitive theory, the curriculum covered the transmission and prevention of STIs, HIV/AIDS, the use of condoms, pregnancy, and particularly, the development of decision-making and resistance/negotiation skills. The program was divided into 10 lessons for 7th-grade students and a 5-lesson booster program for 8th graders. Additionally, several of the homework activities involved parents, and an optional adults-only education session was also held.

Between 1991 and 1993, a field test of the program was conducted with approximately 2,400 students in 15 school districts throughout metropolitan Chicago. Compared to their peers in other areas of the city, students in the participating districts were considered to be at greatest risk for HIV infection. All program activities were originally designed to appeal to high-risk youths, including African Americans, who comprised more than half of the participating teens.

Theoretical Framework

YAPP was guided by social cognitive theory (previously referred to as social learning theory).

Social cognitive theory is based on the idea that knowledge alone is insufficient to produce behavioral change. Instead, the theory points toward four components that must be included in any effective prevention program. The first component is informational, designed to increase knowledge. The second component targets the development of the social and self-regulative skills that a teen needs to translate knowledge into effective behavior. The third component focuses on developing skills and self-efficacy by providing opportunities for practice and corrective feedback in applying skills in high-risk situations. Finally, the fourth component is designed to strengthen the social supports available to help youths carry out the desired changes.

YAPP contained all four of these necessary components. First, the curriculum provided state-of-the-art HIV/AIDS-related information. Second, the program incorporated activities that helped students build their resistance and negotiation skills. Third, role-play exercises provided teens with the opportunity to practice their newly acquired skills. Fourth, *YAPP* created social supports for teens by involving peers, parents, and the entire school in the program.

Program Objectives

As an STI/HIV/AIDS risk-reduction program, the *YAPP* was designed to help teens

1. avoid high-risk behaviors (e.g., drug use, sexual intercourse before one is psychologically ready);
2. increase their AIDS-related knowledge, attitudes, self-efficacy, and intentions;
3. learn protective (e.g., correctly using condoms with spermicides) and avoidance (e.g., avoiding risky situations) behaviors as a result of their improved knowledge, skills, and self-efficacy.

Program Schedule

Description of Program Sessions

The following five components were used throughout *YAPP* classes to reinforce program lessons:

- *Anonymous question box:* Students were given the opportunity to ask any questions they had about STI/HIV/AIDS, sexuality, and other related topics without fear of being identified.
- *Brainstorming:* This technique was used during group discussions to allow students to feel that all opinions and thoughts were valued.
- *Role playing:* Role-play activities encouraged *YAPP* participants to experience real-life situations and practice new skills.
- *Parent interactive homework:* Several homework activities required that students and their parents work together to apply the information and skills taught in the program.

- *Parent workshop:* This optional activity familiarized parents with the curriculum and increased adults' awareness of STI/HIV/AIDS and risky behaviors affecting teens. Although the program developers had originally planned a more extensive series of adult activities to accompany the parent workshop, they found that adults were unwilling or unable to take part.

A brief overview of the sessions appears below.

7th-Grade Curriculum. *Class 1: Decision Making.* At the start of this class, the teacher explained the ground rules that would govern group discussions and invited students to submit any questions they had throughout the program to the anonymous question box. The class then considered the factors that influenced teens' decision making (e.g., family, friends, boy/girlfriend, teachers, media, religion, school). Through role-play exercises, students were introduced to the SAFER method of decision making:

S = *Study* the problem and clarify the decision to be made.

A = List the *alternatives* or choices you have.

F = *Find* the best alternative/choice for you by considering the advantages and disadvantages of each one.

E = *Execute* the plan (do it!).

R = *Review* and consider the outcome of your decision.

For homework, students considered two situations in which they had to make decisions about risk-taking behavior and explained their decision-making process for each. In addition, students and their parents or guardians completed a survey assessing their patterns of communication.

Class 2: Resistance/Negotiation Skills. At the start of this session, the homework was reviewed and questions from the anonymous question box were answered. (These activities occurred at the start of all subsequent lessons.) This class was designed to help teens recognize that the importance of their decisions would vary. Working in small groups, students brainstormed to create a list of decisions and decided whether each was a big or small decision. Then the teacher introduced the six S's—resistance/negotiation skills that could guide one in reaching good decisions:

S = *Stop,* look, and listen.

S = *Say* "no."

S = *State* your response repeatedly, and in different ways.

S = *Suggest* other things to do.

S = *Say* "good-bye."

S = *Stay* away.

Several role-play exercises were used to review the SAFER method of decision making and practice the six S's of resistance/negotiation skills.

Class 3: A is for AIDS. This session provided students with basic factual information about HIV and AIDS, including transmission, infection, and prevention. Students learned that their risk of exposure to the HIV virus would increase as they participated in risky behaviors. The class then watched and discussed the video *HIV and AIDS: Staying Safe,* which introduced facts about HIV and AIDS.

Class 4: Prevention (Abstinence and Safer Sex). During the first part of the class, abstinence was discussed as the only 100% certain method for STI/HIV/AIDS prevention. Together, the group explored alternative ways to express love and romantic feelings apart from sexual intercourse. Then the focus shifted to issues concerning sexuality, methods of contraception, pregnancy, and transmission of STI/HIV/AIDS. At the end of the period, the instructor led a demonstration of the proper way to use condoms and spermicidal foam or lubricant.

Class 5: Whose Decision Is It? Students identified and analyzed the ways various media try to influence their decision making. They looked not only at sexual messages, but also at the ways they were persuaded to buy a product or wear a particular style of clothing.

Class 6: Teen AIDS. A group exercise and the video *AIDS/STIs* showed students how quickly AIDS could be transmitted from person to person.

Class 7: Prevention (Be Safe—Don't Do Drugs). During this lesson, students examined the reasons why adolescents used drugs and the consequences that could result. A series of role-play activities reinforced participants' decision-making and resistance/negotiation skills in real-life situations concerning drugs.

Class 8: STI: Stop That Infection. This lesson provided students with general information about STIs, including transmission and prevention. The group applied the SAFER decision-making method and the six S's of resistance/negotiation skills in role-play activities.

Class 9: Drugs and STIs. Focusing on ways to prevent STIs, the class again used the SAFER decision-making method and the six S's of resistance/negotiation skills in a series of role-play activities. In another activity called "Give me your best jive/line," students learned to negotiate safer sex practices and considered delaying sexual intercourse until they were emotionally and mentally ready. For homework, students wrote a newsletter column for a school newspaper giving advice about risk-taking choices and decisions.

Class 10: Program Review. The final session of the 7th-grade program helped students integrate the information and skills they had learned concerning STI/HIV/AIDS, drugs, and human sexuality. In a group activity, students divided into two teams and answered questions about each of the topics covered in the curriculum.

Optional Parent Workshop. A separate 60- to 90-minute session was held for parents and guardians of 7th-grade students participating in the *YAPP* program. The session introduced parents to the curriculum, discussed current trends in sexual activity and drug use among teens, and encouraged parents to talk about sexuality and risk behaviors with their children. The video *A is for AIDS* was also presented to parents.

8th-Grade Curriculum. *Lesson 1: Making Decisions.* During the first lesson of the 8th-grade booster program, students reviewed the ground rules that would govern each of the class discussions. They were invited to submit any questions they had to the anonymous question box. A poster reviewed the SAFER decision-making method and the six S's of resistance/negotiation skills. These concepts were reinforced through role-play activities concerning pressure to have sex and engage in risky behaviors. Students created their own skits. For homework, students wrote their autobiographies, imagining themselves at a point 5 years in the future.

Lesson 2: Sexuality and STIs (HIV/AIDS). After answering students' questions from the anonymous question box, the instructor summarized key information, including myths and facts about transmission, prevention, and infection of HIV/AIDS and other STIs. The group then divided into two- to four-person teams to review case studies concerning risks for exposure to HIV/AIDS. For each case, the teams answered a series of questions about the decisions the characters would have to make.

Lesson 3: Relationships, Abstinence, and Safer Sex. This lesson aimed to help students understand and manage healthy relationships. The instructor asked students to brainstorm about their various relationships and the reasons for beginning them. The risks of gang involvement were also discussed. In the second part of the class, the instructor led a demonstration of the correct way to use condoms with spermicidal foam/lubricant.

Lesson 4: Preventing Risky Behaviors. In this lesson, the SAFER method of decision making and the six *S*'s of negotiation/resistance skills were reinforced again through several role plays involving sexuality and drugs. Key facts about drugs and STIs were also reviewed by the class.

Lesson 5: Ready for the Future. The final lesson was designed to integrate all of the *YAPP* lessons concerning HIV/AIDS, other STIs, drugs, and human sexuality. Students reconsidered the autobiographies they had written earlier in the program, focusing on factors that might interrupt their plans. Leading a group discussion on the transition to high school, the instructor asked students to think about the new groups of people they would meet and the situations and pressures they would encounter. Teens were reminded to apply the decision-making and resistance/ negotiation skills they had practiced throughout the program.

Program Implementation

During the original field study, a 1-day training session was held to prepare instructors to implement the curriculum. The instructors were all master's-level health educators who also attended a seminar series to remain informed about current developments in the field of HIV/AIDS.

Establishing Ground Rules

Ground rules for group discussions were established at the start of the first 7th-grade lesson and again at the start of the 8th-grade booster program. This helped create an atmosphere of trust and comfort in which students felt free to discuss issues concerning sexuality, drugs, and STIs. The Ground Rules poster was hung in a conspicuous spot in the classroom and on it were listed each of the following rules:

- Everyone has a right to his/her own opinion and feelings.
- Each individual deserves respect and privacy.
- No one is allowed to "put down" or to laugh at another's ideas or opinions.
- Give the speaker a chance to complete his/her statements (don't interrupt others).
- Questions are both encouraged and important.
- One person speaks at a time.
- What is said in the classroom stays in the classroom.

Importance of Role Playing

Practicing newly learned skills was a critical piece of *YAPP*. Because role plays were based on fictional situations, students might have said things as actors that they otherwise would not have said. Therefore, it was important to remind students not to interpret anything said in a role-play situation as a sign of interest in having a relationship or sexual intercourse, or in doing anything else depicted in the exercise.

Additionally, instructors needed to keep students motivated and excited about participating in the role plays. The following points were helpful during the field study:

- Provide structure and direction to students.
- Remind students of the purpose of role-play activities.

- Encourage students to use the SAFER method and the six *S*'s of resistance/negotiation skills.
- Involve the whole class by having them listen to the skit and provide helpful feedback to their peers.
- Following each exercise, invite students to analyze the decisions made and the skills used.
- Limit the time allotted for each skit so that at least two or three teams have a chance to participate in each role play.

Parent Education Session

The optional parent education session was held during the 7th-grade portion of the program. To encourage parents to attend, sites in the field study provided child care and refreshments.

PROGRAM EVALUATION

The Original Evaluation

Design

The effectiveness of *YAPP* was investigated in a field study conducted in 15 school districts in metropolitan Chicago. Research focused on the protective behaviors of students who first became sexually active during the study period. Patterns of parent–child communication, knowledge of HIV/AIDS, and intentions concerning protective behavior were also investigated for the entire sample of participants.

Of 45 school districts in the metropolitan area, students in the 15 districts selected for the study were considered to be at greatest risk for HIV infection based on several behavioral measures, including rates of reported STIs, adolescent pregnancies, school dropouts, minority enrollment, and poverty. Participating districts were randomly assigned to take part in one of three interventions: (a) the *YAPP* curriculum, including both 7th- and 8th-grade lessons, as well as parent-interactive activities (5 districts); (b) the *YAPP* curriculum, 7th- and 8th-grade lessons only, without the parent-interactive component (5 districts); or (c) their own standard AIDS education program (5 districts).

The study began in 7th-grade classrooms during the 1991–1992 school year, and continued through 1992–1993 for the 8th-grade booster program. The five districts assigned to use their standard AIDS education programs during the study period typically provided students with either a short (half-day to 1 day) informational workshop or a field trip to a health museum. These control group districts were given the *YAPP* program once the field study concluded.

Using results from a self-report questionnaire, the researchers compared both groups of *YAPP* participants with students in the control district schools. To assess the impact of the program over time, questionnaires were administered at three points:

- Time 1: at the start of the 7th-grade lessons (pretest)
- Time 2: at the conclusion of the 7th-grade lessons (posttest)
- Time 3: at the conclusion of the 8th-grade booster program (delayed posttest).

Evaluation Materials

Student surveys. The original field study used separate questionnaires for 7th-grade and 8th-grade students. An additional survey, administered to 9th-grade students, was used for subsequent analyses.

The 7th-grade survey was administered at the start of the program (Time 1, pretest) and again at the end of the 7th-grade program (Time 2, posttest). Included were measures of HIV/AIDS knowledge, sexual attitudes, self-efficacy, sexual and protective behavior, drug use by self and peers, and attitudes toward people with AIDS.

The 8th-grade survey was administered to students at the end of the 8th-grade program (Time 3, delayed posttest). It followed a similar structure to the 7th-grade survey.

The researchers administered an additional follow-up survey to about half of the students during their 9th-grade year. This instrument, though somewhat shorter than the others, included comparable measures of sexual attitudes, drug use, and sexual behavior. More than half of the respondents (57%) completed the survey by telephone, and the rest mailed in their surveys.

Parent surveys. The parent questionnaires were completed by the parents of students in the *YAPP* program. Separate surveys were developed for 7th- and 8th-grade parents. Questions measured attitudes and values about AIDS, drug use, and sexual activity, as well parent–child communication and parental involvement.

Evaluation Questions

Focusing on teens who first became sexually active during the study period, the researchers considered the following question:

- What effect does *YAPP* have on teens' actual practice and intention to practice protective behavior (e.g., use condoms and/or condoms with foam or lubricant during intercourse)? Looking at all program participants, the researchers also considered the following questions:
- What effect did the *YAPP* have on parent–child communication?
- What effect did *YAPP* have on teens' knowledge about HIV/AIDS?
- What effect did *YAPP* have on teens' attitudes toward people with AIDS?
- What effect did *YAPP* have on teens' beliefs about their ability to purchase and use condoms and foam or lubricant?

Data Collection Procedures

Approximately 1 week prior to the Time 1 (pretest) assessment, "passive" informed consent forms were mailed to students' parents or guardians in accordance with Illinois law. These forms were to be returned by parents/guardians only if they did not want their child to participate in the program or did not want their child to complete a confidential, self-administered questionnaire. Students were also given the option of nonparticipation in any part of the project. Refusal rates were less than 1%.

All participating students completed a paper-and-pencil survey under the supervision of trained data collectors—first in the 7th grade, and twice more, after they completed the 7th- and 8th-grade interventions. The survey included questions on decision making, refusal skills, estimates of risk-taking behaviors among peers, attitudes toward people with AIDS, knowledge about AIDS, and patterns of communication with parents and peers. Additional questions asked students about their patterns of sexual activity and knowledge and intentions regarding protective behaviors.

Sample

The intervention sample comprised 2,392 7th-grade students (1,459 treatment and 933 control) who completed the pretest survey. Because few parents actually took part in the adult activities that had been planned for the parent-interactive intervention, the researchers combined the two groups of *YAPP* participants in their analyses.

Within the original sample of participants, 67% of the treatment group and 70.4% of the control group completed the delayed posttest during the 8th grade. Approximately 58% of these teens were African American, 21% were White, and 16% were Hispanic. The researchers also noted that about one-third of the students had already become sexually active by the Time 1 (pretest) assessment in 7th grade.

Approximately 19% of the teens became sexually active for the first time between the Time 1 and Time 3 assessments; this group of students comprised the "newly sexually active students" for whom results are reported below.

Evaluation Results

Newly Sexually Active Students

Protective Behavior. Following the intervention, there were no significant differences between newly sexually active *YAPP* participants and their control group peers in terms of the number of sexual partners or the use of condoms. However, the groups did differ in their use of condoms together with contraceptive foam/lubricant. At the 8th-grade posttest, *YAPP* participants were somewhat more likely to have ever used condoms with foam (p < .10). Additionally, on measures of behavioral intentions, 85% of newly sexually active *YAPP* participants, compared to 63% of control group members, reported that they would, or might, use condoms with foam in the future (p < .001). The researchers further observed that within the sample, males and Hispanics were more likely to report ever having used condoms with foam. Also, *YAPP* students had a lower frequency of sexual activity and were more likely to have used condoms with foam/lubricant in the past 30 days, as compared to the control students.

All *YAPP* Participants

Parent–Child Communication. The *YAPP* curriculum appeared to have a positive impact on students' sense of comfort in discussing both drug use and sexuality with their parents. Yet, students also felt that their parents' feelings about whether they should have sex were less important to them than were their parents' feelings about using illicit drugs (marijuana and cocaine). Moreover, students believed that their parents would be less upset about sexual activity, as compared to drug use, by their children.

Attitudes Toward People With AIDS. By the 8th-grade assessment, *YAPP* participants showed more tolerance toward people with AIDS.

Knowledge. *YAPP* participants showed clear gains in their HIV/AIDS-related knowledge following the intervention. In particular, they scored higher than their control group peers on questions about modes of transmission, HIV prevention, the safety of the blood supply, transmission via casual contact, and the reasons for using condoms with foam/lubricant.

Self-Efficacy. Following the intervention, *YAPP* participants expressed greater belief than their control group peers in their ability to obtain protective products, including condoms and contraceptive foam or lubricant, from a store or clinic.

Behaviors and Behavioral Intentions. Analyses revealed that the program had no significant effects on actual STI/HIV/AIDS prevention behaviors, such as carrying condoms or using condoms and foam or lubricant together. Additionally, for the full study sample, no differences were found between *YAPP* participants and members of the control group on the teens' number of sexual partners.

However, the program did appear to have some effect on teens' behavioral intentions. Following the intervention, *YAPP* participants who anticipated being sexually active in the coming year were more likely than their control group peers to intend to use condoms and foam/lubricant.

Summary

YAPP was designed to educate junior high school students about STIs/HIV/AIDS and encourage sexually active teens to practice protective behaviors. The results of the original program evaluation suggested that *YAPP* appeared to have the greatest behavioral impact on newly sexually active students (those who first began having intercourse during the study period). Compared to their peers in control group schools, this subset of *YAPP* participants was more likely to have ever used condoms with foam or lubricant, to have used condoms with foam or lubricant within the past 30 days, and to intend to use condoms with foam or lubricant in the future. *YAPP* students also had a lower frequency of sexual activity in the past 30 days. However, no effects were found on measures of the youths' number of sexual partners or on the use of condoms alone. Additionally, the intervention did not influence the protective behaviors of students who were already sexually active when the program began.

On other outcome measures for the full sample of *YAPP* participants, the program appeared to improve teens' attitudes toward people with AIDS, factual knowledge of HIV/AIDS, feelings of comfort in discussing sexuality and drug use with their parents, belief in their ability to obtain condoms, and intentions to use condoms with foam or lubricant in future sexual encounters.

YAPP IN THE COMMUNITY TODAY

In the past 3 years, *YAPP* has been implemented in four communities in three Eastern states.

NOTE

1. A full set of program materials, including curriculum manuals, student workbooks, activity guides, videos, evaluation materials, and more, is available for purchase from Sociometrics at http://www.socio.com/pasha.htm.

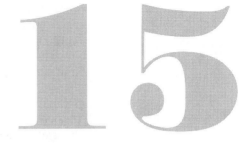

Draw the Line/Respect the Line: A Middle School Intervention to Reduce Sexual Risk Behavior

Tabitha A. Benner

Original Program Developers and Evaluators

University of California, San Francisco
   The Center for AIDS Prevention Studies

ETR Associates
   Scotts Valley, CA

PROGRAM ABSTRACT

Summary

Draw the Line/Respect the Line (DTL) was developed in an effort to provide a school-based prevention program for sexually transmitted infection (STI)/HIV and pregnancy to youths before they begin to engage in risky behaviors. The primary aim of the program was to reduce the number of middle school students who initiate or have sexual intercourse and to increase condom use among students who are sexually active. *DTL* was designed for delivery in regular middle school class settings in 6th through 8th grades. *DTL* helps students define their personal limits (draw the line), think ahead and prepare for sticking to those limits, and respect the limits of others (respect the line).

   DTL was implemented in an urban area of northern California between spring 1997 and spring 1999. The randomized controlled trial involved 19 public middle

Draw the Line/Respect the Line was supported by a grant from the National Institute of Mental Health (#MH51515).

schools in three school districts. Ten schools were randomly assigned to receive *DTL,* while the remaining 9 schools continued with regular classroom activities regarding STI/HIV and pregnancy prevention, as determined by the school district.

Participating students (n = 2,829) were surveyed at baseline in 6th grade (1997) and each spring thereafter through 2000 (1 year after completion of the 8th-grade curriculum, 36 months after baseline). While the intervention had no demonstrable effect on girls' behavior, evaluation results indicated that the intervention delayed sexual initiation among boys (adjusted percentages for intervention vs. control, 1 year postintervention: 17.3 vs. 24.5, *p* = .03). In addition, boys in the experimental group exhibited greater knowledge than their control group counterparts, had more positive attitudes about not having sex, and were less likely to find themselves in situations that could lead to sexual behaviors (adjusted mean score, intervention vs. control: 1.88 vs. 2.06, *p* = .002).

Focus

☑ Primary pregnancy prevention ☐ Secondary pregnancy prevention ☑ STI/HIV/AIDS prevention

Original Site

☑ School based ☐ Community based ☐ Clinic based

Suitable for Use in

DTL is suitable for use in school classrooms as well as in community organization settings.

Approach

- ☑ Abstinence
- ☑ Behavioral skills development
- ☐ Community outreach
- ☐ Contraceptive access
- ☑ Contraceptive education
- ☐ Life option enhancement
- ☑ Self-efficacy/self-esteem
- ☑ Sexuality/HIV/AIDS/STI education

Original Intervention Sample

Age, gender   The original intervention sample consisted of 2,829 students of nearly equal gender proportions. Average age at baseline was 11.5 years.

Race/ethnicity   Most participants (59.3%) self-identified as Hispanic, 15.9% were Asian, 16.5% were White, 5.2% were African American, and 3.1% were Other.

Program Components

- ☐ Adult involvement
- ☐ Case management
- ☑ Group discussion
- ☑ Lectures
- ☐ Peer counseling/instruction
- ☐ Public service announcements

- ☑ Role play
- ☐ Video
- ☑ Other: Homework requiring parent or adult participation

Program Length

Each of the 19 lessons is intended to be given during a 45–50 minute standard classroom time frame. There are 5 lessons for 6th graders and 7 each for 7th and 8th graders.

Staffing Requirements/Training

Family life educators taught the curriculum during the original implementation. Classroom teachers implementing the intervention should be skilled in using interactive teaching methods and guiding group discussions. They should also be comfortable with the program content.

Bibliography

Coyle, K. K., Kirby, D. B., Marín, B. V., Gómez, C. A., & Gregrorich, S. E. (2004). Draw the Line/ Respect the Line: A randomized trial of a middle school intervention to reduce sexual risks. *American Journal of Public Health, 94*(5), 843–851.

Related References by the Developers of *DTL*

Denner, J., Coyle, K. K., Robin, L., & Banspach, S. (2006). Integrating service learning into a curriculum to reduce health risks at alternative high schools. *Journal of School Health, 75*(5), 151–156.

Marín, B. V., Kirby, D. B., Hudes, E. S., Coyle, K. K., & Gómez, C. S. (2006). Boyfriends, girlfriends and teenagers' risk of sexual involvement. *Perspectives on Sexual & Reproductive Health, 38*(2), 76–83.

THE PROGRAM

Program Rationale and History

When *DTL* was developed in the mid- to late-1990s, there were several adolescent sexual-risk-reduction interventions available for high school–aged youths, offered either in school settings or in clinics or community-based organizations.[1] There were fewer multiyear programs available that focused the prevention message on middle school youths—before they began to engage in the risky behaviors. *DTL* was a pioneering 3-year program designed for classroom delivery to 6th, 7th, and 8th graders, with the purpose of reducing the number of students who initiated or engaged in sexual intercourse, and increasing condom use among those students who did have sex. The intervention centered on the theme of discovering/defining one's personal limits for a variety of situations—both nonsexual as well as sexual— and learning to respect the limits of others.

The intervention included 19 sequential lessons. Each lesson built on earlier concepts. The 6th-grade curriculum included 5 lessons that featured limit setting and refusal skills in nonsexual situations. The 7 lessons for 7th graders addressed determining personal limits regarding sexual intercourse, understanding the consequences of unplanned sexual intercourse, using intra- and interpersonal skills to maintain limits, and respecting others' limits. The 7-session 8th-grade curriculum included an HIV-positive guest speaker, a condom demonstration, and practicing of refusal skills in dating situations.

The *DTL* curriculum was developed and pilot tested over a several-year period. Students in focus groups provided information about how youths thought and felt about various topics related to sexuality. They also provided feedback about lesson ideas. Each lesson activity was tested in schools that were not part of the formal evaluation study. Additional pilot testing occurred following activity revisions and organization/creation of lessons. Student feedback was used throughout the development process to improve the lessons and make them more enjoyable.

Theoretical Framework

The primary theoretical underpinnings of *DTL* were social cognitive theory (SCT) and social inoculation theory (SIT). SCT emphasizes that in order to effect change, the learner must have knowledge, motivation to effect the change, expectancy of some positive outcome related to the new behavior, and self-efficacy to perform the behavior correctly and consistently. SIT emphasizes behavioral rehearsal as a way to "inoculate" learners and prepare them for resisting peer pressure and so forth in future risky situations.

Program Overview

DTL is delivered over a 3-year period to 6th, 7th, and 8th graders by classroom teachers or trained family life educators. The intervention incorporates interactive learning techniques, role-play activities, games, small-group exercises, and parent- or other adult-involved homework assignments. The cumulative curriculum is based on several principles:

1. Not having sexual intercourse is the healthiest sexual limit for middle school students.
2. Students can set their own personal limits.
3. Students can be motivated to maintain the limits they set for themselves.
4. Students will invariably encounter challenges (e.g., peer pressure) to their limits.
5. Students can overcome the challenges to their limits.
6. Students who respect the limits of others will be less coercive.
7. Each student has unique needs.
8. Condom use is essential protection for those who are sexually active.

6th-Grade Curriculum

The 6th-grade curriculum was divided into 5 sessions that addressed personal limits and meeting challenges to those limits.

Lesson 1: Draw the Line/Respect the Line. Students were introduced to the program and to the concept of having personal limits. They used a game of "Simon Says" to gain an understanding of where they would draw the line for certain nonsexual behaviors and to learn about peer pressure.

Lesson 2: Steps for Drawing the Line, Part 1. Students learned the first two (of four) steps in drawing the line (saying "No, I don't . . ." and using body language that says "no"), and then they used role-play activities to practice those steps.

Lesson 3: Steps for Drawing the Line, Part 2. Students worked in pairs to practice the refusal skills learned in Lesson 2. In a homework assignment, each student asked an adult about the pressures the adult faced when he or she was the teen's age, and how that adult knows when someone really means no.

Lesson 4: Changing the Subject and Walking Away. Students learned the last two steps in drawing the line: changing the subject and walking away. Using one of three possible scenarios, they wrote responses to pressure lines, using the four steps. Finally, they practiced these refusal skills aloud with partners and discussed how they had used the steps.

Lesson 5: Friends Respect the Line. Students learned that accepting another person's refusal gracefully and respectfully could be tricky. Respecting a friend's line by not pressuring him or her showed respect for the friend.

7th-Grade Curriculum

The 7th-grade curriculum introduced the need for drawing lines with regard to sexual pressures and behaviors.

Lesson 1: Welcome. After developing class rules, students tackled the question of what made it so hard to say no to sex. They also explored possible gender differences in sexual pressures. They explored the need for planning ahead to help them stick to their limits.

In this lesson, the anonymous question box was introduced. It continued to be a part of the program through 7th- and 8th-grade lessons.

Lesson 2: Reasons for Not Having Sex. The story of Tina and Marco, two 8th graders, had two possible endings—one in which they had sex, and one in which they didn't. Students used this story to explore what the characters would have thought/felt and how they would have reacted to one another the next morning; 2 days later; and, in the situation where they did have sex, 3 weeks after the encounter, when Tina's period was late.

Lesson 3: Handling Risky Situations. Continuing with the story of Tina and Marco, students learned to identify warning signs that could lead them to risky behavior. They explored the role of factors such as embarrassment that might have pressured them into crossing their lines or not removing themselves from risky situations. As homework, each student talked with an adult about the Tina and Marco story and solicited the adult's feedback on how the characters' lives would have been changed if they had had a baby at that point in their lives.

Lesson 4: Drawing the Line in Situations That Could Lead to Sex. Using half-scripted role plays, students practiced refusal skills, first by writing responses to pressure lines and then by verbal practice in pairs.

Lesson 5: STI Facts. Students learned the common symptoms of STIs, took an STI quiz, and read a story about a young couple who discovered they had genital warts. Students learned the basics of treating STIs (e.g., going to a clinic). As homework, they called a national STI hotline and solicited answers to STI questions.

Lesson 6: STI and Relationships. Students participated in a scripted talk show (complete with "Applause" cue cards). The "audience" participated in making suggestions on what the talk show guests could have done to stick to their limits. Students then broke out into gender-matched dyads to practice giving advice to a friend who was being pressured.

Lesson 7: Making a Commitment. Students completed a worksheet in which they applied the skills of avoiding risky situations, drawing the line, and respecting someone else's line. In order to protect students' privacy, they completed the worksheet anonymously. The teacher answered any questions from the anonymous question box that had not been addressed.

8th-Grade Curriculum

The 8th-grade lessons addressed determining personal limits and their underlying reasons, identifying situations that could challenge a limit, and practicing strategies to handle those situations.

Lesson 1: HIV and Teens. Students read and discussed the story of a young woman who is HIV-positive. They reviewed information learned in 7th grade about STI transmission and prevention. They then made personal commitments about how they, as 8th graders, would draw the line to reduce their risk for STI/HIV and pregnancy.

Lesson 2: Draw the Line Challenge. Students participated in a game designed to review and present information about preventing STIs. In the "Draw the Line Challenge," teams chose from among four categories of questions and raced against each other to the finish line, advancing as they answered questions correctly.

Lesson 3: Difficult Moments. Students used the story of Trina and Kashid to explore how sexual feelings, disparity of limits, and difficult situations could challenge their ability to stick to their personal limits. Trina and Kashid had very strong sexual feelings for one another and were just discovering that they had different personal limits when Kashid's mother came home.

Lesson 4: Sticking to Your Limit. Students discussed ways to handle difficult situations and then put their suggestions into practice via role plays. They also wrote questions for the HIV-positive guest who would speak with them in Lesson 5.

Lesson 5: Talking With a Person Who Has HIV. An HIV-positive guest speaker shared his/her experience living with HIV or AIDS—his/her life as young person; decisions that had put him/her at risk of HIV; internal and external pressures that had affected his/her decisions; and how HIV had impacted his/her life, relationships and long-term plans. As homework, students completed a worksheet in which they rethought their feelings/impressions of people who were HIV positive.

Lesson 6: Reduce Your Risk. Students discussed which protection methods were effective for STI/HIV prevention and pregnancy prevention. They watched the teacher demonstrate proper condom use (students did not practice using condoms themselves). They then worked in small same-gender groups to identify "dos and don'ts" of condom use.

Lesson 7: Staying Safe. In this final lesson, students identified an image to help them stick to their limit even when tempted to cross their line. They also evaluated the extent to which their limit would protect them against STI/HIV and pregnancy. The teacher answered any questions remaining in the anonymous question box.

Program Implementation

Program Planning

Before delivering *DTL,* review your school district's policies regarding parental consent for participation. In addition, some school districts have strict policies regarding what can and cannot be said about sex in the classroom. You may need to be guided by these policies as you implement this program. Finally, some lessons require the assistance of a second adult.

PROGRAM EVALUATION

The Original Evaluation

Study Design

DTL was implemented over a 3-year period, from 1997 to 1999. The final follow-up assessment was given in spring 2000. Four ethnic and socioeconomically diverse school districts in northern California were selected to participate in the original study, although one district later withdrew.

In the evaluation study design, 10 middle schools were randomly assigned to receive the *DTL* curriculum; the remaining 9 middle schools received the usual classroom activities with respect to STI, HIV, and pregnancy prevention. The research team used a multistep restricted randomization process. First, schools within each district were initially partitioned into matched sets. Then, two matched groups were formed, each consisting of one school set from each district. Finally, these two matched groups were randomized to the intervention or control condition.

Students were tested at baseline, in the spring of 1997, in 6th grade. They were tested again at the end of 7th and 8th grades. The final follow-up was given at the end of 9th grade—3 years after baseline and 1 year after completing the intervention. Trained data collectors administered the pencil-and-paper self-report surveys at each data point. The evaluation instrument was available in both Spanish and English.

Study Population

At baseline, the average participant age was 11.5 years. The sample gender mix was nearly equal (50.1% female). Students reported the following racial/ethnic data: 5.2% African American, 15.9% Asian, 59.3% Latino, 16.5% White, and 3.1% Other. Approximately 4% reported having had intercourse at baseline. Baseline data was collected from 2,829 students.

About 24% of students who returned consent forms were denied participation at baseline by their parents. The majority of parents who refused participation felt their children were too young to complete a survey about sexual behaviors.

Evaluation Questions and Outcome Measures

The survey assessed demographics, sexual behaviors, and sexuality-related psychosocial factors. The instrument assessed the following variables:

- Knowledge about HIV and condoms (6 items)
- Attitudes/reasons for having sex (7 items)
- Attitudes/reasons for not having sex (8 items)
- Beliefs supporting popularity with sex (2 items)
- Peer beliefs favoring sex (6 items)
- Beliefs favoring pressure for sex (1 item per gender group)
- Self-efficacy to refuse sexual activity (4 items)
- Coercive behavior (4 items)
- Situations that could lead to sexual behavior (4 items)
- Unwanted sexual advances (4 items)

Evaluation Results

Repeated measures of logistic and linear regression models were used to estimate the treatment group effects, separately for boys and girls, on study outcomes from baseline to the end of 9th grade. Additional analyses determined whether group membership (treatment vs. control) affected each measured psychosocial construct assessed at the end of 8th grade. When primary regression analyses found treatment effects on sexual intercourse in the last 12 months, subsequent analyses tested whether the psychosocial constructs mediated that event.

Results for Girls

Although there were statistically significant behavioral changes for boys, there were none for girls. The 8th-grade surveys revealed, however, that approximately 30% of the girls had boyfriends who were 2 or more years older. These girls were more likely to report having had sex. It is possible that more instruction on the influence of older partners on sexual behaviors and more skill practice in handling possible coercion may have helped improve the results for girls.

Girls in the intervention group did show significantly greater HIV and condom knowledge than the control group girls ($p < .05$), perceived fewer norms supporting sexual intercourse ($p = .02$), and reported significantly fewer incidents of unwanted sexual advances at the 8th-grade follow-up than did their control group counterparts.

Results for Boys

Boys who received *DTL* were less likely than their control group counterparts to initiate sex (adjusted percentages for intervention vs. control, 1 year postintervention: 17.3% vs. 24.5%, $p = .03$). In addition, at each follow-up, fewer intervention group boys reported having sex than control group boys ($p = .04$, $p = .01$, and $p = .02$ for 6th, 7th, and 8th grades, respectively). Intervention boys demonstrated significantly greater HIV and condom-related knowledge at the final assessment ($p < .001$). They perceived fewer peer norms supporting sex ($p = .001$), had more positive reasons for not having sex ($p = .003$), had stronger sexual limits ($p = .004$), and reported putting themselves in fewer situations that could lead to sexual behaviors ($p < .001$). The intervention may have created a norm within the school environment that made boys more comfortable with the idea of not having sex.

Summary

Evaluation results indicated that *DTL* was successful in delaying sexual initiation among middle school boys over a 36-month period. The study also suggested that a theory-driven, school-based intervention could reduce sexual risks among middle school boys.

DTL IN THE COMMUNITY TODAY

Since the release of the replication kit in 2006, *DTL* has been implemented in communities in 4 states across the United States, as well as in Washington, D.C.

NOTE

1. A full set of program materials—including facilitator's manual for grades 6, 7, and 8; evaluation materials, and more—is available for purchase from Sociometrics at http://www.socio.com/pasha.htm.

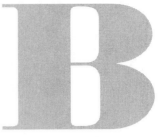

Programs Designed for Youths in High School

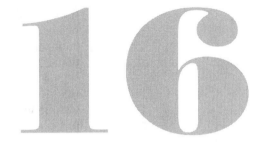

AIDS Prevention for Adolescents in School: A High School-Based STI/HIV/AIDS Prevention Program

Anne Belden, M. Jane Park, and Janette Mince

Original Program Developers and Evaluators

Heather J. Walter, MD, MPH
   Child and Adolescent Psychiatry
   Children's Memorial Hospital
   Chicago, IL

Roger D. Vaughan, MS
   Center for Population and Health
   Columbia University School of Public Health
   New York, NY

PROGRAM ABSTRACT

Summary

This 6-session program for high school students is delivered by regular classroom teachers. Combining principles of the health belief model with social psychology,

AIDS Prevention for Adolescents in School was supported by a grant from the National Institute of Mental Health/National Institute on Drug Abuse (5-P50-MH43520).

the curriculum aims to improve students' knowledge, beliefs, self-efficacy, and risk behaviors concerning HIV/AIDS. The first 2 classes provide general information about transmission and prevention of HIV/AIDS and teach students how to appraise their own risk behaviors. During the next 2 sessions, myths about peers' sexual behaviors are addressed, values clarification is introduced, and students use role-play and negotiation skills to practice delaying sexual intercourse. The final lessons involve discussions of purchasing and using condoms, and students use role-play and negotiation skills to practice consistent condom use.

A field study of the program was conducted with a predominantly African American and Hispanic sample of students attending four New York City public high schools. At the 3-month follow-up assessment, compared with a comparison group of peers, program participants scored significantly better on measures of knowledge, beliefs about the benefits of risk reduction, beliefs about the commonness of risky and preventive behaviors among their peers, and beliefs about one's own ability to effect positive change (e.g., self-efficacy). The program also was found to be effective in reducing sexually active participants' number of total sex partners and number of high-risk sex partners, and in increasing their use of condoms.

Focus

☐ Primary pregnancy prevention   ☐ Secondary pregnancy prevention   ☑ STI/HIV/AIDS prevention

Original Site

☑ School based   ☐ Community based   ☐ Clinic based

Suitable for Use In

Although it was originally implemented in high school classrooms, *AIDS Prevention for Adolescents in School* is equally suitable for use in community-based organizations.

Approach

- ☑ Abstinence
- ☑ Behavioral skills development
- ☐ Community outreach
- ☐ Contraceptive access
- ☑ Contraceptive education
- ☐ Life option enhancement
- ☑ Self-efficacy/self-esteem
- ☑ Sexuality/HIV/STI education

Original Intervention Sample

Age, gender   The field study included 1,201 students ages 12 to 20 years (average age = 15.7 years); 58% of the participants were female.

Race/ethnicity   37% African American, 35% Hispanic, and 28% Other (mostly non-Hispanic, White, or Asian).

Program Components

- ☐ Adult involvement
- ☐ Case management

- ☑ Group discussion
- ☑ Lectures
- ☐ Peer counseling/instruction
- ☐ Public service announcements
- ☑ Role play
- ☑ Video
- ☐ Other

Program Length

The 6-hour program is divided into six class lessons that are delivered on consecutive school days.

Staffing Requirements/Training

Regular classroom teachers implement the program. A 1-day in-service training session is recommended to introduce teachers to the curriculum's objectives and activities.

BIBLIOGRAPHY

DiClemente, R. J. (1993). Preventing HIV/AIDS among adolescents: Schools as agents of behavior change. *Journal of the American Medical Association, 270*(6), 760–762.

Walter, H. J., & Vaughan, R. D. (1993). AIDS risk reduction among a multiethnic sample of urban high school students. *Journal of the American Medical Association, 270*(6), 725–730.

Walter, H. J., Vaughan, R. D., Ragin, D. F., Cohall, A. T., Kasen, S., & Fullilove, R. E. (1993). Prevalence and correlates of AIDS-risk behaviors among urban minority high school students. *Preventive Medicine, 22,* 813–824.

Related References by the Developers of the *AIDS Prevention for Adolescents in School*

Armstrong, B., Cohall, A., Vaughan, R. D., Scott, M., Tiezzi, L., & McCarthy, J. F. (1999). Involving men in reproductive health: The Young Men's Clinic. *American Journal of Public Health, 89*(6), 902–905.

Cohall, A., Cohall, R., Dye, B., Dini, S., Vaughan, R. D., & Coots, S. (2007). Overheard in the halls: What adolescents are saying, and what teachers are hearing, about health issues. *Journal of School Health, 77*(7), 344–350.

Cohall, A., Kassotis, J., Parks, R., Vaughan, R., Bannister, H., & Northridge, M. (2001). Adolescents in the age of AIDS: Myths, misconceptions, and misunderstandings regarding sexually transmitted diseases. *Journal of the National Medical Association, 93*(2), 64–69.

Rickert, V. I., Wiemann, C. M., Vaughan, R. D., & White, J. W. (2004). Rates and risk factors for sexual violence among an ethnically diverse sample of adolescents. *Archives of Pediatric & Adolescent Medicine, 158*(12), 1132–1139.

Vaughan, R. D., McCarthy, Walter, H. J., Resnicow, K., Waterman, P. D., Armstrong, B., et al. (1996). The development, reliability, and validity of a risk factor screening survey for urban minority junior high school students. *Journal of Adolescent Health, 19*(3), 171–178.

THE PROGRAM

Program Rationale and History

AIDS Prevention for Adolescents in School was a six-session, school-based program aimed at reducing transmission of the HIV virus among teenagers.[1] The curriculum was designed to increase students' knowledge about HIV/AIDS, modify their beliefs about the risks of infection, improve their motivation and ability to avoid risky situations, and ultimately, empower teens to reduce their sexual risk behavior.

The program was originally developed to meet the particular needs of multi-ethnic, inner-city teens. A team of health professionals with specialized training in preventive medicine, public health, adolescent psychiatry, and adolescent medicine developed the curriculum, using the results of a needs assessment survey. The survey documented high levels of sexual risk behaviors among the target population of teens, including unprotected intercourse, intercourse with multiple partners, and intercourse with high-risk partners. Additionally, the program developers recognized that adolescents/young adults comprised one of the fastest growing groups of people with AIDS, and that African Americans and Hispanics were disproportionately represented among both urban AIDS cases and urban HIV-positive teens.

A field study of the program was conducted with 1,201 predominantly African American and Hispanic high school students in New York City in 1990–1991.

Theoretical Framework

Two analytic perspectives, social cognitive theory (SCT) and the health belief model (HBM), guided development of the program.

Principles of the HBM suggest that individuals will be likely to engage in health-related behaviors when the following conditions are met:

1. One perceives that the problem (e.g., HIV/AIDS) poses a serious threat to one's well-being.
2. One understands the benefits and barriers to taking preventive action.
3. One feels able to effectively carry out the recommended actions.

Similarly, SCT is based on the idea that knowledge alone is insufficient to produce behavioral change. Instead, the theory points toward four factors that together determine the likelihood of engaging in some action, such as using condoms to protect oneself from HIV/AIDS:

1. A person's understanding of what must be done to avoid infection
2. The belief that one will be able to use condoms
3. The belief that the method will be successful in preventing infection
4. The benefit one anticipates from accomplishing the behavior (e.g., staying healthy)

The original program developers reasoned that adolescents were particularly at risk for HIV infection because they frequently possessed relatively low levels of self-efficacy, or confidence in their ability to perform a particular behavior successfully, such as to negotiate the use of a condom with their partners. The developers also identified personal skills as important factors in determining how (and how successfully) teens would act. For this reason, the *AIDS Prevention for Adolescents in School* curriculum aimed to develop students' resistance and negotiation skills for acting in sexual situations, including correctly using a condom, saying "no," and removing oneself from unsafe situations. Moreover, because SCT links learning to repeated observation and imitation, the program instructor modeled socially desirable behaviors, and students practiced these behaviors through role plays.

Program Objectives

The overall goal of the curriculum was to reduce transmission of HIV among teenagers. Additionally, the program was designed to meet the following objectives:

1. To convey correct facts about HIV transmission and prevention to students

2. To teach students to accurately appraise their risk of getting HIV/AIDS, based on their own behaviors, and to foster an appropriate level of concern based on this appraisal
3. To direct students to appropriate AIDS-preventive resources within their school and local community
4. To help students clarify their personal values relating to involvement in sexual intercourse, and to facilitate an understanding of the effects of outside influences on these values
5. To empower students to develop the negotiation skills necessary to delay sexual intercourse
6. To empower students to develop the negotiation skills necessary to acquire condoms and use them consistently and effectively

Hypothesized Outcomes

It was hypothesized that participation in the *AIDS Prevention for Adolescents in School* program would be associated with

- increased knowledge about HIV/AIDS;
- increased belief in the benefits of risk reduction;
- increased belief in one's ability to change one's own behaviors and reduce the risk of infection;
- fewer sex partners and high-risk partners; and
- increased use of condoms.

The original field study targeted multiethnic, inner-city teens—other groups of participants may have shown more dramatic results following the intervention.

Program Activities

The six-lesson curriculum aimed to effect change in students' knowledge, beliefs, self-efficacy, and sexual risk behaviors through the following three activities:

1. *Lectures.* A lecture format was used during the first session to enable teachers or program leaders to convey important facts about HIV/AIDS to the class. The lecture was informally structured and combined with group discussions.
2. *Group discussion.* Throughout the program discussions were used to address students' questions, explore new concerns, review program activities and out-of-class assignments, share personal values relating to sex, and evaluate role-playing scenarios and negotiation strategies.
3. *Role play.* This powerful learning technique was used extensively during the final sessions to enhance the development of life skills, particularly those that would help teens resist pressures to engage in HIV risk behaviors. Through role play, participants could experience real-life social pressures to engage in unsafe behaviors and react spontaneously to these pressures. Students could also assess their personal reactions and develop the negotiation and assertiveness skills that were necessary to resist such pressures in their daily lives.

Program Schedule

Listed below are brief summaries of the six program lessons. During the field study, lessons were held on consecutive days and led by regular classroom teachers.

Lesson 1

This lesson was designed to increase students' basic understanding of HIV/AIDS, including transmission and prevention. In the field study, a guest speaker delivered this lecture to the class. A few days prior to the start of the lesson, students wrote down their questions about the disease. The guest speaker (or program instructor) addressed these questions during his/her presentation.

Lesson 2

In this lesson, students learned how to appraise their risk of acquiring HIV/AIDS with a "Rate the Risk" worksheet and a series of vignettes about teens. In addition, they were encouraged to stop engaging in any risky behaviors, to explore the reasons why they were involved in such activities, to practice preventive measures, and to consider getting an HIV antibody test. During the second half of the class, the group reviewed the "AIDS Resource Guide." For homework, students searched for an advertisement that appealed to them and determined whether and how it used sexual imagery to promote the product.

Lesson 3

This lesson encouraged students to clarify their personal values about engaging in sexual intercourse. It was also designed to help participants understand the ways in which outside influences (such as peer pressure and the media) could influence their values and beliefs about intercourse. As a group, the class discussed reasons why one might choose to delay sexual involvement, as well as poor reasons for having sex before one was ready. In the next activity, the class considered how the media and other influences could pressure teens into feeling that they should act in ways that conflicted with their personal values. Students shared the advertisements they analyzed for the Lesson 2 homework assignment.

Lesson 4

The purpose of this lesson was to empower students to develop and apply the negotiation skills necessary to delay involvement in sexual intercourse. The session began with a group discussion and role play of "lines" that were used to persuade others to have sex. The group considered circumstances in which it could be difficult to say no. Additional role plays were used to help students practice responding to typical "lines" by saying no persuasively. One pair of students acted out the scenario in front of the class, while the rest of the group offered feedback.

Lesson 5

Helping students develop skills and confidence to use condoms were the goals of this session. At the start of the period, the class viewed the *Tracee and Andy Think It Through* video clip. The video showed a teenage girl who felt ready to begin having sex with her boyfriend. She wanted her boyfriend to use condoms but was unsure how to approach him. Following the video, the class discussed ways that Tracee could have convinced Andy to use condoms.

Additional role-play activities provided students with opportunities to practice their condom negotiation skills. The class also considered other barriers to using condoms, such as the belief that they were unnatural, or that they were unnecessary if neither partner is infected.

Lesson 6

The final lesson was designed to help students feel comfortable buying and using condoms. First the teacher demonstrated the correct way to put on and remove a condom, using a zucchini or banana as a penile model. Then the class discussed where and how to buy condoms.

PROGRAM EVALUATION

The Original Evaluation

Design

The effectiveness of the *AIDS Prevention for Adolescents in School* program was investigated in a field study conducted in four public high schools that were demographically representative of the entire high school population in New York City. Ninth- and 11th-grade students in two schools served as the intervention group (program participants), and 9th and 11th grade students in two other schools served as the comparison group.

The study compared changes in the intervention and comparison group members' HIV/AIDS-related knowledge, beliefs, self-efficacy, and sexual risk behaviors. To assess these changes, self-report questionnaires were administered to all students at two points:

- Time 1: about 2 weeks prior to the start of the intervention (pretest)
- Time 2: 3 months following the conclusion of the program (3-month follow-up)

Evaluation Questions

The researchers examined the effect of participation in the *AIDS Prevention for Adolescents in School* program on several outcome measures. In particular, they considered whether, as predicted, program participants showed

1. increased HIV/AIDS-related knowledge;
2. increased belief in the benefits of risk reduction;
3. more accurate beliefs about the commonness and acceptability of risky behaviors among peers;
4. improved self-efficacy;
5. reduced HIV/AIDS risk behavior.

Data Collection Procedures

A 94-item questionnaire was first administered to students by research staff approximately 2 weeks before the program began, and again about 3 months following the intervention. In addition, to provide a measure of the reliability of the instrument, 10% of the students were randomly selected to complete the survey one extra time, 2 weeks following the Time 1 assessment.

Because the student questionnaire was considered to be part of a customary educational evaluation, the New York City Board of Education waived its usual parental consent procedures. However, students were assured that their responses were voluntary and confidential and would be reported only in the aggregate. To enable the researchers to track the youths for the duration of the study, individual surveys were identified by students' four-digit school identification numbers.

Sample

The full study sample comprised 667 program participants and 534 comparison students; more females than males (58% vs. 42%) participated. Youths ranged in age from 12 to 20; on average, students were nearly 16 years old. Within the sample, 37% of the teens were African American, 35% were Hispanic, and 28% were Other.

Evaluation Results

At the Time 1 assessment, one-third of the sample reported engaging in sexual intercourse during the past 3 months. Of those who were sexually active, more than half said that they used condoms inconsistently or not at all, 20% reported having two or more sexual partners, and 5% reported having intercourse with high-risk (e.g., intravenous drug using) partners. Overall, more than two-thirds of the sexually active students showed some evidence of high-risk behaviors at the start of the study.

At the Time 1 assessment, program participants showed slightly higher behavior risk scores, as well as lower levels of HIV/AIDS-knowledge than their comparison group peers. At the follow-up assessment, program participants scored significantly higher than the comparison group on five of eight outcome measures, as explained below. In addition, none of the effects appeared to vary significantly by students' school, age, gender, race/ethnicity, or classroom teacher. Furthermore, teachers' effectiveness in leading the program was found to be unrelated to the outcome measures.

HIV/AIDS-Related Knowledge

Following the *AIDS Prevention for Adolescents in School* program, participants showed significant gains in their HIV/AIDS-related knowledge. Their scores rose from 75.6 at baseline to 85.5 at the 3-month follow-up assessment, as compared to 78.8 (baseline) and 81.2 (follow-up) for the comparison group students ($p < .0001$).

Beliefs About the Benefits of Risk Reduction

Program participation was associated with significant gains regarding beliefs about the benefits of risk reduction. Participants' scores rose from 3.5 at baseline to 3.8 at follow-up, compared to 3.7 (baseline) and 3.8 (follow-up) for the comparison group ($p < .0001$).

Beliefs About Peer Norms

Program participants showed significant gains in the accuracy of their beliefs about the commonness of peer risk and preventive behaviors. For participants, scores rose from 2.8 to 2.9 following the intervention, while the comparison group's scores remained level at 2.8 ($p < .003$).

Self-Efficacy

Program participants' belief in their ability to successfully perform AIDS-preventive actions rose from 3.7 to 3.9 between the Time 1 and Time 2 assessments. This change was significantly higher than that observed for the comparison group, whose scores rose from 3.7 to 3.8 ($p < .03$).

Sexual Risk Behavior

Program participants showed a significant reduction in an index of sexual risk behavior, with scores declining from 1.5 to 1.3 between the Time 1 and Time 2 assessments. The risk score for the comparison group increased from 1.0 to 1.3 during the same time period ($p < .006$).

In a breakdown of this index, the program was found to be most effective at increasing sexual monogamy and condom use, and in reducing the number of total sex partners and high-risk sex partners. The intervention showed no effect on sexual abstinence.

On the three remaining outcome measures—beliefs about one's susceptibility to HIV/AIDS, beliefs about barriers to using protection, and beliefs about the acceptability of risky and preventive behaviors—no significant differences were found between the two groups of students.

Summary

The 3-month follow-up data provide evidence that the *AIDS Prevention for Adolescents in School* program had a statistically significant effect in reducing teenagers' sexual risk behaviors. Students who participated in the program also showed favorable changes in their knowledge, beliefs, and self-efficacy related to AIDS-preventive actions. It is noteworthy that these effects were found across a broad spectrum of inner-city, largely minority adolescent students, participating in a 6-hour intervention.

In interpreting the results, the researchers offered two caveats. First, they noted that their sample of teens included students sufficiently motivated to attend school. In contrast, such positive outcomes might not be found with teenagers who are habitually absent or who have dropped out of school, or with teens who show riskier sexual behavior profiles. In fact, the program may have limited effectiveness for such youths, who are at the highest risk of acquiring HIV infection.

In addition, the researchers noted that the program was of very limited duration. To produce dramatic behavioral change, it would be important to supplement short-term educational interventions with intensive, broad-based prevention activities.

AIDS PREVENTION FOR ADOLESCENTS IN SCHOOL IN THE COMMUNITY TODAY

In the past 3 years, *AIDS Prevention for Adolescents in School* has been implemented in 11 communities in 6 states—ranging from New York to California to Florida.

NOTE

1. A full set of program materials, including curriculum handbook, activity booklet, evaluation materials, and more, is available for purchase from Sociometrics at http://www.socio.com/pasha.htm.

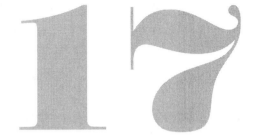

Get Real About AIDS®: A High School-Based STI/HIV/AIDS Prevention Program

Nicole Vicinanza, Starr Niego, M. Jane Park, and Janette Mince

Original Program Developer

Comprehensive Health Education Foundation
    Seattle, WA

Original Program Evaluators

Deborah S. Main, PhD
Donald C. Iverson, PhD
Joe McGloin, MA
    Department of Family Medicine
    University of Colorado Health Sciences Center
    Denver, CO

Stephen W. Banspach, PhD
Janet L. Collins, PhD
Deborah L. Rugg, PhD

The evaluation and development of *Get Real About AIDS*® (Grades 9–12, 2nd ed.) was supported by a contract from the Division of Adolescent and School Health, U.S. Centers for Disease Control and Prevention (200–88–0683).

Lloyd D. Kolbe, PhD

Division of Adolescent and School Health

Centers for Disease Control and Prevention

Atlanta, GA

PROGRAM ABSTRACT

Summary

Get Real About AIDS® a 14-session program for high school students, emphasizes behavioral skill development. During the first several classes, students study transmission and prevention of HIV, teen vulnerability to the virus, and determinants of risky behaviors. In the second half of the program, students learn and repeatedly practice skills to help them identify, manage, avoid, and leave risky situations. The lessons encourage students to delay having sexual intercourse, be monogamous, avoid drugs and alcohol when they do have intercourse, use condoms correctly, get tested for HIV infection if they are at risk, and avoid sharing needles.

A field study of the curriculum was conducted in 17 Colorado high schools serving rural, suburban, and urban populations. In a 6-month follow-up assessment comparing *Get Real About AIDS®* participants with a comparison group of peers, sexually active program participants had fewer sexual partners, purchased and used condoms more frequently, intended to engage in sex less frequently, and planned to use condoms when they did engage in sex. The evaluation data did not record, however, a delay in the onset of sexual activity, a decrease in the frequency of sexual activity, or a reduction in drug and alcohol use prior to sex.

Focus

☐ Primary pregnancy prevention

☐ Secondary pregnancy prevention

☑ STI/HIV/AIDS prevention

Original Site

☑ School based   ☐ Community based   ☐ Clinic based

Suitable for Use In

Although it was originally implemented in high school classrooms, this program is equally suitable for use in community-based organizations.

Approach

- ☑ Abstinence
- ☑ Behavioral skills development
- ☐ Community outreach
- ☐ Contraceptive access
- ☑ Contraceptive education
- ☐ Life option enhancement
- ☑ Self-efficacy/self-esteem
- ☑ Sexuality/HIV/STI education

Original Intervention Sample

Age, gender   A total of 2,849 teens participated in the field study; the average age was 15 years; 51% of participants were male.

Race/ethnicity   65% White, 21% Latino, 6% African American, 3% Asian, 5% Other.

Program Components

- ■ ☐ Adult involvement
- ■ ☐ Case management
- ■ ☑ Group discussion
- ■ ☑ Lectures
- ■ ☐ Peer counseling/instruction
- ■ ☑ Public service announcements
- ■ ☑ Role play
- ■ ☑ Video
- ■ ☐ Other

Program Length

The program is divided into 14 class sessions, each 50 minutes in length; the sessions can be scheduled to suit your own needs.

Staffing Requirements/Training

The program is led by regular classroom teachers, preferably in health or science classes. In the field study, special training was provided to instructors in a 5-day, 40-hour session designed to enhance fidelity to the curriculum. Videotaping and critiques of practice lessons were also included.

BIBLIOGRAPHY

Main, D. S., Iverson, D. C., McGloin, J., Banspach, S. W., Collins, J. L, Rugg, D. L., & Kolbe, L. J. (1994). Preventing HIV infection among adolescents: Evaluation of a school-based education program. *Preventive Medicine, 23*(4), 409–417.

Related References by the Developers of *Get Real About AIDS*®

Basen-Enquist, K., Coyle, K. K., Parcel, G. S., Kirby, D., Banspach, S. W., Carvajal, S. C., & Baumler, E. (2001). Schoolwide effects of a multicomponent HIV, STD, and pregnancy prevention program for high school students. *Health Education & Behavior, 28*(2), 166–185.
Main, D. S. (2002). Commentary: Understanding the effects of peer education as a health promotion strategy. *Health Education & Behavior, 29*(4), 424–426.

THE PROGRAM

Program Rationale and History

The Comprehensive Health Education Foundation (CHEF) originally published this curriculum, aimed at preventing sexually transmitted infections (STIs)/HIV/AIDS, in 1988, using the title *Here's Looking at AIDS and You*™.[1] Following field testing and evaluation of the materials, *Get Real About AIDS*® was introduced as the revised curriculum. The 14-session curriculum for grades 9–12 was designed to educate teens about their vulnerability to HIV/AIDS and teach them the skills necessary to reduce their risk of infection. Separate age-appropriate editions are available for upper elementary (grades 4–6), middle school (grades 6–9), and senior high school students (grades 9–12). This chapter deals solely with the version for high school students.

During the first 5 sessions, participants learned basic facts about transmission and prevention of HIV, including behaviors that would put them at risk of infection. During sessions 6 through 12, students learned how to set limits around risky behaviors.

The final sessions helped students integrate what they had learned in the program into their own lives. The program encouraged teens to delay initiating intercourse, or for those youths who were or who became sexually active, to be sexually monogamous, avoid drugs and alcohol that could cloud one's judgment during intercourse, use condoms, get tested for HIV, and avoid sharing needles. *Get Real About AIDS*® (Grades 9–12, 2nd ed.) was field tested in 10 high schools throughout Colorado.

Theoretical Framework

According to the original evaluators, the program's organization and content could be viewed within the context of two theories for promoting health-related behaviors in youths: social cognitive theory and the theory of reasoned action. Although they use different terminology, both theories assert that knowledge alone is insufficient to produce behavioral change. Rather, four factors together determine the likelihood of engaging in some action, such as using condoms to protect oneself from HIV/AIDS:

1. A person's understanding of what must be done to avoid infection
2. The belief that one will be able to use condoms
3. The belief that the method will be successful in preventing infection
4. The benefit one anticipates from accomplishing the behavior (e.g., staying healthy)

The curriculum was divided into three components: information, skills, and vulnerability and personal impact. The informational component was designed to help teens understand and avoid sexual risk behaviors. Skills training provided instruction and repeated practice in setting and sticking to limits. The final component was designed to help participants understand their own vulnerability to HIV infection, as well as the personal impact of AIDS on their lives.

Key Messages in the Curriculum

Six ideas are reinforced throughout the program sessions:

- AIDS is a serious disease, but it is not easy to get.
- For young people, abstinence from sex and from drugs is the only sure way to prevent becoming infected with HIV.
- Young people have the ability to avoid situations that place them at risk of becoming infected with HIV.
- Young people have the right to have their limits respected.
- Young people have the responsibility to educate others about AIDS.
- People with AIDS deserve our understanding and support.

Program Objectives

Get Real About AIDS® aimed to reduce students' risk of HIV/AIDS and other STIs. Specifically, the curriculum is designed to achieve the following objectives:

1. Increase students' knowledge of STIs and HIV/AIDS
2. Increase students' awareness of their vulnerability to infection
3. Delay the onset of sexual intercourse among students
4. Increase safer-sex behaviors among sexually active students, including
   a. Maintenance of monogamous relationships
   b. Abstinence from drugs and alcohol before intercourse
   c. Consistent and correct use of condoms
   d. HIV testing if one is at risk
5. Increase students' awareness of the risks associated with sharing intravenous (IV) drug needles

Program Schedule

Program Overview

A brief overview of the content and learning objectives for all 14 program lessons appears below. Each lesson is designed to last approximately 50–60 minutes, though the length will vary with the extent of class discussion.

For each lesson, the plan contained

- a "Ready" section summarizing the lesson, learning objectives, and program components addressed in the lesson;
- a "Set" section describing the resources and advance preparation necessary for leading the lesson, as well as new vocabulary terms;
- a "Go" section outlining the steps instructors would follow during the lesson.

Each lesson was organized in a similar manner, beginning with a brief review of the important messages from the previous session, proceeding to the new material and activities, and closing with reinforcement of the day's lessons.

Program Outline

Lesson 1: Teenage Vulnerability to HIV. The introductory lesson established a comfortable environment for learning about AIDS. At the start of the session, the instructor presented the program's methods and goals, discussed HIV/AIDS and teen vulnerability to infection, and established ground rules for the program. A video and group discussion were used to explore the myth that teenagers do not get AIDS. Participants submitted questions to the Question Box. They put their questions in this box at any time throughout the course, and they were given class time to write questions every few sessions. At the end of the period, students were given a newsletter to take home to their parents. The newsletter provided suggestions for parent–child communication regarding HIV/AIDS.

Lesson 2: The Transmission of HIV. In this lesson, teens participated in a simulation that was designed to demonstrate the spread of the AIDS epidemic; they also learned how to assess their own risk of HIV infection. The session concluded with a discussion of HIV testing, including laws about confidentiality.

Lesson 3: All About AIDS and Other STIs. Additional information was provided in this lesson about the ways teens could and could not become infected with HIV and other STIs. Students viewed the video *The Subject Is HIV,* which emphasized two primary messages: (a) AIDS is hard to get, and (b) a person can get AIDS by shooting up or having sex with someone who is infected. Cooperative learning teams were organized to study various STIs using the *STI Facts* pamphlet. These teams continued to work together for the remainder of the program. Finally, the instructor asked participants to interview friends and family members about their knowledge of HIV and to share what they had learned in class with these people.

Lesson 4: Delaying Sex. This lesson provided students with reasons for delaying sexual activity; then, working in small groups, participants considered the ways, both positive and negative, in which relationships change when they become sexual. The instructor asked how the positive changes could be realized without sex. For homework, students asked two or three adults how people know whether they are ready to have sex.

Lesson 5: Preventing HIV Infection. This lesson taught students about the importance of correct and consistent condom use. The instructor first noted that the only sure way to avoid AIDS and other STIs was to abstain from sex and IV drug use. However, since some teens were sexually active and most others would be active eventually, the instructor described condoms as an effective means of preventing transmission. After describing the procedures for correct use, the instructor demonstrated with a penile model. The class considered reasons why many teens failed to use condoms and explored the concepts of responsibility and personal protection. For homework, students visited a store that sold condoms and completed a Point of Purchase data form.

Lesson 6: Limits. The instructor began this lesson by discussing limits teens encounter in everyday life (e.g., driving a car requires a license, holding a job requires getting to work on time). Students then considered the limits that would keep them safe from HIV transmission and explored reasons why it was important to set limits before encountering a risky situation. The barriers that might have kept people from sticking to their limits, as well as the consequences of not sticking to limits were also discussed. Students then participated in a small-group exercise in which they thought of ways to help someone stick to their limits. When finished, the groups shared their ideas with the class. Finally, the class developed a list of limits and consequences concerning sexual behavior; this list was used during the next few lessons.

Lessons 7 and 8: The Refusal Skill™, Days 1 and 2. These two classes introduced The Refusal Skill™, which helped students stick to their limits in risky situations. Students were videotaped during skill practice so that they could receive more specific, in-depth feedback. In addition, it was suggested that the instructor have an assistant model the skill, observe role plays, and offer feedback to students. During the first part of the lesson, students viewed segments of the *Stick to Your Limits* video and discussed how successful the characters had been in maintaining their limits. Then they learned about and practiced The Refusal Skill™, using examples from the list of limits students had developed in Lesson 6. During the second half of the lesson, students continued to practice the skill and explore their feelings in the process.

Lesson 9: Peer Messages. In this lesson, students examined different ways of giving messages about HIV/AIDS to others. They watched the *Public Service Announcements* video and discussed the advantages and disadvantages of receiving information in this format. A worksheet prompted students to consider what messages about HIV/AIDS they wanted to share with others. Students discussed their responses in small groups, sharing their results with the class when they had finished. Finally, the instructor encouraged students to help spread the word about HIV/AIDS to their friends and family.

Lesson 10: Using The Refusal Skill™ Proactively. In this lesson, students applied The Refusal Skill™ to avoid getting into risky situations. Students viewed and discussed segments of the *Stick to Your Limits* videotape and then participated in related role-play exercises. The instructor taught students special techniques to use when they felt pressured to enter into risky situations.

Lesson 11: Becoming Comfortable Using The Refusal Skill™. To help students become more comfortable avoiding risky situations, this lesson included additional role-play exercises. These exercises could also be videotaped to provide participants with in-depth feedback. In conjunction with the activities, the class discussed obstacles to using the skill and ways to overcome them.

Lesson 12: The Refusal Skill for Self-Control™. Students learned a modified version of The Refusal Skill™ that was designed to help them say "no." Using segments from the *Stick to Your Limits* video, students discussed how individuals could stick to their limits, avoid risky situations, and still have fun. These ideas were reinforced with practice exercises. In addition, the instructor encouraged students to think about their own limits and the kinds of situations where they might apply the skills they had learned.

Lesson 13: The Community Meeting. This lesson, built around a large-group role play, required at least 20 participants. Students acted out the parts of community members who met to talk about a high school student, Charles Crawford, who had contracted HIV. Students were assigned to roles (e.g., the principal, school board members, students, and the school nurse) and were given diverse points of view to represent (e.g., people with HIV are dangerous, people with HIV must be homosexual or use drugs, and casual contact with HIV-infected people is not a problem). Certain characters feared that Charles was a danger to other students and should have been removed from school, while others tried to dispel misinformation about HIV/AIDS. After the role play, students discussed their feelings about the exercise, and the instructor asked them to identify incorrect information they had heard during the activity. Finally, students were reminded that it was illegal to discriminate against people who were HIV-positive. For homework, students researched the policy on employees with HIV at one business in their community. (Note: Program developers added Lesson 13 to the program after completion of the field study.)

Lesson 14: Transfer. During the final lesson of the program, students practiced using the knowledge and skills they had acquired. Using "The Next Time . . ." worksheet, students related skills they had learned in the class to their everyday lives. Then they developed and participated in role plays applying The Refusal Skill™ and The Refusal Skill for Self Control™. To bring closure to the lessons, the instructor reinforced the messages that (a) HIV/AIDS was hard to get; (b) a person could get AIDS by having unprotected sex or sharing needles; (c) abstinence from sex and drugs was the only sure way to avoid AIDS and other STIs; and (d) if teens did choose to have sex, they should use latex condoms. Following this review, the instructor asked students to think about what they had learned from the program and what they would do differently now that the program was over. Students shared their answers with the class if they wished.

PROGRAM EVALUATION

The Original Evaluation

Design

The effectiveness of the original *Get Real About AIDS®* curriculum was investigated in a field study carried out in 17 Colorado high schools. In 10 of the schools, trained instructors implemented an intervention that was based on the *Get Real About AIDS®* curriculum. The other 7 schools served as comparison sites.

All participants completed confidential, self-report questionnaires assessing their STI/HIV/AIDS-related knowledge, intentions, and behavior. To assess the impact of the program over time, students' responses were compared across two time periods:

- Time 1: before the start of the intervention (pretest)
- Time 2: 6 months following the intervention (posttest)

Evaluation Questions

The evaluation was designed to assess the program's effect on (a) the initiation of sexual activity among teens, and (b) among teens who were already sexually active at the start of the program, the frequency of sexual risk behaviors.

Specifically, four questions guided the study:

1. Did participation in the *Get Real About AIDS*® program increase teens' STI/HIV/AIDS-related knowledge?
2. Did program participation increase students' intention to engage in safer sexual activities (i.e., be monogamous and use condoms)?
3. Did students who were abstinent at the start of the program continue to postpone sexual intercourse following the intervention?
4. Did students who were sexually active at the start of the intervention reduce the frequency of behaviors that put them at risk of exposure to HIV (e.g., sex with multiple partners and failure to use condoms)?

Data Collection

Schools were recruited for the study from six different school districts located in rural, urban, and suburban settings throughout Colorado. Within each district, comparison and intervention schools were matched as closely as possible with respect to the grade, sex, and racial/ethnic distribution of students. For the duration of the study, comparison schools were encouraged not to implement any new HIV education programs; instead, they were asked to continue using their existing curricula. In four of these schools, no formal HIV/AIDS education was offered. Two of the comparison sites, on the other hand, provided minimal HIV/AIDS instruction to students, including such activities as discussion of infectious diseases in home economics classes and exposure to sexuality materials.

Before the self-report questionnaires were administered, each school followed its district procedures for obtaining parental consent. The surveys, which took about 15 to 20 minutes to complete, were given to students at three points: prior to the intervention, 2 months after the intervention, and 6 months after the intervention. However, only the baseline and 6-month follow-up results were included in the original analysis.

In order to assure students' anonymity, participants were told not to write their names or any identifying numbers on the surveys. Instead, students' Time 1 and Time 2 questionnaires were matched using their responses to the demographic questions.

Sample

Of the 2,844 students who completed the baseline survey, 65% were White, 6% were African American, 21% were Hispanic, 3% were Asian, and 5% were classified as Other. Females made up 49% of the initial respondents, and males 51%. The average age of participants was 15 years. In addition, 44% of this group indicated that they had engaged in sexual intercourse, 25% of students had been sexually active within 2 months of the initial survey, and 1.6% had injected drugs. Matching students' Time 1 and Time 2 surveys yielded a final sample of 979 participants.

Evaluation Results

Get Real About AIDS® appeared to be effective in changing students' knowledge, intentions, and some behaviors, but not in postponing the onset of sexual activity or in reducing the use of injection drugs.

Knowledge

Compared to their peers in the comparison schools, program participants showed significantly greater knowledge of HIV/AIDS at the 6-month follow-up assessment ($p = .004$).

Behavioral Intentions

Program participants also expressed greater intention to engage in safer sexual practices following the intervention. Compared to their comparison group peers, sexually active students were more likely to report their intention to reduce the frequency of intercourse ($p = .017$) and to use a condom when they did have sex ($p = .039$). However, no changes were found either in the teens' intentions to discuss condoms with their partners or in their thoughts about the need to use condoms.

Beliefs

Six months following the intervention, program participants were more likely than comparison group students to believe that engaging in risky behaviors put one at risk for HIV infection ($p = .042$).

Behavior

Behavioral change was observed only among those students who were sexually active. Six months following the program, sexually active *Get Real About AIDS®* participants were more likely than their comparison group peers to purchase condoms ($p = .046$), have fewer sexual partners ($p = .046$), and use condoms more frequently ($p = .048$). No differences were found, however, in their frequency of intercourse or the frequency with which they used drugs and alcohol prior to intercourse.

Summary

The field study showed that the 14-session *Get Real About AIDS®* program was effective in changing students' HIV-related intentions and behaviors that put youths at risk for HIV infection. Six months following the intervention, sexually active program participants had fewer sexual partners, purchased and used condoms more frequently, intended to engage in sex less frequently, and planned to use condoms when they did. However, the onset of sexual activity was not affected by the program in any measurable way. Additionally, although no changes were observed in participants' use of IV drugs, the researchers suggested that the numbers of IV drug–using students were so small that any effect would be hard to detect.

In interpreting their results, the evaluators cautioned that the students who were included in the final sample (e.g., those teens whose Time 1 and Time 2 surveys could be matched) showed lower HIV risk scores at the Time 1 assessment. Similarly, those students who dropped out of the program or the comparison group appeared to be at higher risk for HIV infection. Consequently, the results of this field study, and the effects of the *Get Real About AIDS®* program, might not hold for higher-risk groups of teens, along with those youths who have dropped out or are frequently absent from school.

AWARDS AND RECOGNITION

Get Real About AIDS® has been identified by the Centers for Disease Control and Prevention for inclusion in its Research-to-Classroom Project as a program with credible evidence of reducing sexual risk behaviors.

GET REAL ABOUT AIDS® IN THE COMMUNITY TODAY

In the past 3 years, *Get Real About AIDS*® has been implemented in communities in 3 states: Massachusetts, Arizona, and Ohio.

NOTE

1. A full set of program materials, including *a Get Real About AIDS*® *Kit* for grades 9–12, evaluation materials, and more, is available for purchase from Sociometrics at http://www.socio.com/pasha. htm.

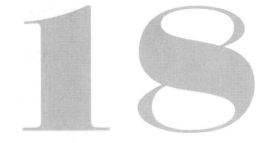

IMB: Information–Motivation–Behavioral Skills HIV Prevention Program

Diana Dull Akers

Original Program Developers and Evaluators

Jeffrey Fisher, PhD
   University of Connecticut
   Center for Health/HIV Intervention and Prevention
   Storrs, CT

William A. Fisher, PhD
   University of Western Ontario
   London, ON, Canada

Stephen J. Misovich, PhD
   University of Hartford
   Hartford, CT

Angela D. Bryan, PhD
   University of Colorado
   Boulder, CO

IMB: Information-Motivation-Behavioral Skills HIV Prevention Program was supported by a grant from the National Institute of Mental Health (#1R01 MH59473).

PROGRAM ABSTRACT

Summary

The goal of the *Information–Motivation–Behavioral Skills HIV Prevention Program (IMB Program)* is to reduce high school students' risk of HIV infection. Program objectives include positively influencing students' HIV prevention knowledge, attitudes, and norms; increasing students' levels of HIV prevention behavioral skills; and increasing students' levels of HIV preventive behavior. The intervention involves a four-session classroom component to be conducted by trained high school teachers. The *IMB Program* is based on the information, motivation, and behavioral skills (IMB) model of health behavior change, which assumes that information, motivation, and behavioral skills are the fundamental determinants of HIV preventive behavior.

An evaluation of the curriculum offered under three intervention delivery formats (classroom-based only, peer-based only, and combination classroom- and peer-based delivery) was conducted by the Center for Health/HIV Intervention and Prevention in 1999. Participants were 1,577 students in four inner-city high schools in Connecticut (61% African American; 28% Hispanic; 11% White, Mixed, or Other). The classroom-based HIV prevention education component effectively promoted risk-reduction behavior change in these urban high school settings at 1 year postintervention.

Focus

☐ Primary pregnancy prevention   ☐ Secondary pregnancy prevention   ☑ STI/HIV/AIDS prevention

Original Site

☑ School based   ☐ Community based   ☐ Clinic based

Suitable for Use In

The *IMB Program* is to be implemented by trained teachers in high school settings. The curriculum is also relevant for other adolescent groups and school settings.

Approach

- ☑ Abstinence
- ☑ Behavioral skills development
- ☐ Community outreach
- ☐ Contraceptive access
- ☑ Contraceptive education
- ☐ Life option enhancement
- ☑ Self-efficacy/self-esteem
- ☑ Sexuality/HIV/AIDS/STI education

Original Intervention Sample

Age, gender   The original intervention sample included 1,577 students in four inner-city schools in Connecticut. The sample was 37% male and 63% female. Participants ranged in age from 13 to 19; the mean age was 14.8 years.

Race/ethnicity   More than half of the participants (61%) were African American; 28% were Hispanic; and 11% classified their race as White, Mixed, or Other.

Program Components

- ☑ Adult involvement
- ☐ Case management
- ☑ Group discussion
- ☑ Lectures
- ☐ Peer counseling/instruction
- ☐ Public service announcements
- ☑ Role play
- ☑ Video
- ☐ Other

Program Length

This classroom-based intervention is implemented over four classroom periods. One period each is devoted to an information and behavioral skills component; two periods are devoted to a motivation component.

Staffing Requirements/Training

High school teachers administer the four-session, classroom-based intervention. You may choose to have one or more teachers offer the *IMB Program,* as your resources allow. All necessary training materials for the intervention are included in this replication kit.

BIBLIOGRAPHY

Fisher, J. D., & Fisher, W. A. (1992). Changing AIDS risk behavior. *Psychological Bulletin, 111,* 455–474.

Fisher, J. D., Fisher, W. A., Bryan, A. D., & Misovich, S. J. (2002). Information–motivation–behavioral skills model-based HIV risk behavior change intervention for inner city high school youth. *Health Psychology, 21*(2), 177–186.

Misovich, S. J. (2002). *Information–Motivation–Behavioral Skills HIV Prevention Program. Program Overview.* Manual produced as part of an overall program of research by J. D. Fisher, W. A. Fisher, S. J. Misovich, and A. D. Bryan, Storrs. University of Connecticut Center for Health/HIV Intervention and Prevention.

New References for the *IMB Program* Since the Release of the Replication Kit

Amico, K. R., Barta, W., Konkle-Parker, D. J., Fisher, J. D. Cornman, D. H., Shuper, P. A., et al. (2007, September). The information–motivation–behavioral skills model of ART adherence in a deep South HIV+ clinic sample. *AIDS and Behavior, 18.* Retrieved March 2008, from http://www.springerlink.com/content/M15446854070784.

THE PROGRAM

Program Rationale and History

In creating and evaluating the *IMB Program,* its developers were responding to several HIV concerns.[1] First, minority adolescents in inner-city areas are at a particularly high risk of HIV infection. Second, while research has shown schools to be efficient and accessible settings for HIV prevention programs, there have been few rigorous evaluations of HIV prevention interventions that have taken place in actual school settings, using existing teaching staff, with the target population of inner-city minority adolescents. As such, the developers of this program sought to create and evaluate a theory-driven, school-based HIV prevention intervention—one designed for inner-city minority adolescents and delivered in actual school settings.

To develop such a program, a multidisciplinary team of educators, psychologists, and public health professionals first conducted needs assessments in ethnically diverse urban high schools. Next, they developed an intervention framework based on the IMB model for changing HIV risk behavior (see below). Finally, they implemented the curriculum in several inner-city high schools in Connecticut during the 1997–98 school year and evaluated the results during the 1998–99 school year. The curriculum was presented in three formats, including a peer-based HIV prevention intervention, a classroom-based intervention, and a combination classroom-based and peer-based intervention. A fourth inner-city Connecticut high school served as a "standard of care" control group.

At the 1-year follow-up, there were significantly increased rates of condom use among sexually active participants in the classroom-based intervention, as compared to participants in the standard-of-care control group. The effects of the two interventions involving a peer-based component failed to be sustained at the 1-year follow-up.

Theoretical Framework

This intervention framework is based on the IMB model of health behavior change (J. Fisher & W. Fisher, 1992). This model assumes that in order to practice HIV preventive behavior, one must possess necessary levels of HIV prevention information, motivation, and behavioral skills. Over the course of the intervention, students' potential deficits in each of these essential HIV prevention elements are identified and corrected through compelling activities and structured discussions.

Program Overview

The *IMB Program* is designed to make optimal use of classroom instruction to promote HIV prevention among adolescents.

Trained high school teachers conducted the classroom-based component of this program, which involved discussions, videotapes, and associated activities to increase students' HIV prevention information, motivation, and behavioral skills.

Program Objectives

There are four main objectives for participants who complete the *IMB Program*. They are

- to increase students' knowledge regarding HIV/AIDS risk and to dispel commonly held myths (e.g., that unprotected sex is safe if one knows one's partner very well);
- to positively influence students' HIV prevention attitudes and norms;
- to increase students' levels of HIV prevention behavioral skills;
- to increase safer sexual practices among students, including abstinence and consistent, correct use of condoms.

Program Schedule

In the original implementation, the *IMB Program* was conducted over four consecutive class periods, preferably over the course of 1 week. The program schedule is listed below.

Day 1: Information Component. *Purpose:* To increase students' HIV prevention information, in part, by challenging and debunking students' misconceptions about HIV transmission and prevention.

Activities: Students viewed the video *Knowing the Facts: Preventing Infection* and completed in-class activities, discussion, and homework assignments associated with the video. *Knowing the Facts* addressed the information component of the HIV prevention intervention. Through concrete examples, the video allowed students to translate the information provided into preventive behaviors in their social environment. *Knowing the Facts* also corrected HIV prevention misinformation widely held by students, such as the belief that known partners were safe partners or that attractive people and similar others were unlikely to be HIV-positive.

Days 2 and 3: Motivation Component. *Purpose:* To motivate students to practice HIV preventive behaviors, such as abstinence or safer sex, by helping them realize that HIV may be a danger for them personally.

Activities: Students viewed the video *Just Like Me: Talking About AIDS* and participated in a classroom discussion focusing on how beliefs and choices led to HIV infection among the interviewees depicted in the video. *Just Like Me* motivated adolescents to practice HIV prevention by showing how HIV can threaten their own lives. The video presented interviews with an ethnically diverse group of six young adults who had believed they were invulnerable to HIV. Each interviewee had engaged in risky behaviors common to adolescents, and as a result, they had become infected with HIV as teenagers. Most had become infected through unprotected sex with a close relationship partner, and they discussed the common misconception that a close partner could never be a source of HIV risk. The negative physical, psychological, and social effects of being HIV-positive or having AIDS were presented in detail and were made relevant to the day-to-day existence of adolescents. Finally, the interviewees emphasized strongly and effectively the importance of protecting oneself from HIV, either by abstaining from sexual intercourse or by consistently and correctly using condoms. (Note: Several of the interviewees in the video died before production of the video was complete. Footage from their funerals is included in the video.)

Day 4: Behavioral Skills Component. *Purpose:* To teach youths behavioral skills for HIV prevention, such as negotiating abstinence and/or correct condom use with a partner.

Activities: Students viewed the video *Stakes Are High: Asserting Yourself* and participated in classroom discussion and activities related to the video's key themes. This video was designed to help adolescents develop the behavioral skills they needed to consistently protect themselves from HIV risk. The video featured a culturally diverse group of adolescents modeling HIV prevention behaviors in an engaging and humorous fashion. In brief vignettes that followed romantic story lines, couples were shown successfully negotiating abstinence and exiting unsafe situations. For couples who decided they were ready to initiate sexual intercourse, the behaviors of purchasing condoms and negotiating their consistent use were depicted.

Program Implementation

Program Planning and Teacher Orientation Activities

Teachers should schedule one or more program orientation meetings at least a month prior to implementing the *IMB Program.*[2] In addition to familiarizing themselves with the content, format, and activities of the curriculum, teachers may want to discuss program implementation issues and strategies relevant to their setting and target audience.

Running the Classroom-Based Component of the Program

The classroom-based component of the *IMB Program* is offered over the course of four classroom sessions. No later than 1 week before the first classroom session, teachers should have

- participated in orientation meetings to review all *IMB Program* materials and brainstormed curriculum delivery efforts;
- created a program calendar, noting the time and dates for the delivery of the four classroom sessions, as well as any scheduled teacher meetings;
- created a sufficient number of Student Workbooks (using the Student Workbook photocopy master included in the replication kit);
- prepared a handout listing the addresses and telephone numbers of nearby HIV-testing facilities and locations where students could obtain condoms;
- obtained required equipment and supplies for the four class sessions (e.g., index cards, condoms, markers, audiovisual equipment, etc.);
- run a last-minute check to ensure proper functioning of the television and VCR/DVD player used to show the three program videos.

No later than 1 day before leading each class session, *IMB Program* teachers should ensure that they understand the

- background and learning objectives for each session;
- procedures for conducting each session;
- time schedule for completing each session's exercises, videos, and discussions;
- materials needed for each session;
- optional "scripts" for each session;
- class exercises, activities, and discussion questions for each session.

PROGRAM EVALUATION

The Original Evaluation

Study Design

The original evaluation study of the *IMB Program* used a quasi-experimental, non-equivalent control group design with four inner-city high schools in Connecticut. The high schools were similar in terms of being located in a major inner-city area, having predominantly minority students, and having approximately equal numbers of students.

In accord with the IMB model, prior to the design of the intervention, elicitation research was first conducted with representative subsamples of the target population to empirically identify critical HIV prevention information, motivation, behavioral skills, and behavior deficits and assets in this population.

Following the design of the intervention, each of the four participating schools was assigned to a particular treatment condition:

Classroom-based intervention: In one high school, regular classroom teachers delivered the *IMB Program* intervention to students. The intervention consisted of HIV prevention information, motivation, and behavioral skills content, targeted to address students' empirically identified deficits in these areas. Teachers were trained to deliver the program content in weekend workshops prior to the delivery of the intervention.

Peer-based intervention: A second high school delivered a peer-based intervention, where selected students interacted with friends and acquaintances outside classroom settings to address HIV prevention information, motivation, and behavioral skills deficits identified in the target population. Peer educators were trained to deliver the program content in weekend workshops prior to the delivery of the intervention.

Combination classroom/peer-based intervention: A third high school offered a simultaneously delivered classroom-based and peer-based intervention.

Comparison group: A fourth high school served as a "standard of care" comparison group. They were exposed to their school's standard HIV/AIDS curriculum, known as "AIDS Week," which included health classes offering HIV prevention information.

Researchers conducted pre-, post-, and follow-up tests 3 months and 1 year after the end of the intervention to assess the effects of the intervention.

Study Population

The participants in this study were 1,577 students located in four inner-city schools. Participants were 37% male and 63% female and ranged in age from 13–19 years, with a mean age of 14.8 years. The racial/ethnic breakdown of the group was 61% African American, 28% Hispanic, and 11% White or Other. At the time of the pretest, the majority of boys in the study (63%) reported being sexually active, whereas only 41% of the girls reported the same.

The mean age of all sexually active individuals was 14.92 years, whereas "never sexually active" individuals had a mean age of 14.63 years. While all four schools had predominantly minority students, there were significant differences in age, racial and ethnic makeup, and gender. The researchers statistically adjusted for all measured variables in which the schools differed.

Evaluation Questions and Outcome Measures

The researchers sought to assess the impact of the intervention on HIV prevention information, motivation, behavioral skills, and behavior. Self-administered measures of these constructs based on extensive earlier research were used.

- To measure participants' *levels of HIV prevention information*, researchers used a 23-item Likert-type instrument that focused on topics such as information about HIV transmission and prevention, correct condom storage, and whether condoms are necessary with a steady partner.
- To assess participants' *attitudes toward HIV prevention*, researchers used four 5-point Likert-type items assessing favorable to unfavorable evaluations of personally performing four HIV preventive behaviors (obtaining condoms, carrying condoms, telling a partner to use condoms, and using condoms).
- Participants' level of *HIV prevention motivation* was a function of attitudes, norms, and intentions.
- To assess participants' *intentions to perform HIV preventive behaviors,* researchers used four 5-point Likert-type items assessing behavioral intentions to engage in these HIV prevention behaviors.
- To assess participants' *HIV prevention behavioral skills*, researchers used five 5-point Likert-type items designed to assess perceptions of the difficulty or ease with which one could perform the four critical HIV preventive behaviors, as well as using condoms while under the influence of drugs or alcohol.

Evaluation Results

The results of the study demonstrate that a conceptually based, empirically targeted HIV prevention intervention delivered in inner-city high school classrooms to minority students had significant effects on precursors of HIV preventive behavior at intervention posttest. Additionally, significant effects on HIV preventive behavior (specifically, condom use during sexual intercourse) were noted over a 1-year follow-up period.[3]

The researchers note the lack of significant HIV prevention intervention effects at the 1-year follow-up in all conditions that involved a peer-influence component, a finding that at first seems perplexing. However, this finding mirrors other research showing that when well-trained and supervised peers are directly involved in attempts at changing others' behaviors, their influence may initially be strong and positive, but may wane over time due to a variety of factors. These can include the departure of influential peers from the scene, the loss of social influence as students' social referent groups change over time, and the potentially negative influence of peers who are seen or believed to be enacting risky behavior themselves or tolerating it in others. The researchers believe that future intervention designs that incorporate long-term supervision of peer educators may moderate these effects.

THE *IMB PROGRAM* IN THE COMMUNITY TODAY

In the past 3 years, the *IMB Program* has been implemented in one community in Rhode Island. It has also been implemented in Hong Kong.

NOTES

1. A full set of program materials, including teacher's manual, student workbook, videos, flash cards, evaluation materials, and more, is available for purchase from Sociometrics at http://www.socio.com/pasha.htm.

2. In the original study, teachers were trained to deliver the program content in weekend workshops prior to the delivery of the intervention. Your program may opt to host a similar weekend workshop or a series of orientation/training meetings held at times that are acceptable to all teachers.

3. *At the 1-month follow-up:* Participants in the intervention exhibited a significantly greater increase in HIV knowledge than members of the standard-of-care control group ($p < .001$). For sexually inexperienced participants, exposure to the classroom intervention resulted in marginal improvement in behavioral skills, whereas exposure to the combined intervention resulted in significant improvement in attitudes, norms, HIV prevention intentions, and behavioral skills, relative to standard-of-care controls. The combined intervention had similar significant positive effects on the behavioral skills of sexually experienced participants.

   At the 3-month follow-up: There were significant increases in condom use in the combined intervention ($p < .04$) and in the peer intervention ($p < .05$) compared with standard-of-care controls.

   At the 1-year follow-up: The classroom-based intervention resulted in significant increased condom use ($p < .01$) for the year following completion of the intervention, in comparison with controls. For the year following completion of the intervention, effects of the combined intervention and the peer intervention were no longer in evidence.

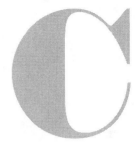

Programs Designed for Young Women

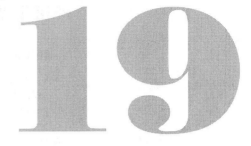

FOCUS: Preventing Sexually Transmitted Infections and Unwanted Pregnancies Among Young Women

Tabitha A. Benner

Original Program Developers and Evaluators

Cherrie Boyer, PhD
Mary-Ann Shafer, MD
Lance Pollack, PhD
Kelli Betsinger, BA
Y. Jason Chang, MS
Julius Schachter, PhD
   University of California, San Francisco, CA

Heidi Kraft, PhD
   Naval Health Research Center, San Diego, CA

Richard Shaffer, PhD
Stephanie Brodine, MD
   Naval Health Research Center, San Diego, CA
   San Diego State University, San Diego, CA

FOCUS was supported by grants from the Department of Defense under the Women's Health Initiative (#DAMD17–95-C-5077) and Leadership Education in Adolescent Health (LEAH), Maternal and Child Health Bureau (#MCH000978).

PROGRAM ABSTRACT

Summary

FOCUS is a four-session cognitive-behavioral group intervention that addresses preventing sexually transmitted infections (STIs) and unintended pregnancies. The program was originally developed for delivery to young women U.S. Marine Corps recruits.

Following a baseline survey and self-administered vaginal swab (for STIs), 2,157 women participants were randomized into either the experimental group (n = 1,062) or the control group (n = 1,095) during their 1st week of recruit training. Baseline pregnancy screening was deemed unnecessary as all women are screened by the Marines prior to beginning recruit training. Both experimental and control groups received interventions of four 2-hour sessions, delivered during the 1st, 2nd, 4th and 12th weeks of recruit training.

Of the original sample, 88.8% (n = 1,916) completed the intervention *and* graduated from the 13-week recruit training (more than 240 were discharged prior to completing the recruit training and were lost to the intervention). At first follow-up, approximately 1 month after completing the intervention, 80.8% (n = 1,743) of the original sample participated. At second follow-up, approximately 14 months after the intervention, 64% (n = 1,381) of the original sample took part.

The evaluation results revealed that a higher proportion of the control group had a postintervention STI or unintended pregnancy (odds ratio [OR] = 1.41, 95% confidence interval [CI] = 1.01–1.98). Among participants who had no history of STIs or pregnancy, but who engaged in risky sexual behaviors just before recruit training, the control group was more likely to acquire a postintervention STI (OR = 2.05, CI = 1.74–4.08), and have had multiple sexual partners (OR = 1.87, CI = 1.01–3.47) postintervention.

Focus

☑ Primary pregnancy prevention ☐ Secondary pregnancy prevention ☑ STI/HIV/AIDS prevention

Original Site

☐ School based ☑ Community based ☐ Clinic based

Suitable for Use In

FOCUS is suitable for use in group or class settings in clinics, community-based organizations, or schools/colleges. *It should be noted, however, that the subject matter is mature and in some cases quite graphic in nature and may not be appropriate for participants under the age of 16.*

Approach

- ☐ Abstinence
- ☑ Behavioral skills development
- ☐ Community outreach
- ☐ Contraceptive access
- ☑ Contraceptive education
- ☐ Life option enhancement
- ☑ Self-efficacy/self-esteem
- ☑ Sexuality/HIV/AIDS/STI education

Original Intervention Sample

Age, gender   The original intervention sample included 2,157 young women, aged 17 or older; approximately 90% of the sample was 22 or younger.

Race/ethnicity   More than half of the participants (56%) were White, 19.7% were Latina, 16.1% were African American, and about 5% were Other.

Program Components

- ■ ☐ Adult involvement
- ■ ☐ Case management
- ■ ☑ Group discussion
- ■ ☑ Lectures
- ■ ☐ Peer counseling/instruction
- ■ ☐ Public service announcements
- ■ ☑ Role play
- ■ ☑ Video
- ■ ☑ Other: PowerPoint slide presentations

Program Length

This four-session intervention was implemented in 2-hour segments. However, each segment is divided into several discrete modules, allowing implementation in shorter segments if necessary.

Staffing Requirements/Training

In the original implementation of *FOCUS*, the intervention was facilitated by two research assistants with groups of 20–25 participants. In your milieu, you may wish to consider conducting the intervention with health educators or other female facilitators who are both familiar and comfortable with the mature subject matter.

BIBLIOGRAPHY

Boyer, C. B., Shafer, M.-A., Shaffer, R. A., Brodine, S. K., Pollack, L. M., Betsinger, K., et al. (2005). Evaluation of a cognitive-behavioral, group, randomized controlled intervention trial to prevent sexually transmitted infections and unintended pregnancies in young women. *Preventive Medicine, 40*, 420–431.

Related References by the Developers of *FOCUS*

Boyer, C. B., Shafer, M. A., Shaffer R. A., Brodine, S. K., Ito, S. I., Yniguez, D. L., Benas, D. M., & Schachter, J. (2001). Prevention of sexually transmitted diseases and HIV in young military men: Evaluation of a cognitive-behavioral skills-building intervention. *Sexually Transmitted Diseases, 28*(6), 349–355.

Sieverding, J., Boyer, C. B., Siller, J., Gallaread, A., Krone, M., & Chang, Y. J. (2005). Youth united through health education: Building capacity through a community collaborative intervention to prevent HIV/STD in adolescents residing in a high STD prevalent neighborhood. *AIDS Education & Prevention, 17*(4), 375–385.

THE PROGRAM

Program Rationale and History

Of the estimated 15 million new cases of STIs diagnosed annually, approximately one-quarter of them are among young people aged 15–24.[1] Although adolescents have a lower rate of contracting HIV/AIDS than adults, the developers of *FOCUS* hypothesized that by reducing the prevalence of STIs among young, sexually active women in the 15–24 age group, the higher HIV infection rates in older age groups could also be reduced. Since the release of this replication kit in 2005, the CDC estimates that the number of new STI cases in the United States has risen to 19 million per year (2005 STI surveillance data), and that nearly half of the diagnosed cases are among young people aged 15–24. In addition, pregnancies and births among teens aged 15–19 decreased slightly (also 2005 data), while births among young women ages 20–24 increased slightly.

Unintended pregnancies are also prevalent among younger women. Studies conducted during the 1990s revealed that approximately 49% of pregnancies among adolescent and young adult women were unintended. Incidence data gathered by the U.S. military revealed that unintended pregnancies were 60%–80% higher among adolescent recruits than their civilian counterparts.

While research has shown that theory-based STI and HIV prevention interventions can be effective, prior to the current study no research had been conducted that focused on preventing STIs and unintended pregnancies simultaneously. Military recruit training, with follow-up during the first year of military service, provided a well-defined, national, nonclinic sample of healthy young women with whom to evaluate the effectiveness of a cognitive-behavioral intervention to prevent both STIs and unintended pregnancies.

FOCUS (or its control equivalent) was presented to 2,157 Marine Corps recruits who were voluntarily randomized into either the experimental group ($n = 1,062$) or control group ($n = 1,095$). Both interventions were delivered over the 12-month period of June 1999 to June 2000, during the 1st, 2nd, 4th, and 12th weeks of recruit training (any women dismissed from Marine recruit training prior to week 12 were lost to the intervention). The experimental intervention sought to reduce postintervention STIs and unintended pregnancies, and the number of self-reported casual partners, multiple partners, and other risky sexual behaviors. The control intervention sought to improve participants' physical performance, reduce their risk of training injuries, and examine the risks and prevention of cervical and breast cancers in young women. Both interventions consisted of four 2-hour interactive sessions.

The research team used the Marine Corps' "lead" and "follow" platoon designations when randomly assigning participant groups to either the control or experimental condition. Platoons were used as the unit of randomization for this study. The random number tables used to determine the group assignations were established before the start of the study. Platoons were informed of their group assignment at the first intervention session, after enrollment and baseline assessment were completed. Each session was cofacilitated by two trained civilian research assistants. Each group had 20–25 participants.

Follow-ups were conducted after the recruits returned from their first leave (average 34.5 days after graduating from the 13-week recruit training) and during their first duty assignment (average 12.8 months after baseline).

Theoretical Framework

The primary theoretical underpinning of the intervention is a cognitive-behavioral approach, focusing on elements of the information–motivation–behavioral skills model (IMB). Cognitive-behavioral therapy seeks to change a person's thinking and behaviors by educating the person and reinforcing positive experiences that will lead to fundamental changes in the way that person behaves. IMB posits that information is a prerequisite to risk-reduction behavior; motivation to change those behaviors determines prevention behaviors, and behavioral skills affect whether a knowledgeable, motivated individual will be able to change his or her behavior.

Program Overview

FOCUS was an 8-hour intervention consisting of four 2-hour sessions. The sessions were broken down into a varying number of discrete modules. Although there were interactive activities (e.g., role-play exercises, visualizations, etc.), the modules were constructed primarily around the PowerPoint slide sets, accompanied by lecture and augmented with discussion and other activities.

Program Design

The program developers set specific goals for each session:

Session 1: Increase knowledge about unintended pregnancies and STIs including HIV/AIDS. Modify values, beliefs, and attitudes that impact sexual behavior.

Session 2: Increase knowledge about hormonal and barrier contraceptives. Build communication skills to prevent risky sexual behaviors and increase condom use.

Session 3: Increase knowledge about the signs, symptoms, and consequences of STIs/HIV/AIDS. Increase knowledge about the transmission and prevention of STIs/HIV. Build communication skills to prevent STIs/HIV.

Session 4: Modify attitudes about the effects of alcohol and its relationship to sexual risk behaviors. Build refusal communication skills. Build condom use skills. Increase awareness about how life choices can impact decision making and health.

In order to accomplish these goals, each session had specific educational objectives.

Session 1

Session Objectives

1. Increase participants' awareness of how their values and attitudes shape their views of themselves as sexual beings.
2. Evaluate how participants' values impact their decisions about unplanned pregnancies and STIs.
3. Educate participants about the risks associated with unplanned pregnancies and STIs.
4. Provide basic facts on female and male reproductive anatomy and physiology.
5. Assist participants in developing and articulating their career and/or life goals.
6. Examine how reproductive health behaviors may impact participants' goals.

Objectives Into Action

The first session began with an ice-breaker values exercise in which participants examined their awareness of their own values and attitudes about themselves as women and as sexual beings. Three slide sets and a DVD followed, providing fundamental information on women's reproductive health care, men's risk for STIs versus women's risk for STIs (and what that difference could mean to a woman who acquired one or more STIs), and the basics of an annual gynecological exam. The DVD *The Basics of Women's Reproductive Health Care* introduced many topics that were covered in greater depth later in the intervention. To conclude the session, participants completed a "life goals" worksheet in which they explored their 2- and 5-year goals, as well as thoughts on future parenting.

Session 2

Session Objectives

1. Provide historical overview of contraceptive methods.
2. Discuss factors that influence women's decisions about contraceptive use/nonuse.
3. Discuss the pros and cons of various contraceptive methods.
4. Increase participants' awareness of the impacts that unplanned pregnancies may have on one's personal life, education, and career.
5. Examine the range of options available in the event of an unplanned pregnancy and sources of social support.
6. Build communication skills regarding sexual behavior and contraceptive use with a sexual partner.
7. Discuss participants' feelings and attitudes about contraceptive use, and communication about those topics with sexual partners.

Objectives Into Action

Following a review of the first session and a brief overview of the second, this session moved into slide sets. "Introduction to Contraception" was first, followed by "Hormonal Contraceptive Methods." Participants then engaged in a visualization exercise in which they imagined themselves going to a doctor or clinic for a pregnancy test.

Before getting their test results, they viewed another slide set, "Barrier and Other Contraceptive Methods." The visualization exercise then resumed. Pieces of candy (such as butterscotch and peppermint) determined the outcome of the pregnancy test. The "Pregnancy Options and Social Support" slide set examined a range of possibilities for a newly pregnant woman to consider.

Participants then approached the topic of communication regarding sexual behavior and contraceptive use with their sexual partners, first through a role-play activity and then in a small-group discussion.

Session 3

Session Objectives

1. Describe the risks and transmission of STIs/HIV.
2. Discuss risky sexual practices.
3. Have participants assess their own STI/HIV acquisition risk.
4. Increase participants' awareness of how assumptions about a potential sexual partner can influence their risk perceptions.
5. Describe the signs, symptoms, and consequences of STIs/HIV/AIDS.
6. Build skills to communicate with potential partners.
7. Discuss how HIV is a reality in the community.
8. Examine the impact of HIV on those who are infected with HIV and on their friends and families.

Objectives Into Action

The first slide set of this session examined STI transmission and strategies for safer sex, including sexual activities ranging from no risk to high risk. The group then participated in a personal risk assessment activity.

The next slide set, "STI/HIV/AIDS Signs, Symptoms & Consequences," contained photographic images that were quite graphic in nature. These were clinical photographs of what to look for and what symptoms might look like for a man or a woman. The session concluded with the *In Our Own Words* DVD in which five ethnically diverse HIV-positive young people talked candidly about their lives and the prospects for their future.

Session 4

Session Objectives

1. Describe the effects of alcohol use.
2. Simulate social and emotional challenges women face early in their careers.
3. Describe the steps required for proper condom use.
4. Examine the barriers to consistent condom use.
5. Provide an opportunity for participants to practice condom-use skills.
6. Build communication skills to enable participants to leave risky sexual situations.
7. Discuss the appropriate time to seek reproductive health care.
8. Discuss barriers and benefits to seeking reproductive health care.

Objectives Into Action

The "Overview of Alcohol Effects and Use" slide set introduced and explored the ways alcohol affects people. The slide set also addressed some of the reasons people drink, drinking patterns, blood alcohol levels, and fetal alcohol syndrome. The DVD *Good to Go* followed the stories of four fictional women Marine recruits who enter the Marines Corps at different stages in their sexual lives. Several of the intervention's themes were woven into this 20-minute DVD.

Participants then engaged in condom-use practice and a condom relay game. A role-play activity delved into the communication skills that might be needed in order to remove oneself from a risky situation. The final slide set addressed access to health care, particularly when relocating to a new job or school.

Program Implementation

Each of the four sessions is divided into several modules. If delivering the intervention in 2-hour segments is unsuitable for your setting, you may wish to divide the established sessions into shorter minisessions. The modules provide natural topical divisions should you need to do this.

PROGRAM EVALUATION

The Original Evaluation

Study Design

The randomized, controlled, behavioral intervention trial of the *FOCUS* program was conducted between 1999 and 2000, when all female Marine Corps recruits (n = 2,288) were approached for voluntary enrollment in the program. Of these young women, 2,157 (94.3%) agreed to participate in the study; 1,062 (49%) were assigned to the experimental condition, and 1,095 (51%) were assigned to the control condition. Those agreeing to participate provided written informed consent.

During a typical 13-week Marine Corps recruit training cycle, two platoons consisting of 50–75 women are formed for training purposes. Platoons are designated by the training command as "lead" and "follow" platoons. The research team used this natural grouping to randomly assign "lead" and "follow" platoons to either the experimental or control group, using a random numbers table that was established before the start of the study. Platoons were informed of their group assignment at the first intervention session, after formal study enrollment and the administration of the baseline assessment and vaginal swabs.

Follow-up instruments were completed at approximately 4 months postbaseline (after their first 3-week leave following completion of recruit training) and approximately 14 months postbaseline.

Study Population

All study participants were female. Most (55.9%) self-identified as White; 19.7% were Latina; 16.1% were African American; 3.1% were Asian/Pacific Islander; 2.5% were Native American; and 2.6% were Mixed or Other. Slightly more than 90% of the sample population was 21 years of age or younger, with over 50% being 17 or 18 years old.

At baseline, 74.6% held a high school diploma or a GED. Most participants were single (93.2%), and 12% had previously had an STI. Less than a quarter of the participants (21.6%) reported using condoms at every sexual encounter. More than 65% reported having had more than one casual sexual partner.

Evaluation Questions and Outcome Measures

Self-administered paper-and-pencil questionnaires assessed behavioral risk factors as well as demographic markers. Participants' sexual risk in the 3-month period before entry into recruit training included the total number of sexual partners, the number of casual partners, frequency of condom use, and frequency of sexual intercourse while under the influence of alcohol or other substances. Questions on alcohol and other substance use covered the month before recruit training. Clinical risk factors included the participants' history of pregnancies and STIs (self-reported).

In addition to the paper-and-pencil questionnaire, laboratory-verified test results for chlamydia, gonorrhea, trichomoniasis, and pregnancy were obtained for each participant. These test results were gathered as part of a reproductive health examination required of all female Marine recruits (independent of this study) and involved endocervical specimens, first morning urine samples, and a self-administered vaginal swab. (Where logistically possible, participants provided urine samples and self-administered vaginal swabs for both follow-ups; however, since the endocervical specimens could be collected only during a pelvic examination, this step was excluded from both follow-up assessments.)

Evaluation Results

Postintervention STIs or Unintended Pregnancies

When postintervention STIs and unintended pregnancies were combined into a single outcome variable, a significant effect for the group was observed ($p = .043$). A significantly higher proportion of the control group (23.9%) than the experimental group (17.9%) tested positive for either an STI or an unintended pregnancy (OR = 1.41, 95% CI = 1.01–1.98).

Postintervention STIs

Among study participants who had no preintervention history of STIs or pregnancy, but who reported having engaged in risky sexual behaviors in the month before starting recruit training, the control group was significantly more likely (21.8%) than the experimental group (8.0%) to acquire a postintervention STI (OR = 3.25, 95% CI = 1.74–6.03).

Postintervention Multiple Sex Partners and Casual Sex Partners

Among study participants who reported not being sexually experienced at baseline, control group participants were significantly more likely than experimental group participants to report having multiple sexual partners postintervention (OR = 1.87, 95% CI = 1.01-3.47). Also among sexually inexperienced participants (at baseline), control group participants were significantly more likely to report having at least one casual sex partner during the follow-up period (OR = 2.05, 95% CI = 1.04–4.08).

Summary

Overall, the intervention was effective in reducing the number of unplanned pregnancies and in reducing STI transmission among the women in the intervention group as compared with their control group counterparts. Intervention participants were also less likely to report having either multiple or casual sex partners.

FOCUS IN THE COMMUNITY TODAY

Since the release of the replication kit in 2006, *FOCUS* has been implemented in Maryland.

NOTE

1. A full set of program materials, including a program guide, DVDs, CD-ROM with PowerPoint slides, brochures, evaluation materials, and more, is available for purchase from Sociometrics at http://www.socio.com/pasha.htm.

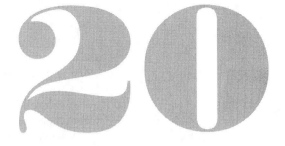

What Could You Do?: Interactive Video Intervention to Reduce Adolescent Females' STI Risk

Tabitha A. Benner

Original Program Developers and Evaluators

Julie Downs, PhD
Wändi Bruine de Bruin, PhD
Claire Palmgren
Baruch Fischhoff, PhD
   Carnegie Mellon University, Pittsburgh, PA

Pamela Murray, MD, MPH
   Children's Hospital of Pittsburgh, PA

Joyce Penrose, DPH, RN-C
   Slippery Rock University of Pennsylvania
   Slippery Rock, PA

PROGRAM ABSTRACT

Summary

What Could You Do? was developed to provide a cost-effective method of delivering a sexually transmitted infection (STI), risk-reduction intervention for adolescent

What Could You Do? was supported by a grant from the National Institute of Allergies and Infectious Diseases (IU19 AI 38513).

girls. The interactive video intervention aims to increase knowledge of STIs, decrease sexual risk behaviors, and decrease STI acquisition.

Participants were recruited from four health care sites in the urban Pittsburgh area: the adolescent medicine clinic of a children's hospital, two community health centers, and a women's teaching hospital. The young women participating in the study were all between 14 and 18 years old and had engaged in heterosexual vaginal sex in the 6 months prior to the study. Written informed consent was obtained from all participants or from their parents/guardians for participants under 18.

Following the completion of baseline measures and a self-administered vaginal swab, participants were randomly assigned to one of three conditions: (a) interactive video (experimental condition), (b) content-matched control condition (a 127-page book containing all of the content of the interactive video), or (c) topic-matched control condition (23 commercially available brochures, with content closely matching that of the video and book). Booster sessions followed at 1, 3, and 6 months after the initial intervention.

At all follow-up points, the participants in all three conditions increased their STI knowledge, both general and specific. Participants in the video condition were more likely than their control condition counterparts to have been completely abstinent in the time from baseline to the 3-month follow-up (odds ratio [OR] = 2.5, $p = .027$). This pattern diminished between the 3-month and 6-month visits (OR = 1.45, $p = .344$). Although there were no significant differences in condom use among the conditions, there was a trend toward more condom use and fewer condom failures among the participants of the video condition.

At the 6-month follow-up, participants in the control conditions were nearly twice as likely as video condition participants to have been diagnosed with an STI (OR = 2.79, $p = .05$). This pattern held for all nine reported diseases.

Focus

☐ Primary pregnancy prevention   ☐ Secondary pregnancy prevention   ☑ STI/HIV/AIDS prevention

Original Site

☐ School based   ☐ Community based   ☑ Clinic based

Suitable for Use In

What Could You Do? is suitable for use in physician and clinic offices. It may be suitable for use in schools provided there is privacy for the viewer (some of the material is graphic in nature).

Approach

- ■ ☐ Abstinence
- ■ ☑ Behavioral skills development
- ■ ☐ Community outreach
- ■ ☐ Contraceptive access
- ■ ☐ Contraceptive education
- ■ ☐ Life option enhancement
- ■ ☑ Self-efficacy/self-esteem
- ■ ☑ Sexuality/HIV/AIDS/STI education

Original Intervention Sample

Age, gender   The original intervention sample consisted of 300 females, aged 14–18.

Race/ethnicity   Most participants (75%) self-identified as African American, with 15% White and 10% Other or Mixed race.

Program Components

- ■ ☐ Adult involvement
- ■ ☐ Case management
- ■ ☐ Group discussion
- ■ ☐ Lectures
- ■ ☐ Peer counseling/instruction
- ■ ☐ Public service announcements
- ■ ☐ Role play
- ■ ☑ Video
- ■ ☑ Other: Cognitive rehearsal

Program Length

Given the interactive nature of the video, the amount of time a viewer spends with it will depend largely on the selections she makes at any of the several decision points. The "structured" version of the DVD permits the viewer to follow a single story line, whereas the "flexible" version allows the viewer to skip or review sections at will. In the original evaluation study of *What Could You Do?*, girls spent an average of 45 minutes viewing the interactive video.

Staffing Requirements/Training

No staffing or training is required for the interactive video. Only a television and DVD player, or personal-sized DVD player are needed. (Note: Although the DVD can be viewed on a computer, it functions more smoothly when viewed with a DVD player.) Headphones, for privacy, are optional.

BIBLIOGRAPHY

Downs, J. S., Murray, P. J., Bruine de Bruin, W., Penrose, J., Palmgren, C., & Fischhoff, B. (2004). Interactive video behavioral intervention to reduce adolescent females' STI risk: A randomized controlled trial. *Social Science & Medicine, 59,* 1561–1572.

Related References by the Developers of *What Could You Do?*

Downs, J. S., Murray, P. J., Bruine de Bruin, W., & Fischhoff, B. (2006). Specific STI knowledge may be acquired too late. *Journal of Adolescent Health, 38*(1), 65–67.

THE PROGRAM

Program Rationale and History

Historically, adolescent girls have faced special risk factors for STI acquisition, including age-related physiological vulnerability, limited disease knowledge, and frequent condom failures.[1] In addition, young women have often felt that they had little control over sexual situations, thereby limiting their ability to act on their knowledge.

For many adolescents, STI prevention has required increased awareness, knowledge, and behavioral change. While several facilitator-led group interventions had demonstrated effectiveness for behavioral change, in some situations those interventions have proven too costly for implementation in patient care or community-based sites. The current study evaluated the effectiveness of an interactive video intervention as compared to both a content-matched control, offering the material in book form, and a topic-matched control using commercially available brochures.

In developing the *What Could You Do?* intervention, the research team sought an alternative means of delivering an effective STI risk-reduction program to young women in a cost-effective format. *What Could You Do?* was designed to deliver in-depth information on STIs, STI prevention, condom use, and condom negotiation in an individualized interactive video format. The advent of user-friendly media technology made it possible for a stand-alone video intervention to deliver a high-quality program in any setting where a television and DVD player could be set up. Such a program eliminated the constraints and logistics of the facilitator-led group model, enabling easier implementation, reduced costs, and improved program fidelity.

In order to develop relevant content, the research team conducted nearly 50 loosely structured interviews, using open-ended questions. The interviews revealed four general trends:

1. Respondents seldom described decision making regarding sexual behavior. Instead, they viewed those behaviors arising from influences beyond their control.
2. Many did not fully understand the concept of risk reduction, dismissing condoms, for example, because they were not 100% effective at pregnancy prevention.
3. Their lack of knowledge of overall reproductive health caused them to use terms, such as *safe sex*, without fully understanding the terms' meanings.
4. They knew little about STIs other than HIV/AIDS, many believing that an annual pap smear provided the test for all STIs.

Various iterations of the intervention were pilot tested to ensure that the final version would address realistic, culturally appropriate, relevant, and useful information to help young women make more informed decisions and better negotiate and implement related risk-reduction strategies.

Theoretical Framework

The developers relied on the mental models approach in developing *What Could You Do?* This approach is theoretically grounded in behavioral research and methodologically grounded in qualitative research. Mental models are representations in the mind of real or imaginary situations—small-scale models of reality used to anticipate events. Mental models can be constructed from perception, imagination, or comprehension. They underlie visual images, but they can also be abstract, representing situations that cannot be visualized. Each mental model represents a possibility. The approach has been used to help people acquire and apply knowledge about a broad spectrum of risks.

Program Overview

As originally designed, *What Could You Do?* offered young women the opportunity to view and/or review (in the case of the "flexible" format) STI risk-related scenarios relevant to them. The DVD was divided into three related story lines, each with a unique set of issues and possible outcomes. Brandi's story focused on reproductive health and STI knowledge. Keisha's and Caitlin's stories both focused on aspects of sexual situations.

In a separate risk-reduction segment, Brandi's older sister taught Brandi about condom use. Condom use was stressed throughout as having positive outcomes (pleasure, reassurance) rather than negative ones (suspicion, disease). Male characters pressed for unsafe sex; female characters modeled less risky behaviors.

In Keisha's and Caitlin's stories, the male narrator broke in at various choice points and asked, "What next?" This was followed by two or three possibilities for how the situation might develop, leading either toward or away from safer sex. If the viewer selected the least risky situation when asked to make a choice ("What could *you* do?"), the narrator later directed the viewer to the more risky options and took her through the potentially unsafe scenarios and their corresponding decision points. "You might think Keisha (or Caitlin) doesn't have any choices in this situation," he said. "But she does. What could you do? . . . Think about it, and practice it in your head." The video would then stop for 30 seconds to encourage cognitive rehearsal.

The video began with four friends gathering at the food court of a mall. After the characters and their corresponding STI-related risk issues were introduced, the viewer chose which character she would follow: Brandi, Keisha, or Caitlin.

Brandi

Brandi recently had unprotected sex with her boyfriend. Having experienced some unusual discharge, she went to see a gynecologist for a pelvic exam and STI tests. At the food court, she was still waiting to hear the results. She was nervous and admitted that she might have felt better if she just knew more about STIs. Ann, a nursing student also at the food court, offered to stop by later with her nursing school textbook so they could look things up together.

In this reproductive health and STI knowledge segment of the video, there were three primary vignettes:

1. Brandi and her doctor discussed the steps involved in a pelvic exam, including what to expect and which STI tests were or were not included as part of a standard annual exam.
2. Brandi and the doctor discussed the difference between viruses and bacteria, treatments, and how to prevent STIs.
3. At Brandi's house, Brandi and Ann (the nursing student) discussed acquiring and preventing STIs, and different types of sex and their risk levels. They focused on nine STIs in some depth (chlamydia, crabs, genital herpes, syphilis, gonorrhea, genital warts, hepatitis B, HIV, trichonomiasis), including symptoms and whether the STIs were viral or bacterial. There were also photographs of external symptoms to look for. (*Note:* Many of the pictures are graphic in nature.)

Keisha

Keisha and her boyfriend, Michael, had been together for a while but had not yet had sex. Michael invited her over to his place when no one would be home. Keisha had to decide what to do next. If she suggested inviting friends to join them, how would she handle Michael's reaction? What if she suggested going to a movie?

If the viewer selected the low-risk option(s), either those above or others that came up later, the narrator would take her through the higher risk options. For example, if the viewer decided that Keisha would go to Michael's place and stay in the living room listening to music, the narrator would return saying, "You selected the option of listening to music. What if Keisha had agreed to go to Michael's room?" The video would then take the viewer to the more risky scenarios, providing decision points (and cognitive rehearsal) for saying no to sex, negotiating condom use, and leaving the situation if no condoms were available or if Michael refused to use one.

Caitlin

Caitlin and Mark had met for the first time at a recent party, and they hit it off really well. As they sat on the couch in the living room, surrounded by friends, he began kissing her. She needed to decide what to do: ask him to stop or encourage him ("What next?").

If she encouraged him, she would be faced with decisions about going to another room to be alone with him, having sex with him, his refusing to use the condom she brought, and having sex without a condom. At each decision point, the viewer was asked about choices in the situation and what she could do if faced with a similar situation.

Tying It All Together

The girls reconvened in the food court to hear Brandi's test results. She and Ann shared what they learned about STIs and STI testing while reviewing the nursing textbook. Brandi offered to teach the other girls what her older sister taught her about putting a condom on a guy in a way that "he'll like it." The video then jumped to that vignette.

Brandi's older sister showed Brandi how to use a condom, using a cucumber as a penis proxy. Not only did the sister encourage Brandi to practice putting the condom on, but she told Brandi why doing it incorrectly could lead to breakage or other condom failure. They discussed carrying condoms (versus expecting the male partner to do so), opening the package so as not to rip it, unrolling the condom correctly with a reservoir tip, and removing the condom. They also discussed appropriate lubricants. Brandi's older sister acted as a role model who bought condoms, carried them, talked with her partner about them, and used them.

Program Implementation

Before implementing *What Could You Do?* in your setting, consider setting aside a private area for viewing the video, thereby enhancing the viewer's privacy. A set of headphones, while not required, will eliminate the sounds and discussions related to the video. Many of the photographs of STI symptoms shown in Brandi's story, and the corresponding dialogue, are quite graphic. No dedicated staff or facilitator is required.

PROGRAM EVALUATION

The Original Evaluation

Study Design

After completing the baseline measures, and providing a self-administered vaginal swab, 300 girls aged 14–18 were randomly assigned to one of three conditions. Girls randomized to the experimental condition viewed an interactive video that addressed sexual situations, risk reduction, reproductive health, and STIs (both general and specific information). Girls in this condition were not only able to choose which sections to watch but also to determine how the story line unfolded. In the first visit, regardless of condition, participants in all groups spent at least 30 minutes with the sexual-situations and risk-reduction sections of the material (DVD, book, or pamphlets) to ensure that all girls received similar intervention doses.

Girls randomized to the content-matched control group viewed a 127-page book that contained transcripts of the materials contained in the video, as well as selected images. Pages of the book were sequenced like a "choose your own adventure" book, with specially designed tabs, colors, and paper size. Anecdotal reports indicated that the adolescents randomized to this group tended to read the information as presented, in page order, rather than follow the story lines.

For the topic-matched control condition, the research team selected 23 commercially available brochures. The brochures were written at a basic level, contained information closely aligned with the video content, and were about the same length as the content-matched book.

A longitudinal, randomized, controlled design compared the three *What Could You Do?* interventions' impacts on sexual behavior and STI acquisition over a 6-month period. The girls returned for follow-up visits at 1-, 3-, and 6-month intervals after completing the intervention. At each follow-up point, participants were allowed to spend 15 minutes with intervention materials, either to view previously unseen segments or to review prior to testing.

Study Population

All of the adolescent study participants were culled from four urban Pittsburgh sites: an adolescent medicine clinic at a children's hospital, two community health centers, and a women's teaching hospital. To be eligible for participation in the study, girls had to be between 14 and 18 years old and have had vaginal sex within the past 6 months. Most participants (75%) classified themselves as African American, with 15% White and 10% Other or Mixed race.

For the purposes of evaluation, the two control groups were collapsed into a single group. At baseline, there were no significant differences between the intervention and control groups in terms of demographic characteristics. There were also no baseline differences between conditions for any of the outcome measures except abstinence, where those in the video condition were more likely to be abstinent than their control group counterparts ($\chi^2 = 5.76$, $p < .05$).

Evaluation Questions and Outcome Measures

The questionnaire used at all measurement points contained 71 questions. The general STI knowledge segment contained 40 true/false questions about reproductive health, disease, and condoms. In the specific STI knowledge segment, respondents indicated whether each of 15 statements applied to each of the nine focal STIs. Self-reported behavior questions asked about sexual behavior in the last 3 months, including number of sexual partners; frequency of condom use; frequency of condom breakage; and self-report of diagnosis with chlamydia, crabs, genital herpes, genital warts, gonorrhea, hepatitis B, HIV, syphilis, or trichomoniasis.

In addition to the self-administered paper-and-pencil questionnaire completed at each follow-up point, participants provided a self-administered vaginal swab at baseline and at the 6-month follow-up.

Evaluation Results

For binary outcomes (e.g., participants reporting an STI diagnosis in the past 3 months), the research team performed logistic regressions to compare those in the video condition to the control groups, controlling for baseline where appropriate. For knowledge and condom use, researchers used analyses of covariance (ANCOVAs) to compare the experimental and (combined) control groups, again controlling for baseline. For condom failure rates, the larger sample had greater variance, precluding the use of standard analysis of variance.

Abstinent participants were omitted from analyses on condom use, as they had had no opportunity to use condoms. Abstinent participants and those who had never used condoms in the past 3 months were also omitted from the analyses on condom failures, as they had had no opportunity for a condom to break, leak, or fall off.

STI Knowledge

The research team hypothesized that all three interventions would improve basic knowledge, owing to the nature of content and the participants' abilities to learn from the materials. This hypothesis held true: There were no effects of intervention condition at any of the follow-up points for general or specific STI knowledge. However, knowledge scores did improve across all conditions over time, revealing significant improvements in both general STI knowledge [$F(1,214) = 69.09$, $p < .001$] and specific STI knowledge [$F(1,214) = 58.62$, $p < .001$].

Self-Reported Sexual Behaviors

Participants in the video condition were more likely than their control group counterparts to report complete abstinence from baseline to the 3-month follow-up (OR = 2.5, $p = .027$). This pattern diminished between the 3- and 6-month visits (OR = 1.45, $p = .344$). The researchers noted that while abstinence in the experimental group was greater during the first 3 months, the lack of a statistically significant effect at the 6-month visit is not due to a decrease in abstinence in this group, but rather to a nonsignificant improvement in abstinence among control group members.

There was no significant difference between conditions in how often participants reported using condoms from baseline to the 3-month follow-up [$F(1, 206) = 0.33$, $p = .57$], or from the 3-month to the 6-month follow-up [$F(1, 213) = 2.13$, $p = .15$], although the trend was toward more condom use among those participants assigned to the video condition.

Condom Failures

Condom failure rates appeared to improve steadily over time for those watching the video, compared to an apparent plateau among the control group. While there was not a significant difference between the groups for reported condom failures at the 3-month point [$F(1, 150) = 0.01$, $p = .92$], condom failure rates improved overall in both conditions among those who used condoms at both intervals [$F(1, 99) = 3.84$, $p = .05$]. At the 6-month follow-up, video condition participants reported fewer condom failures than their control group counterparts [$F(1, 186) = 5.19$, $p = .02$].

STI Acquisitions

At the 6-month follow-up visit, participants in the video condition were less likely to report having been diagnosed with an STI, with control group members nearly twice as likely to report such a diagnosis (OR = 2.79, $p = .05$). This pattern held true for all nine reported diseases (sign test, $p = .004$).

Summary

The sample recruited for this evaluation of *What Could You Do?* represents adolescents at several clinical sites in the Pittsburgh community who were seeking medical care for various reasons. The results may not be generalizable to other settings such as schools or community organizations. However, the evaluation study revealed that the video intervention could be incorporated easily into usual clinic care without the need for a facilitator or the logistics of a group intervention.

NOTE

1. A full set of program materials, including two versions of the *What Could You Do?* DVD, evaluation materials, and more, is available for purchase from Sociometrics at http://www.socio.com/pasha.htm.

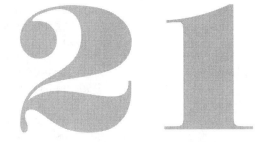

AIDS Prevention and Health Promotion Among Women: An HIV/AIDS Prevention Program for Young Women

Nicole Vicinanza, Starr Niego, and Janette Mince

Original Program Developers and Evaluators

Stevan E. Hobfoll, PhD
Anita P. Jackson, PhD
Paula J. Britton, PhD
James B. Shepherd, PhD
  Kent State University
  Kent, OH

Justin P. Lavin, MD
  Akron City Hospital
  Akron, OH

PROGRAM ABSTRACT

Summary

AIDS Prevention and Health Promotion Among Women is designed to assist participants in developing and following a sound sexual health plan. Based on the

AIDS Prevention and Health Promotion Among Women was supported by grants from the National Institute of Mental Health, Office on AIDS (1R01 MH45669), and Kent State University Applied Psychology Center.

concepts of empowerment, group social support, and culturally sensitive skill building, this program comprises four 1.5- to 2-hour small-group sessions (2–8 participants) conducted over the course of 3 months. Video segments promote group discussion, spark group role plays, and engage participants in cognitive rehearsal and guided fantasy exercises designed to encourage healthy choices about one's body and sexuality.

Specifically, this program encourages women to think about the physical and emotional consequences of unsafe sex. It helps them achieve a sense of mastery and positive expectations when discussing sexual history, HIV/AIDS testing, monogamy, spermicide and condom use, and other health-related concerns with their partners. In addition, the program teaches participants how to effectively negotiate safer sex with their partners and maintain safer-sex goals. This program was field tested with pregnant, low-income African American and White women who were using medical center obstetrics services in Akron, Ohio. Compared to control groups, participants showed significant and sustained increases in HIV/AIDS knowledge, safer-sex goals, and safer-sex behaviors, including spermicide and condom purchase and use.

Focus

☐ Primary pregnancy prevention ☐ Secondary pregnancy prevention ☑ STI/HIV/AIDS prevention

Original Site

☐ School based ☐ Community based ☑ Clinic based

Suitable for Use In

AIDS Prevention and Health Promotion Among Women can be implemented in clinics and community-based organizations. Although the original field study was conducted with pregnant women, the program is also appropriate for older adolescents and young adult women (ages 16 +). In addition, because the program contains explicit information regarding intravenous (IV) drug use, it may be most suitable for groups engaging in high-risk behaviors.

Approach

- ■ ☐ Abstinence
- ■ ☑ Behavioral skills development
- ■ ☐ Community outreach
- ■ ☑ Contraceptive access
- ■ ☑ Contraceptive education
- ■ ☐ Life option enhancement
- ■ ☑ Self-efficacy/self-esteem
- ■ ☑ Sexuality/HIV/STI education

Original Intervention Sample

Age   The field-test participants included 206 unmarried women in their second trimester of pregnancy who were using obstetric clinic services. Their ages ranged from 16 to 29 years; the average age of participants was 21.

Race/ethnicity The field test population was 57% African American, 40% White, 3% Other.

Program Components

- ■ ☐ Adult involvement
- ■ ☐ Case management
- ■ ☑ Group discussion
- ■ ☐ Lectures
- ■ ☐ Peer counseling/instruction
- ■ ☐ Public service announcements
- ■ ☑ Role play
- ■ ☑ Video
- ■ ☑ Other: Guided imagery, group social support, cognitive rehearsal

Program Length

This program is designed to last a total of 6–8 hours. The program schedule is fairly flexible and can be adjusted to suit the particular site. However, it is recommended that the four program sessions be conducted over a period of 2 to 3 months, with participants attending a single 1.5- to 2-hour session every 2 or 3 weeks.

Staffing Requirements/Training

A female master's-level psychologist or health educator should deliver the interventions. One facilitator is recommended for each group of up to eight women. The facilitator should have the ability to empathize with participants, a good working knowledge of HIV/AIDS and health concerns, and the ability to communicate a positive health message. Training should include group process skills, role-playing and associated skills, and multicultural psychology. Video feedback on a practice session, if possible, is also suggested.

BIBLIOGRAPHY

Hobfoll, S. E., Jackson, A. P., Lavin, J., Britton, P. J., & Shepherd, J. B. (1994). Reducing inner-city women's AIDS risk activities: A study of single, pregnant women. *Health Psychology, 13*(5), 397–403.

Levine, O. H., Britton, P. J., James, T. C, Jackson, A. P., Hobfoll, S. E., & Lavin, J. P. (1993). The empowerment of women: A key to HIV prevention. *Journal of Community Psychology, 21*, 320–334.

Related References by the Developers of *AIDS Prevention and Health Promotion Among Women*

Hobfoll, S. E., Jackson, A. P., Lavin, J., Johnson, R. I., & Schroder, K. E. (2002). Effects and generalizability of communally oriented HIV-AIDS prevention versus general health promotion groups for single, inner-city women in urban clinics. *Journal of Consulting & Clinical Psychology, 70*(4), 950–960.

THE PROGRAM

Program Rationale and History

AIDS Prevention and Health Promotion Among Women is intended to help women incorporate safer-sex practices into their lives.[1] This 2- to 3-month program uses four small-group discussion sessions to engage women's thoughts and feelings concerning the consequences of unsafe sex. Guided visualizations are used to motivate women to adopt and maintain safer-sex practices. In addition, role play and cognitive rehearsal exercises help participants achieve a sense of mastery and positive expectations when discussing sexual history, HIV/AIDS testing, monogamy, spermicide/lubricant and condom use, and other health-related concerns with their partners. This program also directly addresses the relationship between drug and alcohol use and the risk of HIV infection. Specific instruction is given for cleaning IV drug works. Increased knowledge, confidence, and skills provide a basis for participants to effectively negotiate safer sex with their partners. Furthermore, the group format provides support in setting and keeping safer-sex goals.

This program was developed by researchers from Kent State University, the Akron City Hospital, and John Carroll University, with a grant from the National Institute of Mental Health and support from the Kent State University Applied Psychology Center. The program was initially field tested with a group of pregnant adolescents and women in Akron, Ohio, between 1990 and 1993.

Theoretical Framework

The program is rooted in ideas of participant empowerment, socially sensitive skill building, and research, indicating that a successful HIV/AIDS prevention program

- provides accurate information on transmission and safer-sex options, particularly condom use;
- raises participants' sense of their personal risk of infection;
- increases participants' belief that they can successfully perform safer-sex behaviors;
- increases social support for safer-sex behaviors;
- increases participants' social and cultural acceptance of safer-sex behaviors.

The program is based on Bandura's social learning theory (SLT) and Hobfoll's conservation of resources (COR) theory. SLT elaborates the processes through which intentions can be translated into behavioral change, and postulates that learning occurs through practice and observation of social models. Learning is mediated by internal beliefs about one's ability to succeed, as well as others' evaluation of one's own performance.

According to the theory, the likelihood of engaging in some action, such as using birth control, is determined by four factors:

1. A woman's understanding of what must be done to avoid pregnancy
2. The belief that she will be able to use the method
3. The belief that the method will be successful at preventing pregnancy
4. The benefit she anticipates from accomplishing the behavior (e.g., preventing pregnancy through effective contraception)

Another important tenet of SLT is that people learn skills by observing others' behavior and then imitating them. In *AIDS Prevention and Health Promotion Among Women,* teachers and peers first model socially desirable behaviors, such as using birth control, and then participants practice those behaviors in role plays.

COR theory suggests that the threat of AIDS is an additional stressor facing women who are already overtaxed in their coping efforts. In such situations, COR theory posits that an intervention must increase both the personal and social resources of women. COR theory further suggests that target groups must see the intervention as both adding new resources and building on their current resource strengths.

Program Objectives

The overall goal of the program is to empower women to develop and employ a sound sexual health plan. Specifically, women will

1. know what behaviors put them at risk of exposure to HIV;
2. understand methods for preventing exposure;
3. achieve a sense of mastery and positive expectations when discussing sexual history, HIV/AIDS testing, monogamy, spermicide and condom use, and other health-related concerns with their partners;
4. develop safer-sex plans and practices.

Hypothesized Outcomes

It is hypothesized that program participants will increase:

1. their knowledge about HIV/AIDS;
2. their intention to adopt safer-sex practices, specifically spermicide and condom use;
3. their actual practice of safer sex.

Program Schedule

AIDS Prevention and Health Promotion Among Women was composed of four 1.5- to 2-hour small-group sessions. Each session had several content themes incorporating role plays, cognitive rehearsal, guided fantasy, and short video segments containing information and examples. During the original field study, the program developers identified four elements critical to the translation of program material into behavioral change. To be successful, the developers reasoned, the program should

1. integrate real and important issues from the participants' lives into the discussions;
2. use the group format to encourage cohesiveness and support among participants;
3. engage group facilitators (as opposed to group leaders) to promote mutuality and equality;
4. promote ongoing and authentic relationships among the participants and staff members.

These four elements served as goals in each program session. The content of each session is summarized below.

Session 1: Drug Use, Alcohol Use, and AIDS

Participants gained a sense of comfort in the group setting and discussed general health concerns, including drug and alcohol use and HIV/AIDS. They were also introduced to role play, cognitive rehearsal, and guided visualization exercises. This session used the five video segments on the *Session 1: Drug Use, Alcohol Use, and AIDS* tape.

Session 2: Condom and Spermicide Use and Controlling the Conditions of Sexual Encounters

Participants learned the importance of using condoms and spermicide/lubricant. They learned appropriate condom use and had the opportunity to practice correct condom application with a penis model. Following this exercise, they discussed potential barriers to safer-sex practices. Role play and cognitive rehearsal exercises helped participants gain a sense of confidence and positive expectations when purchasing condoms and spermicide/lubricant, and in discussing their use with sexual partners. A guided fantasy exercise helped participants understand the emotional consequences of safer- and nonsafer-sex plans. This session used the five video segments on the *Session 2: Condom and Spermicide Use and Controlling the Conditions of Sexual Encounters* tape.

(Note: At the time the research for this program was conducted, the use of spermicides containing nonoxynal-9, or condoms treated with nonoxynol-9, was strongly encouraged. However, since the release of this replication kit, clinical research has shown that repeated use of spermicides containing nonoxynol-9 can cause irritation and microscopic tears in the vaginal and/or rectal membranes, leaving a woman or man more susceptible to contracting sexually transmitted infections (STIs), including HIV. Current science indicates that the use of water-based lubricants, while not effective deterrents of infection in and of themselves, may help to prevent irritation caused by the use of unlubricated condoms and thus help to minimize the risk of infection.)

Session 3: Sexual History, Saying No to an Unwanted Intensive Sexual Proposition, and Developing a Mutual Sexual Behavior Plan

This session provided participants with information about communicating safer-sex behaviors with their partners, as well as opportunities to practice these skills. It covered issues such as discussing one's sexual history, HIV/AIDS testing, and developing a mutual safer-sex plan. Role plays and cognitive rehearsal were used to practice discussing these topics with partners and to help participants discover potential barriers in these discussions. A guided visualization exercise helped participants realize the physical and emotional outcomes from following/not following a safer-sex plan. This session used the five video segments on the *Session 3: Sexual History, Saying No to an Unwanted Intensive Sexual Proposition, and Developing a Mutual Sexual Behavior Plan* tape.

Session 4: Relapse Prevention, Postintervention Sexual Life, Alternatives to Intercourse, Mutual Monogamy, and Cleaning Drug Works

In the final session, women discussed their postintervention sexual options and strategies for maintaining their safer-sex plans after the program. In addition, they received information on how to clean IV drug works. Role plays and cognitive rehearsals helped participants gain a sense of mastery and positive expectations when discussing the maintenance of their safer-sex plan with their partners. A guided visualization exercise helped them realize the consequences of maintaining/not maintaining their safer-sex action plan. This session used the five segments on the videotape *Session 4: Relapse Prevention, Postintervention Sexual Life, Alternatives to Intercourse, Mutual Monogamy, and Cleaning Drug Works.*

PROGRAM EVALUATION

The Original Evaluation

Design

The effectiveness of *AIDS Prevention and Health Promotion Among Women* was originally assessed in a field study in Akron, Ohio. The study compared the HIV/AIDS knowledge, safer-sex plans, and safer-sex practices of three groups of women. One group received the intervention described above (AIDS prevention group). A second group participated in a comparable health program (general health promotion group) in which they were taught identical skills (i.e., negotiation in sexual situations, making a general sexual health plan), using identical methods (information, role play, cognitive rehearsal, and guided fantasy exercises) in the same amount of time, but which did not include AIDS-specific information. A third group, which received no intervention, was used as a control (control group). Data were collected from all participants at three points:

Time 1: before the start of the program (preintervention)

Time 2: immediately following the end of the program (postintervention)

Time 3: 6 months after the end of the program (6-month follow-up)

The 206 original study participants were all single women in their second trimester of pregnancy who sought obstetrical care at one of three inner-city clinics for low-income women.

Evaluation Questions

Three questions guided the field study.

1. What effect did the intervention have on participants' knowledge about AIDS?
2. What effect did the intervention have on participants' intent to adopt safer-sex practices?
3. What effect did the intervention have on participants' actual practice of safer sex?

Data Collection Procedures

Participants were recruited when they sought obstetrical services at one of three clinics serving low-income women in Akron, Ohio. Eighty percent of those asked agreed to participate in the study. Preintervention data were collected at the initial contact. Participants were paid $10 for completing the first survey, $15 for the postintervention survey, and $20 for the follow-up. To help offset the cost of transportation and child care, women in both the AIDS prevention and general health promotion groups also received $5 for each group session they attended.

At each assessment period, participants completed a questionnaire with the following measures:

- *Safer-sex knowledge.* This 13-item scale measures knowledge of AIDS transmission and prevention.
- *Condom and spermicide usage.* This 4-item scale measures condom and spermicide use during vaginal and anal sex in the few weeks preceding the study.
- *Abstinence and number of partners.* These items assess women's sexual behavior over the past year, including the number of partners.
- *Discussion with partners.* One item probes whether women discuss AIDS-related behavior with their partners.
- *Intention to purchase, and purchase of condoms and spermicide.* In this 4-item scale, women report on their intent to purchase condoms and/or spermicide in the future and whether they have recently obtained condoms and/or spermicide.

In addition to the self-report items, the evaluators measured the actual condom and spermicide purchases by participants. At the start of the study, participants received credit cards containing their photo and an ID number, but not their name. These credit cards could be used to purchase condoms and spermicide at pharmacies near their clinic. The evaluators obtained reports of the women's purchases from local pharmacies.

Original Intervention Sample

Study participants were single women in their second trimester of pregnancy who had not lived with a partner steadily during the last 6 months. Women who were under treatment for a chronic illness, such as diabetes or kidney disorders, were excluded. Minors needed parental consent for their participation. Slightly more than half (57%) of the participants in this study self-identified as African American, 40% were White, and the remaining 3% were Other. Most of the participants (75%) had incomes under $10,000 per year.

For the two intervention groups, all participants who completed three or more sessions were included in the sample. Thirty-seven women began the study but did not complete it. The only difference between participants who were included and excluded from the study was that those who attended fewer than three sessions were slightly better educated.

Evaluation Results

Compared to their peers in the general health promotion and control groups, members of the AIDS prevention group showed the most favorable outcomes, particularly on measures of safer-sex intentions and practices. Although most of the changes were moderate in magnitude, they were maintained at the 6-month follow-up. The intervention was equally effective for African American and White women. The AIDS prevention participants showed the following outcomes:

1. *Increased AIDS knowledge.* Participants in the AIDS prevention group had significantly greater AIDS knowledge than the no-intervention controls on the 13-item safer-sex questionnaire.
2. *Increased discussion of AIDS with a partner.* AIDS prevention group members were significantly more likely than the no-intervention group to discuss AIDS-related behavior with a sexual partner.
3. *Safer-sex intentions and practices.* The AIDS prevention group showed greater increases in safer-sex intentions and practices than either the general health promotion or the control groups.
4. *Increased reported usage of condoms and spermicide.* Participants in the AIDS prevention group reported a greater increase in their use of condoms and spermicide compared to the no-intervention group.
5. *Increased acquisition of condoms and spermicide.* Compared to their peers in the other two groups, AIDS prevention participants showed the most significant gains in condom and spermicide acquisition.

All of the results reported above were significant at the $p < .05$ level.

Overall, the intervention showed no effect on abstinence or the number of sexual partners. The evaluators observed that because few of the participants had had more than five partners in the year preceding the study, significant change might be difficult to measure.

Summary

The results of this evaluation showed that *AIDS Prevention and Health Promotion Among Women* could produce significant changes in women's safer-sex behavior. The combination of HIV/AIDS-related information and skills practice was more effective in getting women to develop healthy sexual plans than the health-only intervention. Women in the AIDS prevention group demonstrated significant, lasting change in their knowledge of HIV/AIDS prevention, communication about HIV/AIDS, intentions and actual behaviors concerning safer-sex behaviors, as well as condom and spermicide acquisition and use.

AIDS PREVENTION AND HEALTH PROMOTION AMONG WOMEN IN THE COMMUNITY TODAY

In the past 3 years, *AIDS Prevention and Health Promotion Among Women* has been implemented in 24 communities in six states. A single state, Florida, accounts for half of the implementation sites for this program.

NOTE

1. A full set of program materials, including program manual, videotapes, evaluation materials, and more, is available for purchase from Sociometrics at http://www.socio.com/pasha.htm.

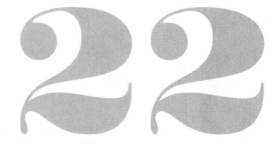

A Clinic-Based AIDS Education Program for Female Adolescents: An HIV/AIDS Prevention Program for Young Women

J. Barry Gurdin, Starr Niego, Margaret S. Kelley, and Janette Mince

Original Program Developers and Evaluators

Vaughn I. Rickert, PsyD
  Department of Obstetrics & Gynecology
  University of Texas Medical Branch at Galveston
  Galveston, TX

Anita Gottlieb, RNP
  Department of Pediatrics
  Arkansas Children's Hospital
  Little Rock, AK

M. Susan Jay, MD
  Loyola University School of Medicine
  Maywood, IL

A Clinic-Based AIDS Education Program for Female Adolescents was supported by grant from the Arkansas Department of Health.

PROGRAM ABSTRACT

Summary

This is a single-session group intervention originally targeted toward sexually active girls between 13 and 21 years of age. The session includes a brief lecture on transmission and prevention of HIV/AIDS (based on Centers for Disease Control and Prevention [CDC] guidelines), followed by a video demonstrating the purpose and use of condoms. As the session ends, participants receive an educational booklet reinforcing the program's lessons and coupons that may be redeemed anonymously for an unmarked box of condoms at a local pharmacy. The redemption rate of the coupons provides a measure of the program's impact. A field study of the intervention was conducted with 75 White and African American females, all of whom were sexually active. Among prior purchasers of condoms, girls who took part in the intervention were significantly more likely to redeem the coupons than were control groups of their peers. Overall, 60% of program participants obtained condoms, a rate 2.5 times greater than that recorded in a comparable program without a confidential coupon redemption procedure.

Focus

☐ Primary pregnancy prevention   ☐ Secondary pregnancy prevention   ☑ STI/HIV/AIDS prevention

Original Site

☐ School based   ☐ Community based   ☑ Clinic based

Suitable for Use In

This program can be implemented in a variety of medical or reproductive health clinic settings, providing that arrangements can be made with a local pharmacy for confidential coupon redemption.

Approach

- ☐ Abstinence
- ☑ Behavioral skills development
- ☐ Community outreach
- ☑ Contraceptive access
- ☑ Contraceptive education
- ☐ Life option enhancement
- ☑ Self-efficacy/self-esteem
- ☑ Sexuality/HIV/STI education

Original Intervention Sample

Age, gender   The original sample included 75 females, ages 13 to 21 years.
Race/ethnicity   52% African American, 48% White.

Program Components

- ☐ Adult involvement
- ☐ Case management
- ☐ Group discussion

- ☑ Lectures
- ☐ Peer counseling/instruction
- ☐ Public service announcements
- ☐ Role play
- ☑ Video
- ☑ Other: Coupons for confidential condom redemption

Program Length

The single 1-hour session includes a lecture and video presentation, along with distribution of an educational booklet and coupons for confidential condom redemption.

Staffing Requirements/Training

A medical or health services professional should lead the educational sessions with groups of up to four teens.

BIBLIOGRAPHY

Rickert, V. I., Gottlieb, A., & Jay, M. S. (1990). A comparison of three clinic-based AIDS education programs on female adolescents' knowledge, attitudes, and behavior. *Journal of Adolescent Health, 11*(4), 298–303.

Related References by the Developers of the *Clinic-Based AIDS Education Program for Female Adolescents*

Harrykissoon, S. D., Rickert, V. I., & Wiemann, C. (2002). Prevalence and patterns of intimate partner violence among adolescent mothers during the postpartum period. *Archives of Pediatric & Adolescent Medicine, 156*(4), 325–330.

Rickert, V., Davis, S., & Ryan, S. A. (1997). Rural school-based clinics: Are adolescents willing to use them and what services do they want? *Journal of School Health, 67,* 144–148.

Rickert, V. I., Pope S. K., Tilford, J. M., Scholle, S., Wayne, J., & Kelleher, K. J. (1996). The effects of mental health factors on ambulatory care visits by rural teens. *Journal of Rural Health, 12*(3), 160–168.

Wiemann, C., Aguarcia, C., Berenson, A., Volk, R., & Rickert, V. (2000). Pregnant adolescents: Experiences and behaviors associated with physical assault by an intimate partner. *Maternal and Child Health Journal, 4*(2), 93–101.

THE PROGRAM

Program Rationale and History

In 1986 the U.S. surgeon general issued a report emphasizing that health education could help control the HIV/AIDS epidemic by promoting changes in individual behavior.[1] Drawing upon that report, *A Clinic-Based AIDS Education Program for Female Adolescents* is designed to promote the use of condoms by sexually active girls between 13 and 21 years of age. The brief, single-session intervention combines a lecture covering transmission and prevention of HIV/AIDS with a humorous video demonstrating the purpose and use of condoms for protection from sexually transmitted infections (STIs). Finally, participants receive an educational booklet reinforcing the program messages, along with a coupon that may be redeemed anonymously for a box of condoms.

A field study of the program was conducted in a medical clinic in Little Rock, Arkansas. Participants included 75 sexually active females visiting the clinic for primary health care.

Theoretical Framework

Most middle and high school students want to increase their knowledge of HIV/ AIDS. They would also prefer to receive this information from a doctor or nurse, and in person rather than in printed form. However, when this program was developed, most school-based HIV/AIDS education programs focused exclusively on providing teens with biomedical information, rather than on encouraging the development of preventive behaviors. The original program developer asserted that HIV/AIDS education could be provided in clinics without the need for the kind of broad-based community support required to launch school-based programs. A medical clinic serving adolescent patients was chosen as a potentially effective site for educating sexually active females about HIV infection and preventive behaviors.

Program Objectives

As an HIV/AIDS risk reduction program, *A Clinic-Based AIDS Education Program for Female Adolescents* is designed to meet the following educational objectives:

1. Increase female adolescents' understanding of transmission and prevention of HIV/AIDS
2. Improve female adolescents' attitudes toward condoms as a method of STI protection
3. Promote the use of condoms by sexually active females

Program Schedule

The educational intervention was designed to fit into a single 1-hour clinic visit. In the field study of the program, the session was delivered to small groups of teens, ranging in size from one to four participants.

Description of Session Components

Part I: AIDS Education. The session began with a brief lecture about HIV/AIDS, based on health education guidelines issued by the CDC. In particular, the guidelines emphasize that HIV/AIDS is very difficult to contract, and that the risk of becoming infected can be virtually eliminated by not engaging in sexual activities or using intravenous drugs.

Part II: Video Presentation. When the lecture concluded, the teens viewed a 25-minute video, *Condom Sense*. The video used humor to explain the purpose and correct use of condoms.

Part III: Wrap-Up. At the conclusion of the session, participants were given an educational pamphlet to take with them: *What Everyone Should Know About AIDS*. The pamphlet reinforced basic principles about HIV/AIDS transmission, treatment, and prevention in simple, easy-to-understand language. In the field study, teens also received a coupon that they could redeem confidentially at the hospital pharmacy for a box of condoms. The coupons were also used in conjunction with the evaluation of the program.

Program Implementation

A Clinic-Based AIDS Education Program for Female Adolescents was led by health professionals who were knowledgeable about HIV/AIDS and risk behaviors, particularly as they pertained to adolescents. The leaders were also comfortable discussing sexuality and contraception with teens. It was important that staff thoroughly reviewed all program materials prior to the start of the session.

Consider Local Needs and Values

Values vary across communities, so the appropriate grades at which to discuss HIV infection and sexuality must be determined locally, on a program-by-program basis. Because *A Clinic-Based AIDS Education Program for Female Adolescents* was aimed at teens who had already become sexually active and was provided in a clinical setting, there was less variance among participants than there might have been in broader school or community settings. However, it is still important to consider which information is appropriate for your teens and your community.

PROGRAM EVALUATION

The Original Evaluation

Design

The effectiveness of *A Clinic-Based AIDS Education Program for Female Adolescents* was investigated in a field study conducted with 75 sexually active females attending medical clinics at Arkansas Children's Hospital in Little Rock, Arkansas. The study compared teens who were randomly assigned to take part in one of three interventions: (a) the control group, who received only an educational pamphlet about HIV/AIDS; (b) the education group, who received the pamphlet along with a brief lecture on HIV/AIDS; and (c) the enhanced-education group who received the pamphlet and lecture and viewed a video explaining the purpose and use of condoms for STI protection. Additionally, at the conclusion of all three interventions, each teen received a coupon that could be redeemed, confidentially, for a box of condoms at the hospital pharmacy.

Two sets of measures were included in the evaluation. At Time 1, after the interventions concluded, the researchers compared the three groups' HIV/AIDS-related knowledge and attitudes, as well as their use of condoms. At Time 2, the condom redemption rate for each group of teens was used as a measure of the programs' effect on behavior.

Evaluation Questions

The researchers hypothesized that enhanced-education group participants would show the most positive outcomes as compared to their peers in the other two groups. In particular, program participants were expected to show

1. greater gains in their HIV-related knowledge;
2. greater improvement in their HIV-related attitudes;
3. higher rates of confidential condom redemption using the program coupons.

Data Collection Procedures

The researchers recruited teens who sought routine medical care at Arkansas Children's Hospital. They explained the purpose of the study, obtained written informed consent, and randomly assigned the teens to one of the three conditions: control (n = 25), education (n = 25), or enhanced education (n = 25). Professional medical staff then carried out the appropriate intervention with small groups of youths, ranging in size from one to four participants.

Adolescents in the control (i.e., pamphlet only) group were first asked whether they had questions about HIV/AIDS. Staff addressed any questions, distributed the educational pamphlets and condom coupons, and then administered all Time 1 measures. A similar procedure was followed with the education and enhanced-education groups. That is, Time 1 measures were taken after the educational activities concluded and participants had received the confidential condom coupons.

Although no names were written on the coupons, each was marked with an identification number, and the researchers privately recorded the identification number printed on the coupon each teen received. To calculate the Time 2 (follow-up) measures, the researchers matched the identification numbers to the teens recorded in their roster.

Research Sample

The researchers recruited 82 teens for the study, of whom 77 agreed to participate. Of this group, 36 were White and 41 were African American. Because two teens failed to provide complete data for the study, the final sample included 75 adolescent females. All described themselves as sexually active and had a history of sexual activity in their medical records.

Evaluation Results

On the Time 1 measures, taken immediately following the interventions, the researchers found no significant differences among the three groups on background measures (e.g., age, race, insurance status), previous condom purchases, or personal experience practicing HIV/AIDS-preventive behaviors.

AIDS-Related Knowledge

The evaluators found that none of the teens in the control group asked any questions about AIDS when prompted to do so, and this group scored significantly lower than the two groups receiving the brief HIV/AIDS education lecture ($p < .001$). However, the two education groups did not differ in their knowledge scores.

AIDS-Related Attitudes

Following the interventions, the three groups showed no significant differences in their attitudes toward people with AIDS, their feelings toward preventive behaviors, or their beliefs about the severity of the disease.

Condom Redemption

The researchers found that 60% of the enhanced-education group participants redeemed their coupons for condoms at the hospital pharmacy, while 44% of the education group and 48% of controls did so. This difference was not statistically significant. However, when the researchers focused on the subset of teens who had previously purchased condoms, enhanced-education group participants showed significantly better outcomes. In particular, among sexually active females who had purchased condoms before the intervention began, enhanced-education group participants were significantly more likely than their peers in the two other groups to obtain condoms at the hospital pharmacy ($p < .05$).

Summary

The results of the evaluation suggest that a brief, single-session intervention can motivate sexually active females who have previously obtained condoms to do so again. The 60% condom-redemption rate for the enhanced-education group was not significantly higher than that of the other two groups; however, it was nearly two and a half times greater than that recorded (25%) in a previous study lacking a confidential redemption procedure. The evaluators also noted that the intervention—consisting of a brief lecture, video, and provision of an educational pamphlet and condom coupon—proved fast, easy to implement, and inexpensive. Moreover, because the program is designed for use in a medical clinic, it may reach high-risk teens who do not regularly attend school.

In interpreting the data, the researchers noted that the enhanced-education treatment appeared to be no more effective than the education (i.e., lecture) treatment alone. However, the small number of teens in each group reduced the statistical power of tests for significant outcomes. Additionally, though the two education groups showed greater understanding of HIV/AIDS relative to their control group peers, the data must be viewed cautiously. In the absence of longer-term follow-up measures, it is not possible to determine whether the differences resulted from exposure to the intervention.

A CLINIC-BASED AIDS EDUCATION PROGRAM FOR FEMALE ADOLESCENTS IN THE COMMUNITY TODAY

In the past 3 years, this program has been implemented in two communities in Texas.

NOTE

1. A full set of program materials, including booklets, videotape, school health education guidelines, evaluation materials, and more, is available for purchase from Sociometrics at http://www.socio.com/pasha.htm.

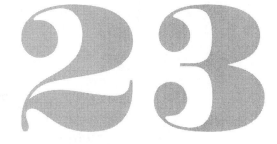

SiHLE: Health Workshops for Young Black Women

Tabitha A. Benner

Original Program Developers and Evaluators

Ralph DiClemente, PhD
Gina Wingood, ScD
Delia Lang, PhD
Richard Crosby, PhD
Vicki Stover Hertzberg, PhD
Angelita Gordon, MS
Alyssa Robillard, PhD
    Emory University
    Atlanta, GA

Kathy Harrington, MPH, MAE
Susan Davies, PhD
Edward Hook III, MD
M. Kim Oh, MD
    University of Alabama
    Birmingham, AL

James Hardin, PhD
    University of South Carolina
    Columbia, SC

SiHLE was supported by a grant from the Center for Mental Health Research on AIDS National Institute of Mental Health (1R01 MH54412).

Shan Parker, PhD
University of Michigan
Flint, MI

PROGRAM ABSTRACT

Summary

The *SiHLE* intervention was developed specifically to address the STI/HIV/AIDS prevention needs of African American adolescent girls. Research has shown that this subgroup of the general population is at higher risk than their White or Hispanic peers. *SiHLE* was originally implemented in the South, where adolescent HIV prevalence was higher than any other geographic region in the United States. The 2005 HIV/AIDS surveillance data from the Centers for Disease Control and Prevention (CDC) indicate that while African American teens aged 13–19 made up only 17% of the population in that age group, 69% of HIV/AIDS cases in the United States that year among 13- to 19-year-old teens were African American teens.

Participants were culled from girls seeking health services at four community health agencies. To be eligible to participate, girls needed to be African American between the ages of 14 and 18 and have engaged in vaginal intercourse within the previous 6 months. At baseline, 522 sexually active African American girls, aged 14–18, completed the baseline survey and were randomized into either the HIV-prevention intervention (n = 251) or the general health control group (n = 271). Each group received a four-session, 16-hour intervention that was offered on consecutive Saturdays.

The HIV-prevention intervention was grounded in social cognitive theory and the theory of gender and power. Participants explored issues related to ethnic and gender pride, risk reduction strategies (including correct and consistent condom use), negotiating safer sex, and healthy relationships as they relate to practicing safer sex.

At the 6-month follow-up point, intervention girls reported using condoms more consistently in the previous 30 days than did their control group counterparts (intervention, 75.3% vs. control, 58.2%). At the 12-month follow-up, intervention girls continued to report more consistent condom use both in the previous 30 days (intervention, 73.3% vs. control, 56.5%) and during the entire 12-month review period (adjusted odds ratio [OR], 2.30; 95% confidence interval [CI] = 1.51–3.5; $p < .001$). In general, at the 12-month point, girls in the intervention group were more likely to have used a condom at last intercourse, and less likely to have had a new sexual partner in the last 30 days. They also had better condom application skills and a higher percentage of condom-protected sex acts than their control-group peers. Promising effects were also observed for chlamydia infections and self-reported pregnancy.

Focus

☐ Primary pregnancy   ☐ Secondary pregnancy   ☑ STI/HIV/AIDS
   prevention   prevention   prevention

Original Site

☐ School based   ☐ Community based   ☑ Clinic based

Suitable for Use In

SiHLE is suitable for use in community based organizations and clinics that provide services to adolescent African American girls.

Approach

- ■ ☐ Abstinence
- ■ ☑ Behavioral skills development
- ■ ☐ Community outreach
- ■ ☑ Contraceptive access
- ■ ☑ Contraceptive education
- ■ ☐ Life option enhancement
- ■ ☑ Self-efficacy/self-esteem
- ■ ☑ Sexuality/HIV/AIDS/STI education

Original Intervention Sample

Age, gender   The baseline sample was 100% female, ranging in age from 14 to 18.

Race/ethnicity   All participants were African American.

Program Components

- ■ ☐ Adult involvement
- ■ ☐ Case management
- ■ ☑ Group discussion
- ■ ☑ Lectures
- ■ ☑ Peer counseling/instruction
- ■ ☐ Public service announcements
- ■ ☑ Role play
- ■ ☐ Video
- ■ ☐ Other

Program Length

SiHLE is delivered in four 4-hour sessions for a total of 16 contact hours.

Staffing Requirements/Training

In the original implementation, a female African American health educator delivered the intervention, assisted by two African American peer educators. There was no formal training for either the health educator or the peer educators; however, you may wish to develop a training program for future health educators in your milieu.

BIBLIOGRAPHY

DiClemente, R. J., Wingood, G. M., Harrington, K. F., Lang, D. L., Davies, S. L., Hook, E. W., et al. (2004). Efficacy of an HIV prevention intervention for African American girls. *JAMA, 292*(2), 171–179.

Related References by the Developers of *SiHLE*

Wingood, G. M., & DiClemente, R. J. (2006). Enhancing adoption of evidence-based HIV interventions: Promotion of a suite of HIV prevention interventions for African American women. *AIDS Education & Prevention, 18*(4 Suppl. A), 161–170.

Wingood, G. M., DiClemente, R. J., Harrington, K. F., Lang, D. L., Davies, S. L., Hook, E. W., et al. (2006). Efficacy of an HIV prevention program among female adolescents experiencing gender-based violence. *American Journal of Public Health, 96*(6), 1085–1090.

THE PROGRAM

Program Rationale and History

Among adolescents, African American girls comprise a subgroup of the U.S. population that is at especially high risk of HIV infection.[1] The CDC's 2005 HIV/AIDS surveillance data indicate that while African American teens aged 13–19 made up only 17% of the population in that age group, 69% of HIV/AIDS cases in the United States that year among 13- to 19-year-old teens were African American teens. That's more than four times the number of cases reported for Hispanic or White teens of the same age. In slightly more than 85% of the cases reported in 2005, the young women contracted HIV by having unprotected sex with an infected male sex partner.

Despite the fact that research has shown that these girls are disproportionately impacted by the HIV epidemic, no intervention designed specifically for African American girls had demonstrated effectiveness in reducing HIV-related risk behaviors. The *SiHLE* program was developed to address this issue in a gender-, culture-, and age-appropriate manner.

The original implementation of *SiHLE* was conducted between 1996 and 1999. Participants were culled from girls seeking health services in four community health agencies in the Birmingham, Alabama, area. The program was delivered to small groups of 10–12 participants on four consecutive Saturdays at a family medicine clinic. *SiHLE* was implemented by an African American, female health educator and two African American peer educators. The peer educators were instrumental in modeling skills and creating group norms supportive of HIV prevention.

Girls randomized into the control condition received a program of equal length that addressed anger and stress management, healthy eating and exercise, and preparing for the professional world. Prior to implementing the trial of *SiHLE*, the research team field-tested both the intervention and control programs with adolescents from the study population.

Theoretical Framework

Social cognitive theory (SCT) and the theory of gender and power (TGP) provided the theoretical framework for *SiHLE*. SCT posits that providing information alone is insufficient to change behavior. Sustained behavioral change requires skills to engage in these behaviors and the ability to use the skills consistently, possibly under difficult circumstances. TGP argues that self-protection by women is often adversely influenced by economic factors, abusive partners, and the socialization of women to be sexually passive or ignorant.

Program Overview

SiHLE was a hands-on, interactive intervention, requiring that the participants take part in the activities and discussions. In the first session, participants signed a "*SiHLE* Pact" in which they committed to participate actively and be supportive of their Sistas in the program.

The first *SiHLE* workshop focused largely on logistics and on ethnic and gender pride. The "*SiHLE* Motto" was introduced, as were ground rules. The session then moved on to explore the joys and challenges of being an African American female, and to examine some of the contributions made by other African American women in the arts and sciences. Session 1 included the poem, "A Room Full of Sisters," by Mona Lake Jones, to help the participants appreciate Black women's inner and outer beauty. Also in the first session, the concept of personal values was introduced through the "Personal Values Clarification" exercise. The importance of personal values was a recurring theme in the remaining three sessions. At the close of the first session, participants completed a pictograph depicting their vision for their lives at age 25.

Workshop 2 opened with "Call Me Black Woman," a poem by Priscilla Hancock Cooper. The poem served to remind participants that Black women can be found worldwide, speaking a variety of languages, wearing their hair in many different ways, yet still connected through their heritage. Participants then shared their thoughts on the personal values exercise they completed in the first session. This discussion highlighted the concept that personal values are personal, and that individuals rank the importance of values based on their individual system of thoughts and beliefs. An examination of the influence of personal values on the pictograph exercise followed. The discussion then moved to the subject of sexually transmitted infections (STIs): what they are, how they are transmitted, and the impacts of undiagnosed STIs on a woman, and potentially on her baby. A card swap game demonstrated how quickly and easily STIs can be spread among partners. Participants explored a few STI-related myths and facts before moving on to the concept of risk and risk reduction. The session also introduced OPRaH: the four-step method for putting on condoms (open, pinch, roll, and hold). Participants practiced with condoms, using penis models (or other proxies) and water-based lubricants. Workshop 2 closed with a game of "*SiHLE* Jeopardy" to test participants' STI/HIV knowledge.

Nikia Braxton-Franklin's poem, "For Free," opened the third workshop as participants revisited the theme of pride in being a Black woman. In this session, participants delved deeper into the concept of risk with the "Luv & Kisses" activity, in which they rated the risk level of activities such as massage, showering together or anal sex without a condom. They explored reasons/excuses why other people and they themselves did not use condoms (and why they would start using condoms). The "Keep It Simple Sista" activity introduced the role of communication and communication styles in negotiating safer sex. The group practiced their assertive communication skills with role plays. More condom practice followed. The "Alcohol & Sex—Not a Good Mix" activity demonstrated how safer sex intentions can be impaired by alcohol.

In workshop 4, the *SiHLE* Sistas practiced their assertive communication skills by drawing "He says . . ." cards (condom excuse lines) and providing spontaneous "She says . . ." responses. Their workshop peers rated the assertiveness level of the response by holding up numbered cards. An in-depth look at healthy and unhealthy relationships followed, including discussion on domestic violence and seeking help when in unhealthy situations. Working in groups for the "Pieces & Parts" exercise, the participants determined whether statements represent aspects of healthy or unhealthy relationships. "The Power Pie" activity examined eight facets of abuse, and invited participants to revisit their own relationships for evidence of power and control issues. Additional workshop time was devoted to potential dangers of breaking up with an abusive partner, and seeking help. In the final activity, "Your Time to Shine," the health and peer educators changed places with the *SiHLE* Sistas: the Sistas "taught" four specific exercises while the educators "learned."

Program Implementation

As noted earlier, there was no formal training program developed for the peer educators in the original implementation of *SiHLE*. However, their roles and scripts can be discussed prior to implementing the program. You may wish to develop a program in your setting that would combine learning about STI/HIV/AIDS prevention with community service via a peer educator program.

PROGRAM EVALUATION

The Original Evaluation

Study Design

Of the 609 girls who met the eligibility criteria, 522 (86%) agreed to participate in the study. After completing the baseline measures, they were randomized into either the intervention (n = 251) or the control (n = 271). Baseline measures included: (a) a paper-and-pencil questionnaire to assess sociodemographics and psychosocial mediators of HIV-preventive behaviors; (b) an interview with an African American female interviewer to assess sexual behaviors and observe condom application skills; and (c) two self-provided vaginal swabs for STI testing. At baseline, significant differences were found for several variables associated with sexual behaviors (and were included as covariates in subsequent analyses). No differences were observed for sociodemographic characteristics.

Follow-up assessments were conducted at 6 and 12 months postintervention. Of the 251 girls allocated to the intervention at baseline, 226 (90%) completed the 6-month assessment, and 219 (87.3%) completed the 12-month assessment. Of the 271 girls allocated to the control condition, 243 (89.7%) completed the 6-month evaluations, and 241 (88.9%) completed the 12-month evaluation. No differences were observed in baseline variables for either study condition in participants retained in the trial compared with those unavailable for follow-up.

Study Population

All participants in the study were African American females between the ages of 14 and 18. All reported having had vaginal sex in the last 6 months. At baseline, 45 (18%) intervention participants and 50 (19%) control participants were receiving public assistance; 60 (24%) and 63 (23%), respectively, had children; 74 (29%) and 79 (29%), respectively, used a condom at last intercourse; 48 (19%) and 43 (16%), respectively, tested positive for chlamydia; and 126 (50%) and 119 (44%) tested positive for depression.

Outcome Measures

The primary outcome measure was defined as self-reported condom use at every episode of vaginal intercourse. Consistent condom use was assessed for the 30 days and the 6 months prior to baseline and at the 6- and 12-month assessments. Other outcome measures included self-reported sexual behaviors (e.g., condom use at last vaginal intercourse, percentage of condom-protected vaginal intercourse acts in last 30 days, new vaginal sex partners in last 30 days, number of times participant applied condoms on their sex partners in past 6 months, self-reported pregnancy), STI status (e.g., positive laboratory test for a new chlamydia, gonorrhea, or trichomoniasis infection), and psychosocial mediators of sexual behavior.

Evaluation Questions

The survey instrument contained 296 questions. Participants were asked to report their behaviors over relatively brief time intervals to enhance accurate recall. Constructs were assessed using scales with satisfactory psychometric properties previously used among African American adolescents. HIV prevention knowledge was measured using a 16-item scale (α = .68). Perceived partner-related barriers to condom use were measured using a six-item scale that assessed attitudes that impeded participants' ability to use condoms effectively (α = .82). Attitudes toward using condoms were measured using an eight-item scale (α = .68). Frequency of sexual communication was measured using a five-item scale assessing the frequency with which participants discussed HIV-preventive practices with sex partners (α = .8). Condom use self-efficacy was measured using a nine-item scale that assessed participants' confidence in their ability to use condoms properly (α = .88). Participants' condom application skills were rated by interviewers (blind to condition) using a structured scoring protocol that ranged from zero to six, with higher ratings reflecting greater proficiency.

Participants also provided two self-administered vaginal swabs at each assessment point. One swab was tested for gonorrhea and chlamydia, the other for trichomoniasis. (Participants who tested positive for an STI were provided with single-dose treatment and risk-reduction counseling.)

Evaluation Results

Effects of the intervention were analyzed separately at the 6-month assessment (baseline to 6-month assessment), at the 12-month assessment (6- to 12-month assessment), and over the full 12-month period from baseline to 12-month assessment.

Overall Condom Use

Intervention participants were more likely than their control counterparts to report using condoms consistently in the 30 days preceding the 6-month follow-up (unadjusted analysis, intervention, 75.3% vs. control, 58.2%; adjusted odds ratio [OR], 1.77; 95% CI, 0.97–3.2; p = .06) and the 12-month follow-up (unadjusted analysis, intervention, 73.3% vs. control, 56.5%; adjusted OR, 2.23; 95% CI, 1.17–4.27; p = .02) and over the entire 12-month period (adjusted OR, 2.01; 95% CI, 1.28–3.17; p = .003). Intervention participants were also more likely than their control counterparts to report using condoms consistently during the 6 months prior to the 6-month assessment (unadjusted analysis, intervention, 61.3% vs. control 42.6%; adjusted OR, 2.48; 95% CI, 1.44–4.26; p = .001) and the 12-month assessment (unadjusted analysis, intervention, 58.1% vs. control, 45.3%; adjusted OR, 2.14; 95% CI, 1.20–3.84; p = .01) and over the entire 12-month period (adjusted OR, 2.30; 95% CI, 1.51–3.5; p < .001). In addition, intervention participants were more likely to report using a condom at last vaginal intercourse, and to report a significantly higher percentage of condom-protected sex acts at all reporting periods. Intervention participants also reported a higher frequency of putting condoms on their partners, and fewer episodes of unprotected sex. Intervention participants demonstrated greater proficiency in using condoms at the 6- and 12-month follow-up periods and over the entire 12-month period.

STIs

The crude STI incidence, by condition, was calculated for chlamydia (intervention, 2.1 vs. control, 2.0 per 100 person-months), trichomoniasis (intervention, 0.9 vs. control, 1.2 per 100 person-months), and gonorrhea (intervention, 0.09 vs. control, 0.7 per 100 person-months). Results of STI-specific analyses, adjusting for the corresponding baseline variable and covariates indicate a treatment advantage in reducing chlamydia infections (OR, 0.17; 95% CI, 0.03–0.92; p = .04). Intervention effects were not observed for trichomoniasis (OR, 0.37; 95% CI, 0.09–1.46; p = .16) or gonorrhea (OR, 0.14; 95% CI, 0.01–3.02: p = .21).

Other Results

In general, intervention participants reported fewer perceived partner-related barriers to condom use, more favorable attitudes toward using condoms, more frequent discussions with male sex partners about HIV prevention, higher condom use self-efficacy scores, and higher HIV prevention knowledge scores. In addition, they were less likely to self-report a pregnancy or have a new vaginal sex partner in the 30 days prior to assessment.

SiHLE IN THE COMMUNITY TODAY

Since 2006, *SiHLE* has been implemented in 31 communities, in 11 states and the District of Columbia. In one state, Iowa, the program is being used in 12 communities.

NOTE

1. A full set of program materials, including facilitator's manual, poster, participant handbook, handouts, evaluation materials, and more, is available for purchase from Sociometrics at http://www.socio.com/pasha.htm.

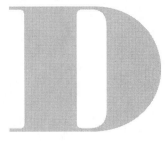

Programs Designed
for Young Men

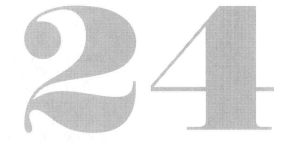

Rikers Health Advocacy Program (RHAP): An STI/HIV/AIDS Prevention Program for Young Men

J. Barry Gurdin, Starr Niego, M. Jane Park, and Janette Mince

Original Program Developers and Evaluators

Stephen Magura, PhD

Janet L. Shapiro, MA

Sung-Yeon Kang, PhD

 National Development and Research Institutes

 New York, NY

PROGRAM ABSTRACT

Summary

This program was originally developed for use with incarcerated male adolescent drug users, who may be detained in custody only briefly. The intensive, short-term intervention consists of four 1-hour, small-group sessions focusing on health education issues, particularly HIV/AIDS. Adapting techniques of problem-solving therapy, the facilitator guides eight-person groups in discussing the following topics: general health, HIV and AIDS, drug abuse and its consequences, sexual behavior, health

Rikers Health Advocacy Program (RHAP) was supported by a grant from the National Institute on Drug Abuse Grant #RO1 DA05942 in cooperation with the New York City Department of Correction.

and AIDS risk behaviors and strategies for seeking health and social services. The discussions provide opportunities for participants to define high-risk attitudes and behaviors, suggest alternative actions and complete challenging "thought teaser" exercises that are designed to help the teens reflect on the reasons underlying their high-risk behaviors.

A field study of the program compared changes in the attitudes and behaviors of *Rikers Health Advocacy Program (RHAP)* participants with those of a comparison group of teens, selected from a waiting list for the program. Both samples were predominantly African American and Hispanic. Following the intervention, program participants expressed more favorable attitudes toward condoms, and were more likely to use condoms during intercourse, as compared with the comparison group of teens.

Focus

☐ Primary pregnancy prevention   ☐ Secondary pregnancy prevention   ☑ STI/HIV/AIDS prevention

Original Site

☐ School based   ☑ Community based   ☐ Clinic based

Suitable for Use In

RHAP is appropriate for school- or community-based programs serving high-risk teens, especially drug users and incarcerated youths. Although it was initially targeted toward males, the curriculum could be used with females. Single-sex discussion groups are recommended.

Approach

- ☐ Abstinence
- ☑ Behavioral skills development
- ☐ Community outreach
- ☐ Contraceptive access
- ☑ Contraceptive education
- ☐ Life option enhancement
- ☑ Self-efficacy/self-esteem
- ☑ Sexuality/HIV/STI education

Original Intervention Sample

Age, gender   The original sample included 110 incarcerated, drug-using males, ages 16 to 18 years (average = 17.8).

Race/ethnicity   64% African American, 33% Hispanic, 3% White.

Program Components

- ☐ Adult involvement
- ☐ Case management
- ☑ Group discussion
- ☑ Lectures
- ☐ Peer counseling/instruction
- ☐ Public service announcements
- ☐ Role play
- ☐ Video
- ☐ Other

Program Length

This is a 2-week, 4-hour intervention. Two 1-hour group sessions are held each week.

Staffing Requirements/Training

One leader is required for each group of approximately eight participants. Leaders should be the same sex as the teens in their group; they must also be comfortable working with high-risk youths and knowledgeable about HIV and drug use/abuse. For training, a thorough review of the curriculum and strategies for facilitating group sessions is recommended.

BIBLIOGRAPHY

D'Zurilla, T. J. (1988). Problem-solving therapies. In K. S. Dobson (Ed), *Handbook of cognitive behavioral therapies* (pp. 85–135). New York: Guilford.

Magura, S., Kang, S. Y., & Shapiro, J. L. (1994). Outcomes of intensive AIDS education for male adolescent drug users in jail. *Journal of Adolescent Health, 15*(6), 457–463.

Related References by the Developers of *RHAP*

Magura, S. Blankertz, L., Madison, E. M., Friedman, E., & Gomez, A. (2007). An innovative job placement model for unemployed methadone patients: A randomized clinical trial. *Substance Use & Misuse, 42*(5), 811–828.

Magura, S., Kang, S. Y., Shapiro, J. L., & O'Day, J. (1995). Evaluation of an AIDS education model for women drug users in jail. *International Journal of Addiction, 30*(3), 259–273.

Magura, S., Laudet, A., Kang, S. Y., & Whitney, S. A. (1999). Effectiveness of comprehensive services for crack-dependent mothers with newborns and young children. *Journal of Psychoactive Drugs, 31*(4), 321–338.

Magura, S., Staines, G. L., Blankertz, L., & Madison, E. M. (2004). The effectiveness of vocational services for substance users in treatment. *Substance Use & Misuse, 39*(13–14), 2165–2213.

THE PROGRAM

Program Rationale and History

RHAP focuses on health education issues, especially HIV/AIDS, relevant to incarcerated, drug-using teenagers.[1] Based on problem-solving therapy, the curriculum introduces knowledge about general health, transmission and prevention of HIV/AIDS, drug abuse and sexual behavior, and teaches teens how to seek health, social and drug treatment services. The four-session program is structured around small group discussions with up to eight inmates.

A field study of the program was conducted between 1991 and 1992 at the New York City Department of Correction's Adolescent Reception and Detention Center on Rikers Island. Participants were predominantly African American and Hispanic, heterosexual, and 16–18 years of age. Over one-half had been arrested at least once before, and one-fifth reported five or more arrests. Funding for the study was provided by the National Institute on Drug Abuse.

Theoretical Framework

Problem-solving therapy is the multistep approach used to structure *RHAP's* group discussions (D'Zurilla, 1988). It appears to be relatively effective when applied in rapidly changing populations—including incarcerated, drug-using adolescents detained for varying periods of time—to reduce drug use and other high-risk activities.

The therapeutic process begins with problem orientation. Group members share and discuss facts and beliefs about the relevant problem, which in this case was HIV/AIDS. The next steps are to define and formulate the problem and then pinpoint specific attitudes and behaviors that must be modified to protect oneself and others from HIV/AIDS. At this stage of the therapy, participants generate alternative solutions by suggesting potential courses of action. Then, during the decision-making step, group members evaluate the strengths and weaknesses of these alternative solutions.

The closing phase of problem-solving therapy is solution implementation. Usually this step is carried out through role plays and rehearsal techniques. However, in *RHAP*, a cognitive reframing exercise is used. The facilitator introduces a situation that is relevant to the everyday lives of high-risk adolescents, and the youths are asked to consider their solutions. Typically, the youths are asked to think about a common event among abusers of illicit, highly addictive substances that results in high-risk behavior. Later, the facilitator helps participants identify the contradiction between their values and actions. It is hoped that reflecting on this contradiction will lead participants to make positive changes in their behavior.

Program Objectives

RHAP aimed to reduce the risk of HIV/AIDS and increase knowledge about health, drug use, and sexuality among incarcerated teenagers. Specifically, the curriculum addressed the following five objectives:

1. To help participants examine the concept of health and determine what they could do to maintain and improve their health and prevent disease in their own lives
2. To learn the basics about HIV and AIDS and how they could affect one's life
3. To learn about HIV and AIDS transmission
4. To learn why people begin and continue using drugs; to recall positive and negative aspects of drug use; to outline options to drug use and summarize safer methods of using drugs, if one "must" continue to use
5. To explore the meanings of sex in one's life, including both positive and negative aspects; to learn how sex-related health problems could be avoided

Program Schedule

The curriculum was delivered in a small-group format with up to eight inmates in each group. Four small-group sessions were held for 1 hour each, twice a week. Although a longer intervention might have been helpful, it was impractical in most jails owing to detention periods of only a few weeks.

Description of Program Sessions

Session 1: Introduction. In the first session, the educator introduced the goals of the *RHAP* program and established ground rules for the group. Participants were encouraged to introduce themselves by relating the first quality about themselves they would like a stranger to know. Although the group discussion may vary with participants' concerns, the facilitator made certain to address the topics of general health, HIV/AIDS, drug use, and sex and sexuality. Toward the end of the discussion, participants classified various types of health and considered how their health concerns affected their individual lives. The facilitator set aside 10 minutes to summarize the content of the discussion and invited participants to discuss their goals for the next three sessions.

Session 2: HIV and AIDS. This session was designed to assess participants' knowledge about HIV/AIDS and to determine the changes that participants and their peers are making in response to the epidemic. The facilitator encouraged the youths to be as specific as possible in discussing the impact of HIV/AIDS on their drug-using subculture. The first part of this session concluded with a "thought teaser." Participants reflected back to the day before they first used drugs. Had they thought they would begin using drugs at that time?

Basic facts about HIV/AIDS were explained during the second half of the session, using analogies to (a) a foreign army's invasion and (b) crowd behavior during a riot. Together the group discussed specific symptoms of the virus, comparing them to similar responses that arise from drug use. Routes of transmission were also explained. The session concluded with a review of modes of HIV transmission, including sharing needles, using a needle already used by someone else, an accidental needle stick, tattooing, and ear and nose piercing.

Session 3: Drug Use. At the beginning of this session, participants shared their responses to the thought teaser introduced in Session 2. The rest of the session was devoted to a discussion of drugs, the consequences of their use and ways to quit or use more safely. After probing how and with whom the youths started using drugs, and how experimentation turned into regular use, the facilitator asked which specific drugs were refused and how people resisted them. Then the facilitator listed reasons why people continued to use drugs and the negative consequences of drug use. At this point, the discussion shifted to the impact of drugs on health, and the problems associated with quitting. After indicating that there were two options—either continuing or stopping use—the facilitator reviewed the safest strategy if a participant felt he must continue to use drugs. The facilitator then summarized the options for those who wanted to stop using. Finally, the facilitator introduced a new thought teaser. In this scenario, each participant imagined that his sister (or mother or girlfriend) had performed oral sex on a friend in exchange for crack cocaine.

Session 4: Sex. Returning to the thought teaser introduced in Session 3, the facilitator asked how participants would have responded to the scenario. From this discussion group members explored the meanings and experiences of sex, including both positive and negative aspects. The facilitator emphasized practical ways to avoid sex-related health problems and asked whether participants or their acquaintances had encountered difficulties with condoms. Finally, the group considered whether drugs and sex met some of the same human needs.

PROGRAM IMPLEMENTATION

Establishing Ground Rules

Facilitators are advised to convey the principles listed below.

1. *Confidentiality.* To ensure that participants feel safe and comfortable sharing their thoughts and feelings, all comments are confidential. Neither the staff nor inmates should ever divulge any information to the correctional staff or anyone else. Nevertheless, in the original field study, a guard was stationed outside the room. Participants were reminded that the grate in the middle might allow sounds to pass, and they were discouraged from discussing specific infractions that may have occurred in the facility.
2. *Everyone's thoughts and feelings are okay.* As long as they are not trying to hurt anyone, participants have a right to their own opinions. No one should be criticized or judged for their feelings.

3. *It is okay not to talk.* A participant can say "I pass," if that individual does not want to share something with the group. At the same time, the more people share, the more everyone will learn from the discussions.

4. *Participants talk one at a time.* They should not interrupt others or start side conversations. They should pay attention to whoever is speaking. Such behavior will encourage all participants to pay attention and show respect to one another.

5. *Participants should be encouraged to express their emotions.* When participants support one another, the whole group can feel supported. Teens should not be afraid to let others know what they need from them.

PROGRAM EVALUATION

The Original Evaluation

Design

The effectiveness of the original *RHAP* program was investigated in a field study conducted with adolescent drug users in jail. The study was carried out in 1991 and 1992 at the New York City Department of Correction's Adolescent Reception and Detention Center (ARDC) on Rikers Island.

From a pool of volunteer inmates, the researchers constructed two empirical groups: (a) program participants and (b) youths who were put on a waiting list for the program. *RHAP*'s effectiveness was investigated by comparing the two groups' scores on several measures of risk behavior, including use of alcohol and noninjecting drugs, frequency of sex with multiple and high-risk sexual partners, frequency of anal sex and frequency of condom use in various contexts.

To assess the impact of the program over time, individual face-to-face interviews were conducted with all teens at two points:

- Time 1: at the start of the intervention (pretest)
- Time 2: about 10 months later (5 months after release from jail) (follow-up)

Evaluation Questions

Two empirical questions guided the field study.

1. Does participation in *RHAP* reduce the frequency of alcohol and noninjecting drug use among teens?
2. Does program participation reduce the frequency of risky sexual behaviors among teens?

Data Collection Procedures

Participants in this study were all recruited from the New York City Department of Correction's Adolescent Reception and Detention Center on Rikers Island. At the start of the field study, the correctional authorities directed the researchers to 11 diverse dormitories housing young men who (a) had recently been admitted to the facility, (b) were in protective custody, (c) had already been sentenced, or (d) were awaiting judicial action.

In a series of visits to each dormitory, the research staff introduced the study to the inmates in residence. They explained that participation was voluntary, all information would be confidential and the project was completely independent of the correctional system. Youths who were interested in participating were asked to sign an informed consent form that was consistent with federal human subjects regulations for prisoners and minors in custody. Additionally, the research plan had been approved by the evaluators' Institutional Review Board, and the data were protected by a Federal Certificate of Confidentiality.

All volunteers were interviewed. Two African American and one Hispanic paraprofessional, who were in recovery from addiction and had personal prison experience, conducted both the Time 1 and Time 2 interviews. The researchers believed that the similar cultural backgrounds and detention experiences of the interviewers and inmates might promote greater honesty by the youths. The semistructured interviews included questions about socio-demographics and family background, alcohol/drug use patterns, drug dealing, involvement with criminal justice, sexual behaviors, psychological status and attitudes toward crime, drug use and AIDS; typically they lasted about 90 minutes.

Following the Time 1 interviews, the two groups of teens—*RHAP* participants and comparison group members—were constructed. Because prison officials were concerned about youths' reactions if they were not offered the opportunity to participate, random assignment to the groups was not employed. Instead, a convenience sample was constructed; the first set of interviewees served as program participants while the remainder were put on a waiting list. Many on this list were released from jail or were transferred within the detention facility before they could participate in the program.

Participants received $10 for completing the Time 1 interview, $5 for attending each group session and $30 for the final, Time 2 interview. The in-jail payments were credited to the participants' commissary accounts.

Sample

The research staff completed Time 1 interviews with 411 incarcerated youths. Of this sample, 110 became program participants. Due to budgetary constraints follow-up data were collected only for 58 early program participants and 99 comparison group members.

The median age of the final sample was 17.8 years. In addition, participants were primarily African American or Hispanic, heterosexual, living with parents or grandparents and not attending school at the time of their arrest. More than half of the participants had been arrested at least once before, and about one-fifth reported five or more arrests. Their offenses included drug dealing and possession, murder, attempted murder, robbery, assault, arson and rape, but property offenses and possession of weapons were the most common charges at arrest.

Since youths who were sentenced and transferred to state prison were not eligible or available for follow-up, the final sample probably underrepresents the most serious or persistent offenders in the population. Overall, the follow-up completion rate was 66% (i.e., number interviewed/number targeted); the researchers found no statistically significant differences on background variables between the youths who participated in the *RHAP* program and those who did not.

Evaluation Results

Time 1 Assessment

At the Time 1 assessment, the youths reported a high degree of involvement in risky behavior, including frequent use of alcohol and marijuana. Twenty-four percent had used cocaine in some form during the month before arrest, although only 3% reported heroin use and none had used intravenous drugs. Also during the month prior to their arrest, 98% of the youths engaged in heterosexual intercourse an average of 3.7 days a week. Three-fourths had multiple sex partners, 10% had high-risk sexual partners and about 30% engaged in heterosexual or homosexual anal sex. About one-fifth never used a condom during sex, and two-thirds used condoms inconsistently, though most (about 66%) carried them regularly.

At the start of the study, the researchers found no statistically significant differences between the behaviors of *RHAP* participants and members of the comparison group.

Follow-Up Assessment

Effects on Condom Use. Ten months after the intervention, *RHAP* participants used condoms significantly more often than their comparison group peers. This outcome was observed for condom use in general, and specifically during vaginal intercourse, oral and anal penetrative sex. The magnitude of the differences between the two groups ranged from 0.6 to 1.0 points on a six-point scale.

Effects on Number of High-Risk Sexual Partners. Program participants reported slightly fewer high-risk sexual partners at the follow-up assessment ($p = .06$), as compared with members of the comparison group.

Effects on Condom Acceptability. The researchers hypothesized that changes in the youths' attitudes toward condoms would parallel changes in their actual condom use. After constructing a measure of condom acceptability, they confirmed this supposition. That is, program participants expressed more favorable attitudes toward condoms than did their comparison group peers.

Effects on Other Risky Behaviors. On measures of the teens' use of alcohol and non-injecting drugs, number of sex partners and frequency of sex, no significant differences were found between the two groups following the intervention.

Summary

RHAP, a four-session HIV/AIDS prevention program incorporating techniques of problem-solving therapy, was found to be effective in reducing some of the high-risk behaviors of incarcerated adolescent drug users. In particular, program participants reported significantly greater use of condoms, both in general and during high-risk acts. In addition, the reduction in high-risk sexual partners fell just short of significance. However, no change was found in other high-risk behaviors practiced by these teens, including the use of alcohol and drugs and sex with multiple partners.

Although *RHAP* proved effective in increasing youths' preventive behaviors and attitudes, open-ended responses to the interview questions revealed that concerns about contraception and other (non-HIV) sexually transmitted infections (STIs)—particularly in contacts with casual partners—helped motivate the youths' increases in condom use. In interpreting their results, the researchers concluded that the youths did not personalize AIDS as a threat, but rather saw it as a problem among other groups, such as gays, adult "crackheads" and "junkies."

Consequently, to prevent HIV from expanding into this highly vulnerable population of teens, the researchers called for intensive, community-based interventions that are designed to integrate the youths into the larger society.

RHAP IN THE COMMUNITY TODAY

In the past 3 years, *RHAP* has been implemented in six states, ranging from New Jersey to Iowa to California.

NOTE

1. A full set of program materials, including a protocol handbook, evaluation materials, and more, is available for purchase from Sociometrics at http://www.socio.com/pasha.htm.

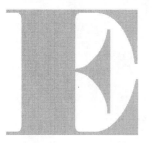

Programs Designed
for College Students

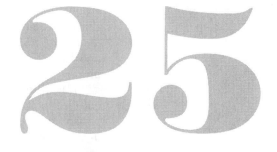

Safer Sex Efficacy Workshop: An Adolescent STI/HIV/AIDS Prevention Program for College Students

J. Barry Gurdin, Starr Niego, M. Jane Park, and Janette Mince

Original Program Developer and Evaluator

Karen Basen-Engquist, MPH, PhD
   Department of Behavioral Science
   University of Texas M.D. Anderson Cancer Center
   Houston, TX

PROGRAM ABSTRACT

Summary

This 3-hour workshop is designed to increase college students' self-efficacy, or belief in their own ability to act successfully to prevent HIV/AIDS and other sexually transmitted infections (STIs). Drawing upon social learning theory, the program includes numerous role-play and skill-building exercises, and is led by peer educators who are trained to serve as persuasive models. To give students the knowledge necessary to practice preventive behaviors, the leaders begin by facilitating a

Safer Sex Efficacy Workshop was supported by a dissertation award from the American Psychological Association.

group discussion about HIV/AIDS and STIs, including transmission and prevention. During the next section, participants discuss personal experiences of and feelings about HIV/AIDS and other STIs. Finally, the students role play safer-sex discussions and learn about correct condom use, gaining confidence in their abilities in the process.

A field study of the workshop was conducted with 209 undergraduate students enrolled in a health education class at the University of Texas. Compared to comparison groups of their peers, program participants showed significant increases in self-efficacy at the 2-month follow-up assessment. Sexually active students also showed an increase in their frequency of condom use.

Focus

☐ Primary pregnancy prevention   ☐ Secondary pregnancy prevention   ☑ STI/HIV/AIDS prevention

Original Site

☑ School based   ☐ Community based   ☐ Clinic based

Suitable for Use In

Although it was originally implemented in a college setting, this program is also suitable for use with young adults ages 18–22 in other educational settings or community-based organizations.

Approach

- ■ ☐ Abstinence
- ■ ☑ Behavioral skills development
- ■ ☐ Community outreach
- ■ ☐ Contraceptive access
- ■ ☑ Contraceptive education
- ■ ☐ Life option enhancement
- ■ ☑ Self-efficacy/self-esteem
- ■ ☑ Sexuality/HIV/STI education

Original Intervention Sample

Age   Among the 209 college students participating in the study, the average age was 22 years.
Gender   67% Female.
Race/ethnicity   82% White.

Program Components

- ■ ☐ Adult involvement
- ■ ☐ Case management
- ■ ☑ Group discussion
- ■ ☐ Lectures
- ■ ☑ Peer counseling/instruction
- ■ ☐ Public service announcements
- ■ ☑ Role play
- ■ ☐ Video
- ■ ☐ Other

Program Length

The single-session workshop is designed to last between 2.5 and 3 hours.

Staffing Requirements/Training

Two peer educators are recommended to lead each 10- to 15-person group. During the original field study, a 20-hour training program was held to introduce the peer educators to basic concepts of the curriculum, as well as HIV/AIDS, STIs, and group process skills.

BIBLIOGRAPHY

Basen-Engquist, K. (1994). Evaluation of a theory-based HIV prevention intervention for college students. *AIDS Education and Prevention, 6*(5), 412–424.

Related References by the Developer of *Safer Sex Efficacy Workshop*

Basen-Engquist, K., Coyle, K., Parcel, G. S., Kirby, D., Banspach, S., Carvajal, S. C., et al. (2001). Schoolwide effects of a multicomponent HIV, STD, and pregnancy prevention program for high school students. *Health Education & Behavior, 28*(2), 166–185.

Basen-Engquist, K., Masse, L. C., Coyle, K., Kirby, D., Parcel, G. S., Banspach, S., et al. (1999). Validity of scales measuring the psychosocial determinants of HIV/STD-related risk behavior in adolescents. *Health Education Research, 14*(1), 25–38.

THE PROGRAM

Program Rationale and History

The *Safer Sex Efficacy Workshop* was a college-level intervention designed to prevent HIV/AIDS and STIs by increasing students' self-efficacy, or belief in their ability to protect themselves from infection.[1] Adapted from the "Eroticizing Safe Sex" guide by the Gay Men's Health Crisis, the 3-hour workshop included small-group discussion, role-play activities and review of basic facts about HIV/AIDS transmission and prevention. The program was guided by social learning theory and used specially trained peer leaders to communicate the importance of safe sexual practices.

A field study of the program was conducted with 209 undergraduate students enrolled in a health education class at the University of Texas. Funding for the study was provided by the American Psychological Association.

Theoretical Framework

The *Safer Sex Efficacy Workshop* was grounded in social learning theory. This theory is based on the idea that knowledge alone is insufficient to produce behavioral change. Instead, the theory points toward four factors that together determine the likelihood of engaging in some action, such as using condoms to protect oneself from HIV/AIDS: (a) a person's understanding of what must be done to avoid infection, (b) the belief that he/she will be able to use condoms, (c) the belief that the method will be successful in preventing HIV/AIDS, and (d) the benefit he/she anticipates from accomplishing the behavior (e.g., staying healthy).

To enhance participants' self-efficacy, the program includes mastery experiences, or practice in successfully completing a task (e.g., negotiating with one's partner and using condoms); role modeling, or watching others perform the task successfully; and social persuasion, which refers to information received from others that one can perform a task successfully. Following principles of social learning theory, the workshop is led by peer educators who are trained to serve as persuasive and appealing models.

Program Objectives

As an STI/HIV/AIDS risk-reduction program, the *Safer Sex Efficacy Workshop* was designed to help participants

1. acquire the information they would need in order to make informed choices about protecting themselves from HIV/AIDS and other STIs;
2. acquire the skills needed to act on those choices;
3. feel more comfortable talking to their sexual partners about safer sex;
4. discover that safer sex does not have to be boring or much trouble—instead, it could be fun and allow participants to be creative.

Underlying Principles of the Workshop

All workshop activities and lessons reinforced three principles:

- Sex is healthy.
- The way in which individuals protect themselves from HIV/AIDS and other STIs should be an informed choice, not one made out of fear and ignorance.
- Changing sexual behavior is not easy, but it can be done if individuals develop the necessary skills and receive support in the process.

Teaching Strategies

Activities in the *Safer Sex Efficacy Workshop* emphasized mastery experiences, role modeling, and social persuasion, as explained below.

- *Mastery experiences:* Students repeatedly practiced negotiating and discussing issues regarding safer sex. The program was premised on the idea that after gaining confidence in their abilities, students would be able to apply these skills in their own relationships.
- *Role modeling:* Peer instructors served as role models, demonstrating techniques for using condoms, comfortably conversing about safer sex and negotiating safer sex with a partner. In addition, students also served as models to one another as they participated in role plays.
- *Social persuasion:* Throughout the workshop, the peer instructors encouraged participants, offered feedback, and discussed the importance of safer sex.

The 3-hour workshop was divided into six segments. Brief overviews of the segments appear below.

Program Schedule

Description of Workshop Segments

I. Introduction. After the facilitator reviewed the goals and guidelines of the workshop, each student paired off with someone he or she did not know. The participants spent about 5 to 10 minutes getting to know one another, and then introduced their new acquaintance to the group.

II. AIDS Information, STI Information, and Personal Risk. The facilitator led the group in a discussion of basic facts about HIV/AIDS and other STIs, focusing on how the infections are and are not transmitted, and the best way individuals can protect themselves from contracting HIV, gonorrhea, chlamydia, and other infections.

Discussion then shifted to students' vulnerability to infection, even if they were not a member of a high-risk group. This section of the workshop concluded with an activity designed to help participants calculate their risk for STIs by adding or subtracting points for various sexual behaviors in which they might have engaged.

III. Discussion of AIDS and Safer Sex. During this segment of the workshop, participants discussed the impact of HIV/AIDS and other STIs on their own lives. Shifting to disease prevention, the facilitator first listed various preventive behaviors (e.g., abstinence, using condoms). Then students considered the five most significant barriers that hamper individuals from following prevention strategies. Working in small groups, participants brainstormed ways they might overcome each of the barriers.

IV. Talking About Safer Sex With Partners and Others. After a brief break, the focus shifted to strategies for negotiating safer sex with one's partner. The instructor divided participants into four-person teams; these teams enacted various role plays involving sexual decision making. Following the role plays, the facilitator brought the groups together to discuss and review what they had learned.

V. Making Safer Sex Fun. The next section of the workshop began with a demonstration of the correct way to use a condom. The participants explored ways of having safer sex in a satisfying manner. Finally, the instructor reminded students about the importance of maintaining confidentiality concerning the workshop discussions.

VI. Closing. Before participants left, the facilitator answered any remaining questions and handed out educational brochures on HIV/AIDS and safer sex.

Program Implementation

During the original field study, a 20-hour training program was held to prepare educators to lead the workshop. The training included a discussion of basic facts about HIV/AIDS and other STIs, as well as the specific skills required to lead the program.

Establishing Ground Rules

Ground rules for group discussions were established at the start of the workshop session. This helped create an atmosphere of trust and comfort in which students would feel free to discuss issues concerning sexuality and protection from STIs, with a particular focus on HIV/AIDS. Ground rules used in the original implementation included the following:

1. Confidentiality. Participants should not repeat outside of the workshop any of the comments offered by students during the session. However, they are free to discuss with friends the content of the program itself.
2. Use "I" statements during group discussions. This type of statement helps people appear more warm and personable to others.
3. Remember that sexual behavior represents a personal choice—there will be a wide range of sexual experiences and practices among group members. For this reason, it is best not to be judgmental about others' behaviors.
4. Participants should be discouraged from censoring anything they may be thinking. In this way, the workshop will be more spontaneous and meaningful for students.

Importance of Role Playing

Practicing newly learned skills is a critical piece of the *Safer Sex Efficacy Workshop*. The role-play activities are designed to encourage participants to talk more easily with their partners and others. Participants are divided into teams of four. In each team, two people role-played four scenarios, while the other two people remained silent and observed. After enacting the scenarios, the whole group discussed several questions probing their feelings, observations and evaluation of the strategies used to negotiate safer sex. This process reinforced participants' ability to communicate clearly and forcefully in romantic encounters.

EVALUATING THE PROGRAM

The Original Evaluation

Design

The effectiveness of the *Safer Sex Efficacy Workshop* was investigated in a field study conducted with 209 students enrolled in an undergraduate health education class at the University of Texas. Volunteers were randomly assigned to take part in one of three interventions: (a) the *Safer Sex Efficacy Workshop*; (b) a didactic lecture on HIV that contained the same information as the workshop, but without mastery experiences, role modeling, or social persuasion; or (c) a lecture on an unrelated topic, family violence.

The study compared the three groups of students on measures of self-efficacy, behavioral intentions and actual behaviors. To measure the impact of the workshop over time, a series of self-report questionnaires was administered to all participants. Behavioral outcomes were measured at all three points listed below, but the cognitive outcomes were measured at Times 1 and 2 only.

- *Time 1:* before the intervention began (pretest)
- *Time 2:* at the conclusion of the intervention (posttest)
- *Time 3:* 2 months following the intervention (follow-up)

Evaluation Questions

The study was designed to examine the effects of the *Safer Sex Efficacy Workshop* on students' self-efficacy, behavioral intentions and actual behaviors regarding safer sex. The researcher hypothesized that workshop participants, compared to their peers attending the HIV and family violence lectures, would show higher self-efficacy and stronger intentions to practice safer sex following the intervention. Additionally, it was predicted that workshop participants would show higher levels of actual safe sex behavior at the follow-up assessment, 2 months later.

Data Collection Procedures

All students enrolled in an undergraduate health education class at the University of Texas were given the option of participating in the study, or writing a short paper to fulfill a course requirement. All opted to participate in the study.

The students were randomly assigned to take part in the *Safer Sex Efficacy Workshop*, or either of the two comparison interventions: the didactic HIV lecture or the family violence lecture.

Data collection was anonymous and confidential. Each participant's pretest, posttest and follow-up questionnaires were linked by a code number formed by combining digits from the student's social security and telephone numbers.

Sample

Of the 209 participants who completed the pretest, 174 (83%) attended the intervention and provided complete data for the remaining two assessments. The sample included more female than male participants, and was predominantly White and heterosexual. On average, participants were slightly under 22 years of age.

Analysis of the behavioral measures was conducted only for those participants who provided complete data at all three assessment periods. After the participants with incomplete data were dropped, the final sample for the behavioral analysis included 67 participants who had sex in the previous 2 months at pretest, posttest, and follow-up. Those who had not had sex at any of the time points were not included in the behavioral analysis.

Evaluation Results

At the Time 1 assessment, there were no significant differences among the three groups on any of the cognitive measures. However, students in the family violence lecture group did report more frequent use of condoms than did their peers assigned to take part in the *Safer Sex Efficacy Workshop*.

Effects on Self-Efficacy

Compared to their peers attending the family violence lecture, participants attending the *Safer Sex Efficacy Workshop* and the HIV lecture both showed significant increases on measures of self-efficacy from the Time 1 to Time 2 assessments.

Effects on Intention to Use a Condom

Again, compared to their peers attending the family violence lecture, both the *Safer Sex Efficacy Workshop* and the HIV lecture participants showed significant gains from the Time 1 to Time 2 assessments.

Effects on Intentions to Communicate About Safer Sex

The *Safer Sex Efficacy Workshop* did not appear more effective than the other interventions in increasing students' intentions to discuss AIDS and their sexual history with their current sexual partners. During the brief (less than 2-week) period from the Time 1 to Time 2 assessments, students in all three groups showed increases on these measures.

Effects on Safer Sex Behavior

During the 2-month follow-up period, workshop participants increased their frequency of condom use more than their comparison group peers. But the degree of improvement was small—on a five-point scale it rose from a mean of 1.7 (between never and rarely) at Time 1 to a mean of 2.2 (between rarely and occasionally) at the Time 3 assessment ($p < .019$).

Summary

Immediately following the intervention, participants in the *Safer Sex Efficacy Workshop* showed increased self-efficacy and intention to use condoms in future sex acts. However, the same material, when delivered in a traditional, didactic format, appeared to have the same effect on students' self-efficacy and intentions concerning safer sex. The comparable results for the workshop and HIV lecture may be attributed to the presence of efficacy-boosting elements in both interventions. Because the same peer instructors delivered all of the interventions, they may have unintentionally served as role models to students. Although present to a lesser degree in the HIV lecture, such role modeling could have been sufficient to strengthen the participants' self-efficacy and intentions regarding safer sex.

The workshop did appear to be more effective in increasing students' actual use of condoms, though only modestly. The small degree of change may have been due to the limited, single-session structure of the program. A similar approach, applied over a longer period of time, might have shown greater effect on participants.

Moreover, in interpreting the results, the researcher noted that at the time of the field study, there was growing awareness of the risk of HIV/AIDS for those outside of high-risk groups. Consequently, the importance of safer sex communication might have already been salient for students, regardless of the intervention in which they took part.

SAFER SEX EFFICACY WORKSHOP IN THE COMMUNITY TODAY

In the past 3 years, *Safer Sex Efficacy Workshop* has been implemented in Maryland.

NOTE

1. A full set of program materials, including instructor's handbook, pamphlets, evaluation materials, and more, is available for purchase from Sociometrics at http://www.socio.com/pasha.htm.

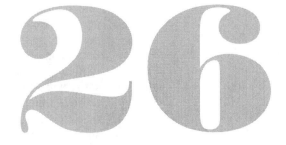

AIDS Risk Reduction for College Students: An STI/HIV/AIDS Prevention Program

William S. Farrell, Kathryn L. Muller, and Janette Mince

Original Program Developers and Evaluators

Diane L. Kimble Willcutts
Jeffrey D. Fisher, PhD
Stephen J. Misovich, PhD
    University of Connecticut
    Storrs, CT

William A. Fisher, PhD
    University of Western Ontario
    London, ON

PROGRAM ABSTRACT

Summary

Designed as a workshop for college students, *AIDS Risk Reduction for College Students* consists of three 2-hour sessions that are based on Fisher and Fisher's information, motivation, and behavioral skills approach to AIDS risk reduction.

AIDS Risk Reduction for College Students was supported by grants and awards from the National Institute of Mental Health (Grant Number MH46224–05), Health and Welfare Canada, and Janssen-Ortho.

The informational component includes "AIDS 101," a slide show that explains transmission and prevention of HIV, testing for the virus and the need for sexually active individuals to use condoms for protection against HIV/AIDS. In the motivational component, small-group discussions are led by a peer health educator, and participants view a video narrated by persons who contracted HIV through unsafe sexual intercourse. Finally, the development of behavioral skills is encouraged through role plays of safer sex communication.

In a field study of the program with 744 college students, participants showed significant gains in knowledge, motivation, and behavior. In particular, sexually active participants were more likely than similar control students to purchase and use condoms during a 2- to 4-month period following the intervention.

Focus

☐ Primary pregnancy prevention   ☐ Secondary pregnancy prevention   ☑ STI/HIV/AIDS prevention

Original Site

☑ School based   ☐ Community based   ☐ Clinic based

Suitable for Use In

This program is most appropriate for older adolescents and young adults, ages 18–22. It can be used in a college setting or a community-based setting.

Approach

- ☐ Abstinence
- ☑ Behavioral skills development
- ☐ Community outreach
- ☐ Contraceptive access
- ☑ Contraceptive education
- ☐ Life option enhancement
- ☐ Self-efficacy/self-esteem
- ☑ Sexuality/HIV/STI education

Original Intervention Sample

Age, gender   A total of 744 college students, 49% male, 51% female, participated in the study; their median age was 20.

Race/ Ethnicity   88% White, 3% African American, 3% Latino, 4% Asian, 1% Other.

Program Components

- ☐ Adult involvement
- ☐ Case management
- ☑ Group discussion
- ☑ Lectures
- ☑ Peer counseling/instruction
- ☐ Public service announcements
- ☑ Role play
- ☑ Video
- ☑ Other: Slide show

Program Length

The program consists of three 2-hour sessions spaced (about) a week apart.

Staffing Requirements/Training

The program is led by a health educator and several peer educators (one peer educator for approximately five to six students). Peer educators take part in an extensive training session covering basic facts about HIV/AIDS, as well as strategies for leading role plays and facilitating small-group discussions.

It is recommended that the health educator have a master's degree in psychology, public health or a related field, as well as significant experience leading HIV prevention programs.

BIBLIOGRAPHY

Fisher, J. D., & Fisher, W. A. (1992). Changing AIDS risk behavior. *Psychological Bulletin, 111,* 455–474.

Fisher, J. D., & Fisher, W. A. (1992). Understanding and promoting AIDS preventive behavior. A conceptual model and educational tools. *The Canadian Journal of Human Sexuality, 1,* 99–106.

Fisher, J. D., Fisher, W. A., Misovich, S. J., Kimble, D. L., & Malloy, T. E. (1996). Changing AIDS risk behavior: Effects of an intervention emphasizing AIDS risk reduction information, motivation, and behavioral skills in a college student population. *Health Psychology, 15*(2), 114–123.

Misovich, S. J., Fisher, W. A., & Fisher, J. D. (2004). A measure of AIDS prevention information, motivation, behavioral skills, and behavior. In C. M. Davis, W. H. Yarber, R. Bauserman, G. Schreer & S. L. Davis (Eds.), *Sexuality-related measures: A compendium* (2nd ed., pp. 328–337). Beverly Hills, CA: Sage.

Related References by the Developers of *AIDS Risk Reduction for College Students*

Fisher, J. D, Fisher, W. L., Bryan, A. D., & Misovich, S. J. (2002). Information-motivation-behavioral skills model-based HIV risk behavior change intervention for inner-city high school youth. *Health Psychology, 21*(2), 177–186.

Malloy, T. E., Fisher, W. L., Albright, L., Mishovich, S. J., & Fisher, J. D. (1997). Interpersonal perception of the AIDS risk potential of persons of the opposite sex. *Health Psychology, 16*(5), 480–486.

THE PROGRAM

Program Rationale and History

Because college students have tended to engage in exceedingly high levels of unprotected sexual intercourse, often with multiple partners in a serially monogamous pattern, they have been at considerable risk for infection with HIV and other sexually transmitted infections (STIs).[1] *AIDS Risk Reduction for College Students* was designed using Fisher and Fisher's information-motivation-behavioral skills (IMB) model of AIDS risk behavior change to reduce HIV risk-related behaviors among male and female college students. The intervention curriculum was specifically designed to address deficits in AIDS risk reduction information, motivation, and behavioral skills that were common among university students.

The program consisted of three 2-hour workshop sessions, which were conducted by a health educator and a team of peer educators. Workshop sessions provided students with accurate knowledge regarding HIV transmission and prevention, motivation to adopt HIV preventive behaviors, as well as the behavioral skills and confidence to execute and maintain risk reduction behaviors. This intervention was originally implemented and field tested with a group of undergraduate dormitory residents at the University of Connecticut.

Theoretical Framework

AIDS Risk Reduction for College Students was based on Fisher and Fisher's IMB model of AIDS risk behavioral change. The IMB model holds that the critical determinants of AIDS risk behavior change are AIDS risk reduction *information, motivation,* and *behavioral skills.* In order to initiate and maintain changes in AIDS risk behavior, individuals must have the following: (a) accurate information regarding AIDS transmission and prevention; (b) motivation—based on social norms and expectations, or feelings of personal vulnerability—to utilize that information; and (c) the necessary behavioral skills and confidence in one's ability (self-efficacy) to perform specific preventive acts.

Program Objectives

The goal of *AIDS Risk Reduction for College Students* was to reduce college students' risk of infection with and transmission of HIV/AIDS and other STIs. Specifically, the program was designed to achieve the following objectives:

- To increase students' knowledge regarding HIV/AIDS risk and transmission and dispel commonly-held "myths" (e.g., unprotected sex is okay if you know your partner's sexual history)
- To increase students' awareness of their personal vulnerability to HIV infection
- To positively influence students' AIDS prevention attitudes and perceived social norms
- To increase students' levels of AIDS prevention behavioral skills
- To increase safer sexual practices among sexually active students, including consistent and correct use of condoms and HIV antibody testing

Program Overview

The *AIDS Risk Reduction for College Students* program consisted of three 2-hour workshop sessions designed to be implemented approximately 1 week apart. The program included three components—informational, motivational, and behavioral skills—which were interspersed across the three sessions. An overview of the program appears below.

Health and Peer Educators

In the original field study, the intervention was implemented in a workshop entitled "Sex in the Age of HIV: Pleasures, Problems, and Prospects." Sessions were conducted in a dormitory setting by a team of one health educator and five peer educators. Peer educators were selected for their ability to act as natural opinion leaders and influence norms and attitudes about HIV prevention; they were also expected to serve as role models. All peer educators took part in an intensive 4-day training session.

During the intervention, the peer educators guided small-group discussions. The discussions addressed

- attitudes toward preventive behaviors (e.g., buying, carrying and using condoms; communicating with partners about HIV-preventive behavior; undergoing HIV antibody testing);
- ways to address negative aspects of preventive behaviors (e.g., using a lubricant to improve sensation with condoms);
- HIV prevention norms, expectations, and behavior.

Informational Component

The information component of the intervention consisted primarily of a slide show ("AIDS 101") addressing college students' performance of AIDS preventive behavior. The slide show, narrated by the health educator, utilized considerable humor, and was heavily illustrated. It included information on HIV transmission and prevention, the relative risk of different behaviors, the effectiveness of condoms, where to get condoms and HIV antibody testing. The slide presentation also debunked incorrect AIDS prevention strategies and risky safer sex decision rules (e.g., not needing to use a condom if you are monogamous or only have sex with "nice" partners). Following the slide presentation, the health educator addressed and corrected "myths" about HIV prevention and transmission, including faulty decision rules and assessments of partner risk.

Motivational Component

This component was designed to influence students' attitudes and perceived social norms regarding AIDS preventive behaviors, as well as perceptions of their personal vulnerability to HIV infection. Peer educators led discussions with small groups (four to six students) that were designed to influence attitudes and social norms regarding HIV prevention behaviors. Large group discussions, led by the health educator, were designed to promote social expectations and support for safer sexual behavior.

Also included in this component was the video *People Like Us*, designed to heighten students' perceptions of personal vulnerability to HIV infection. Interviews with six attractive young men and women introduced viewers to HIV-positive individuals who were similar to the program participants in terms of age, appearance, sexual history and sexual orientation. All had contracted HIV due to unsafe sexual behavior. The video also attempted to influence attitudes toward safer sexual behaviors by stressing that the discomforts of condom use are minor relative to the consequences of contracting HIV/AIDS.

Behavioral Skills Component

The final program component taught students how to effectively initiate and maintain safer sexual behavior, even in particularly challenging situations. Program participants viewed a video (*Sex, Condoms, and Videotape*) produced especially for this intervention. The video used a soap opera format to humorously depict four types of couples (ranging from a several-month relationship to an inebriated couple planning a one-night stand) who successfully practiced safer sex and overcame common impediments to safer sex. A discussion and role play of specific scripts for effective safer sex communication followed the video presentation. All students—male and female—took turns putting a condom on a lifelike model of an erect penis. Finally, participants were given a behavioral homework assignment.

Program Implementation

Using the *Session Guides*, a health educator and several trained peer educators effectively implemented the *AIDS Risk Reduction for College Students* program in the original implementation.

Selecting a Health Educator

The health educator had a master's degree in psychology, public health, or a related field. However, an individual with significant training and experience presenting AIDS education programs would have been be equally suitable for the position. The following knowledge, skills, and abilities were also essential:

- Extensive experience and training in facilitating group sessions
- Training in or understanding of behavioral science research
- High level of comfort speaking about sexual issues

- Strong organizational and supervisory skills
- Ability to communicate ideas with energy and charisma
- In-depth knowledge of HIV transmission and prevention, including awareness of current research and controversies
- Ability to be nonjudgmental and remain focused on HIV prevention issues during group discussion

Moreover, the health educator needed to support the peer educators in feeling excited about the *AIDS Risk Reduction for College Students* program; believing they could succeed in making a difference; feeling (and working as) part of a team; and seeing through difficulties that would inevitably arise during the intervention. In the original implementation, patience, a sense of humor, and flexibility proved tremendously helpful.

Selecting and Training Peer Educators

The peer educators were trained well in advance of the first program session. The training spanned four 1-day sessions; however, holding these sessions on four consecutive days proved to be grueling for peer educators and trainers in the original field study. Therefore, it is advisable to hold sessions once a week over a month, or even once every 2–3 weeks over the summer.

In the original field study, the peer educators took written and oral exams based on the materials and concepts covered in the curriculum. You may also want to do this in your training program.

The original implementation had one trained peer educator for every five to six students participating in your program. Though unfortunate, not all who volunteered to serve as peer educators completed the training satisfactorily. Recruit more trainees than you will need and expect that some will drop out or not adequately master the required skills.

Addressing Relationship Issues

During the original field study of *AIDS Risk Reduction for College Students,* many participants feared that their relationships would be threatened by discussions of safer sex. The program developers found that it was important to confront students' concerns about relationship conflict that may be precipitated by discussion or institution of safer sexual practices. The psychological discomfort associated with viewing one's sexual partner as a potential health threat also needed to be addressed. Including both members of the couple and providing concrete examples of ways in which to deal with relationship issues enhanced the effectiveness of the program.

EVALUATING THE PROGRAM

The Original Evaluation

Design

The field study of *AIDS Risk Reduction for College Students* was conducted with a group of undergraduate dormitory residents at the University of Connecticut. Individual dormitories were randomly assigned to serve as experimental and control dormitories. Dormitories assigned to the treatment condition received the three-session intervention over a 3-week period; floors assigned to the control condition received no intervention. Both treatment and control groups were assessed at three points in time:

Time 1: immediately preceding the program (pretest)

Time 2: 1 month following the program (posttest)

Time 3: 2 to 4 months following the program (follow-up)

Evaluation Questions

The evaluation was designed to assess the program's effects on AIDS information, motivation, behavioral skills, and risk behaviors.

Specifically, the field study addressed the following questions:

1. Did participation in the *AIDS Risk Reduction for College Students* program increase students' STI/HIV/AIDS-related *knowledge*?
2. Did program participation increase students' *motivation* to implement safer sexual practices?
3. Did participation in the program increase students' AIDS risk reduction *behavioral skills*?
4. Did program participation increase students' performance of AIDS risk reduction *behaviors*?

Intervention and Control Groups

Four quadrangles of high-rise dorms with alternating floors of males and females were randomly selected to participate in the field study. Within each quadrangle, individual dormitories were randomly assigned to serve as experimental or control dorms. Within each type of dorm, a female floor was randomly selected for research participation and paired with the male floor above or below with which residents had the closest social ties. The sets of linked female-male floors composed the experimental and control group units.

This design allowed the intervention to be delivered in a mixed sex context and among groups of students who already knew and interacted with one another. In this way, it was hoped that participation would encourage students to change their perceptions (and behaviors) within their natural social networks.

Data Collection Procedures

Students in the experimental and control group units were recruited and paid $10 to complete a pretest that assessed preintervention levels of AIDS risk reduction information, motivation, behavioral skills and behavior. The pretest was distributed at organizational meetings held by each dormitory floor at the beginning of the semester. Students were told that the pretest was part of a longitudinal survey of college sexual behavior sponsored by the National Institute of Mental Health (NIMH). Later in the year, the researchers added, the students would be re-contacted asked to complete additional NIMH surveys.

Students residing on treatment floors were later recruited to participate in the intervention, which was described as a dormitory workshop on sexuality and relationships. Investigators attempted to minimize the possibility that program participants would connect the intervention to the evaluation measures by having separate sets of individuals describe the pretest and workshop. All treatment floor residents who completed the pretest were invited to complete subsequent questionnaires, although not all of them chose to participate in the program. The intervention consisted of three 2-hour sessions held 1 week apart.

Students living on control floors received no intervention, but they were asked to complete the identical pretest, posttest, and follow-up measures at the same time as treatment floor students. The posttest, which assessed risk reduction information, motivation, behavioral skills and AIDS preventive behavior, was administered independently to experimental and control dormitory floors 4 weeks after the final intervention session. Two to 4 months following the final intervention session, participants completed the follow-up assessment, focusing on AIDS risk reduction behavior.

Sample

A total of 744 undergraduate dormitory residents (362 males and 382 females) at the University of Connecticut completed the pretest. Students' median age was 20, and 88.3% were White, 2.7% African American, 3.4% Hispanic, 4.3% Asian, and 1.2% Other. The sample was predominantly heterosexual, with 4% of the males and 2% of the females reporting a history of same-sex sexual behavior. Of those who completed the pretest, 658 completed the posttest, and 570 completed the follow-up measure.

Measures

The Time 1 and Time 2 assessments included measures of AIDS risk reduction information, motivation, behavioral skills, and engagement in AIDS risk and AIDS preventive behavior. The follow-up assessment focused on levels of AIDS risk and AIDS preventive behavior. All of the instruments were self-administered (see Misovich, Fisher, & Fisher, 2004).

Analytic Method

In the original field study, university students living on adjacent male and female dormitory floors composed units that were randomly assigned to treatment and control conditions. Because individuals within particular treatment or control group units were likely to interact with one another socially between the pre-, post-, and follow-up measures, they may have influenced one another's responses to the surveys. Therefore, it could not be assumed that the data points for individual participants within a group would be independent of the data from other participants within the same group. As a result, the program evaluators adopted a data analysis strategy that could estimate the intervention effects at both the individual and group levels (see Fisher, Fisher, Misovich, Kimble, & Malloy, 1996).

Evaluation Results

To be included in the analysis, treatment group participants had to have attended all three intervention sessions and to have completed both the pre- and posttest measures; control participants had to have completed the pre- and posttest measures. In all, 521 participants met these requirements. At the start of the program, no significant differences were found between treatment and control participants on levels of AIDS risk reduction information, motivation, behavioral skills, or behavior.

In addition, the researchers found no significant differences between treatment floor residents who completed all intervention sessions and those who either refused to participate or who dropped out. Similarly, no significant differences were found between treatment and control students who completed the posttest and follow-up measure and those who did not.

Measures of Information, Motivation, and Skills

AIDS Risk Reduction Information. Participation in the *AIDS Risk Reduction for College Students* program produced significant increases in AIDS prevention information. Postintervention scores on both measures of the information construct were significantly higher than those prior to the intervention. This increase was apparent at both the individual ($p < .001$) and group levels ($p < .001$).

AIDS Risk Reduction Motivation. The intervention had a significant effect on two of three measures of AIDS risk reduction motivation. While attitudes toward the performance of AIDS preventive behavior and intentions to engage in such behavior were significantly improved among program participants 1 month following the intervention, the intervention had no reliable effect on social norms. The intervention effect for attitudes was significant at both the individual ($p < .0001$) and group ($p < .005$) levels, while the effect for behavioral intentions only approached significance ($p = .059$) at the group level.

Thus, while the intervention significantly improved attitudes toward performing AIDS preventive behavior and intentions to engage in such behavior, it had no reliable effect on students' perceptions of social norms. Program evaluators offered two possible explanations why the intervention had no impact on participants' perceptions of social support for safer sexual behavior. First, the intervention may not have been successful at actually changing students' social norms. Alternatively, it is possible that the evaluation measures did not adequately assess perceived changes in peer social norms.

AIDS Risk Reduction Behavioral Skills. *AIDS Risk Reduction for College Students* significantly increased participants' perceptions of the effectiveness and ease with which they could enact critical AIDS preventive behaviors. Compared to control group members, program participants showed significantly higher scores on both indicators of behavioral skills. For the efficacy construct, the scores were significant at both the individual level ($p < .0001$) and the group level ($p < .005$); for the difficulty construct, the scores were significant both at the individual ($p < .0001$) and group level ($p < .05$), as well.

Measures of AIDS Risk Behavior

To be included in the analysis of intervention impact on AIDS risk behavior change, treatment students had to have attended all three intervention sessions and completed the pretest, posttest, and follow-up measures of AIDS preventive behavior. In addition, students had to be individuals for whom self-initiated behavioral change or maintenance of such change was necessary (i.e., they had to have been sexually active; to have had a partner who had not already insisted on the practice of safer sex; could not have indicated that both they and their partner had been each other's only lifetime sexual partner; and could not have indicated that both they and their partner had tested negative for HIV). Each of these criteria had to have been met at each of the three measurement intervals. In all, 134 students met these criteria.

The intervention produced consistent, positive changes in almost every indicator of AIDS risk prevention behavior, as explained below.

Safer Sex Discussion. Program participants reported higher levels of discussing AIDS preventive behavior with a sexual partner. This effect was significant at both the individual and group levels 1 month following the intervention; however, this effect was not significant at either level at the 2- to 4-month follow-up assessment. A potential explanation for this finding is that intervention participants may have discussed safer sex with their partners early on, decided upon behavior change, and therefore did not need to discuss the matter further at the time of the follow-up assessment.

Condom Accessibility and Use. The intervention also had a significant effect on condom accessibility and use. Compared to their peers in the control group, program participants were more likely to buy condoms and have them available at the

1 month postintervention and 2–4 months postintervention. This effect was significant at both the individual and group levels.

In addition to increasing condom accessibility, the intervention also produced sustained increases in condom use. Program participants showed significantly greater levels of condom use than control group participants at both the 1 month posttest assessment and the 2- to 4-month follow-up. The posttest indicator of condom use can only be interpreted at the group level, and it was significant ($p < .05$), showing that the intervention increased condom use. At the 2- to 4-month follow-up, condom use can be interpreted at the individual level, and was significant ($p < .005$). Thus, the intervention resulted in an increase of the critical AIDS preventive behavior of condom use, which was sustained over the follow-up period.

HIV Antibody Testing. Finally, while the intervention had had a significant effect at the individual level on increasing HIV antibody testing behavior at the follow-up, program evaluators asserted that this effect should be interpreted with caution. Because individual data did not appear to be independent from group data, this effect was more reliably interpreted at the group level.

Summary

The evaluation showed that the three-session *AIDS Risk Reduction for College Students* program can be effective in changing risky sexual behavior in a college student population. The IMB model-based intervention produced increases in multiple indicators of AIDS risk reduction information, motivation, and behavioral skills, as well as sustained increases in AIDS preventive behavior.

One month following the intervention, program participants showed significant increases in AIDS risk reduction knowledge, motivation and behavioral skills, as well as significant increases in AIDS preventive behaviors, such as having condoms accessible, using them and engaging in safer sex negotiations, all relative to their control group peers. At the follow-up assessment (2 to 4 months after completion of the intervention), program participants again showed significant increases in AIDS risk reduction behaviors, including keeping condoms accessible and using them during intercourse.

An important observation from the field study concerned the potential obstacles to safer sexual practices that were posed by relationship partners. The program evaluators noted that participants often reported that it was a major challenge to initiate and maintain AIDS risk behavior changes with their relationship partners (who were not participants in the intervention). Concern about relationship conflict precipitated by discussion or institution of safer sexual practices and the dissonance, or psychological discomfort, associated with viewing one's sexual partner as a potential health threat were significant obstacles for students. In future implementations of the program, it may be helpful to include couples and explicitly address factors in relationships that may impede AIDS risk behavior change.

AIDS RISK REDUCTION FOR COLLEGE STUDENTS IN THE COMMUNITY TODAY

In the past 3 years, *AIDS Risk Reduction for College Students* has been implemented in communities in 3 states: North Carolina, Michigan, and Maryland.

NOTE

1. A full set of program materials, including session guides, peer educator training manual, videotapes, pamphlets, and more, is available for purchase from Sociometrics at http://www.socio.com/pasha.htm.

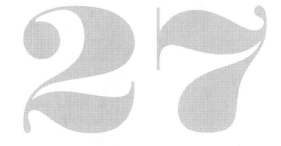

ARREST: AIDS Risk Reduction Education and Skills Training Program

Anne Belden, Starr Niego, and Janette Mince

Original Program Developer and Evaluator

Michele D. Kipke, PhD
Division of Adolescent Medicine
Childrens Hospital Los Angeles
Los Angeles, CA

PROGRAM ABSTRACT

Summary

Principles of the health belief model and social learning theory form the framework for *ARREST,* together with strategies previously found to be effective in changing such adolescent health-risk behaviors as cigarette smoking and early pregnancy. Originally targeted toward high-risk teens between 12 and 16 years of age, the curriculum spans three 90-minute, small-group sessions. Participants receive the following: (a) information about transmission and prevention of HIV/AIDS; (b) instruction and demonstration of purchasing and using condoms with spermicide; (c) guidance in self-assessment of risk behaviors; (d) training in decision making,

ARREST was supported by grants from the Carnegie Corporation, Health Resources and Service Administration, The Rockefeller Brothers Fun, The Fund for the City of New York, Morgan Guaranty Trust Company, W.T. Grant Foundation, Design Industries Foundation for AIDS, and The Samuel and May Rudin Foundation.

291

communication, and assertiveness skills; and (e) peer group support for HIV/AIDS prevention and risk reduction. The teens complete role plays, skill-building exercises, and homework activities. For the duration of the program, they are also asked to record their HIV/AIDS-related thoughts, feelings, and behaviors in a confidential log book.

A field study of the program was conducted with 87 African American and Latino youths who were recruited from three New York City community-based organizations providing alternative education and after-school programs for high-risk teens. Comparing 4-week follow-up measures of program participants with a control group of peers, participants showed significant gains in knowledge and attitudes about AIDS, as well as in sexual refusal and negotiation skills. However, no differences were found between the groups' risk-related sexual behaviors.

Focus

☐ Primary pregnancy prevention ☐ Secondary pregnancy prevention ☑ STI/HIV/AIDS prevention

Original Site

☐ School based ☑ Community based ☐ Clinic based

Suitable for Use In

Although it was originally implemented in a community-based organization, this program is equally suitable for use in schools.

Approach

- ☐ Abstinence
- ☑ Behavioral skills development
- ☐ Community outreach
- ☐ Contraceptive access
- ☑ Contraceptive education
- ☐ Life option enhancement
- ☐ Self-efficacy/self-esteem
- ☑ Sexuality/HIV/STI education

Original Intervention Sample

Age, gender   The field study included 87 at-risk participants, ages 12 to 16 years (average = 13.8); 55% of the sample was female.
Race/ethnicity   59% Latino, 41% African American.

Program Components

- ☐ Adult involvement
- ☐ Case management
- ☑ Group discussion
- ☑ Lectures
- ☐ Peer counseling/instruction
- ☑ Public service announcements
- ☐ Role play
- ☑ Video
- ☑ Other: Peer support groups

Program Length

The 4.5-hour program is divided into three 90-minute training sessions.

Staffing Requirements/Training Program Materials

One skilled HIV/AIDS educator is recommended to lead each group of 10 to 12 students.

BIBLIOGRAPHY

Kipke, M. D., Boyer, C., & Hein, K. (1993). An evaluation of an AIDS risk reduction education and skills training (ARREST) program. *Journal of Adolescent Health, 14*(7), 533–539.

Related References by the Developers of *ARREST*

De Rosa, C. J., Montgomery, S. B., Hyde, J., Iverson, E., & Kipke, M. D. (2001). HIV risk behavior and HIV testing: A comparison of rates and associated factors among homeless and runaway adolescents in two cities. *AIDS Education & Prevention, 13*(2), 131–148.

Kipke, M. D., O'Connor, S., Palmer, R., & MacKenzie, R. G. (1995). Street youth in Los Angeles. Profile of a group at high risk for human immunodeficiency virus infection. *Archives of Pediatric & Adolescent Medicine, 149*(5), 513–519.

Kipke, M. D., Unger, J. B., Palmer, R. F., & Edgington, R. (1996). Drug use, needle sharing, and HIV risk among injection drug-using street youth. *Substance Use & Misuse, 31*(9), 1167–1187.

Schneir, A., Kipke, M. D., Melchior, L. A., & Huba, G. J. (1998). Childrens Hospital Los Angeles: A model of integrated care for HIV-positive and very high-risk youth. *Journal of Adolescent Health, 23*(2 Suppl.), 59–70.

THE PROGRAM

Program Rationale and History

Designed for use with high-risk adolescents ages 12 to 16, *ARREST* aimed to (a) provide teens with information and instruction on HIV/AIDS; (b) enhance their ability to assess the risk level of their own behaviors; and (c) foster the decision-making, assertiveness, and communication skills required for effective prevention and risk reduction.[1] The three-session program was originally targeted toward African American and Latino youths, who were especially vulnerable to HIV infection. Survey data suggested that these groups of teens initiated sexual intercourse at earlier ages, and they showed higher rates of unplanned pregnancies and sexually transmitted infections (STIs). Yet, the curriculum is equally suitable for use with adolescents of all races and ethnicities.

Despite reports that teenagers were well-informed about HIV transmission and prevention, the program developers found that most teens did not think they were at risk of becoming infected. Moreover, many younger adolescents had not developed the kinds of skills that needed for HIV prevention and risk reduction. Typically, for example, these teens were not prepared to negotiate with sexual partners or resist peer pressure in situations where HIV infection was a risk. They were also likely to lack the confidence and skills required to purchase and properly use condoms. To address these issues, the *ARREST* curriculum provided explicit instructions, role modeling, and repeated practice in purchasing and putting on condoms, negotiating safer sex with one's partner and removing oneself from risky situations involving alcohol, drugs, and unprotected sex.

A field study of the program was conducted in 1989 in New York City. The researchers recruited 87 African American and Latino teens from three community-based agencies serving high-risk youths.

Theoretical Framework

ARREST integrated two theories for promoting healthy behavior in youths: the health belief model and social learning theory.

These theories are premised on the idea that knowledge alone is insufficient to produce behavioral change. Instead, they suggest that individuals are likely to reduce their HIV risk-related behaviors when the following conditions are met:

1. One perceives that the problem (e.g., HIV/AIDS) poses a threat to one's well-being.
2. One understands what must be done to avoid infection.
3. One understands the benefits and barriers to taking preventive action.
4. One feels able to effectively carry out the recommended actions.

Drawing upon these principles, *ARREST* first educated teens about HIV infection and risk-related behaviors and then fostered the development of risk reduction skills. Additionally, because social learning theory linked learning to repeated observation and imitation, the program instructor served as a model of socially desirable behaviors. After students observed their instructor engaging in successful communication and decision making, they practiced these skills in a series of role-play exercises.

Program Objectives

As an HIV/AIDS risk reduction program, *ARREST* was designed to meet the following educational objectives:

1. To provide information about HIV transmission and prevention
2. To teach youths how to purchase and properly use condoms with nonoxynol-9 spermicide (Note: Since the time of this study, newer research has indicated that the use of nonoxynol-9 may irritate the vaginal lining and cause microscopic tears to the tissue, leaving the young woman more susceptible to STIs.)
3. To teach youths how to evaluate their level of risk and identify situations associated with risk behaviors
4. To foster the development of decision-making, communication, and assertiveness skills for coping effectively with peer pressure and high-risk situations
5. To establish peer support groups encouraging HIV prevention and risk reduction behaviors

Program Schedule

During the original field study, *ARREST* participants met for five 90-minute sessions, but the first and final meetings were dedicated to the pre- and posttest evaluation assessments. Each training module began with a 30-minute discussion of students' questions, followed by review and reinforcement of the material and take-home exercise from the previous session. During the remainder of the lesson, new material was presented. In the field study, participants were paid $5 at the conclusion of each of the sessions, and an additional $5 if they attended all of the meetings.

Each participant was given a blank notebook that served as a reflective journal. Although the curriculum included a few assigned exercises, teens were encouraged to use the journal for recording their thoughts and feelings outside of the program as well. They also expressed themselves by drawing pictures or writing poetry. Modify or expand the use of the journals in your own implementation of *ARREST* to fit your milieu.

Description of Training Modules

Training Module 1: AIDS Education. This session provided participants with basic information about AIDS and HIV infection, including transmission, prevention, treatment, and testing. By the end of the lesson, participants had an understanding of four essential concepts:

1. AIDS is an infectious disease that has reached epidemic proportions within the United States and throughout the world. AIDS is caused by the human immunodeficiency virus.
2. AIDS is a very difficult disease to contract. There are specific ways in which people become HIV infected—through unprotected sexual intercourse with an infected person, sharing intravenous drug use equipment with an infected person or perinatally, from an infected mother to her newborn child.
3. There is no effective form of treatment or vaccine against HIV infection. Prevention and risk reduction are the only means for protecting oneself.
4. Effective prevention requires either abstinence from sexual intercourse and needle sharing, or risk reduction by consistent use of condoms during sexual intercourse and sterilizing equipment before drug use.

Training Module 2: Instruction on How to Properly Use and Purchase Condoms. This session provided participants with specific information about risk-related behaviors and preventive measures, including the effectiveness of various condoms, how and where to buy condoms, how to prevent condoms from breaking, leaking, or slipping off, and how to effectively use condoms and spermicide or lubricant. Participants learned that effective prevention required that they either delay or abstain from risk-related sexual and drug use behaviors, including the use of condoms and lubricant each time they engaged in oral, vaginal or anal intercourse, and the avoidance of needle sharing. By the end of the session, participants have an understanding of their own risk-related behaviors and have set goals for future prevention and risk reduction.

Training Module 3: Decision-Making, Communication, and Assertiveness Skills Training. Adolescents' desires to be liked by their peers and uncertainty about their own feelings and beliefs have historically made it all the more difficult for them to resist peer pressures. This *ARREST* module was designed to help participants learn how to discuss HIV prevention and risk reduction with friends or sexual partners and how to resist peer pressure. Through role play and group discussion, the program leaders first demonstrated and then invited students to practice avoiding sexual pressures by communicating positively and assertively. The following communication skills were discussed:

- *Assertive talk:* how to assertively communicate one's rights.
- *Expressing feelings:* how to recognize and express feelings in an appropriate and skillful manner.
- *Making a request:* how to be clear, direct, and positive.
- *Coping with refusal:* how to handle situations when requests result in refusals, such as when one's boyfriend refused to use a condom during intercourse.
- *Refusing a request:* when someone makes an unreasonable request (e.g., for unprotected sex or sharing unclean needles), one acknowledged the person's needs, but said "no."
- *Showing appreciation:* how and when to reinforce appropriate behaviors, such as requests to use STI protection.
- *Skills for resisting peer pressure:* how to respond to peer pressure using effective assertiveness and communication techniques.

Program Implementation

ARREST was taught by skilled AIDS educators, with one teacher leading each group of 10 to 12 students. Educators were experienced in leading group discussions, facilitating role-play interactions and conducting demonstrations. They were also able to effectively model the communication and assertiveness skills they were teaching.

Ground Rules for Group Discussions

Listed below are five ground rules to guide your group discussions. Following these rules helped to establish an atmosphere of mutual trust and support during the field test of *ARREST*.

- Everything that is mentioned during the sessions is confidential.
- All participants can choose what thoughts and actions they wish to share and which ones they prefer to keep private.
- All questions are good questions, and all comments are worthy of consideration.
- All participants are expected to listen actively to one another.
- At the same time, all students are expected to show respect for one another. Talking about others' comments outside of the group discussion, or teasing or insulting others will not be tolerated. Different opinions should be respected.

The Use of Journals

At the start of the program, each participant was given a blank journal. The journals were theirs to keep even after the program ended. In the original implementation, the journals were presented with the following introduction:

- Many teens already record their thoughts and feelings in journals or diaries. For others, this will be a new experience.
- Journals provide a safe, private place to express your thoughts. Keep your book in a place where others will not find it.
- People often write in their diaries, but you can also draw pictures or compose music or poetry. Some teens write letters to relatives, friends, or pets. Use whatever method works best for you!

PROGRAM EVALUATION

The Original Evaluation

Design

The effectiveness of *ARREST* was investigated in a field study conducted in New York City in 1989. The study compared participating teens with a control group of youths on a waiting list for the program. The researchers investigated the two groups' HIV/AIDS-related knowledge, attitudes, perception of risk, self-efficacy about avoiding risky situations, as well as their actual sexual behavior. Surveys and role-play assessments were administered to all teens at two points:

- Time 1: at the start of the intervention (pretest)
- Time 2: immediately after the intervention (posttest)

Evaluation Questions

The researchers hypothesized that *ARREST* participants would show significant gains in HIV/AIDS-related attitudes, knowledge, and behavior, relative to their control group peers. In particular, program participants were expected to show

1. increased knowledge and understanding of HIV/AIDS, including perceptions of their own risk of infection;
2. greater self-efficacy, or belief in their own ability to follow preventive behaviors;
3. enhanced assertiveness and communication skills for negotiating prevention and risk reduction and resisting peer pressure.

Data Collection Procedures

Teens were recruited for the study from three agencies providing alternative education and after-school programs for at-risk youths, ages 12 to 16, in New York City. To attract participants, program staff posted flyers, sent letters home, and met with students and teachers to describe the study. The only requirements for eligibility were the ability to speak English and written consent from parents.

Potential participants were assured that all information provided during the study would be confidential. In addition, each teen would receive $5 at the end of each session, plus an additional $5 if they attended all five sessions, for a maximum of $30. Following recruitment, volunteers were randomly assigned either to an *ARREST* intervention group or to a waiting list for the program. The assessments took place during the first and final program sessions.

Research Sample

The final sample included 87 teens, ages 12–16, who were considered to be at elevated risk for HIV infection. Of this group, 39 were male (45%) and 48 were female (55%). More than half of the youths were Latino (59%), and the remainder were African American (41%).

Evaluation Results

Time 1 Assessment

At the start of the study, the researches found no significant differences between the two groups of teens. Overall, 28 of the 87 teens were sexually active. Of this group, 12 reported having had sex during the month before the pretest, with an average of five sexual encounters and two sexual partners during that time. Males were significantly more likely than females to be sexually active. In addition, two females reported having been pregnant and one male had contracted an STI.

Time 2 Assessment

One month after the intervention, program participants showed a significant increase in their knowledge about HIV/AIDS ($p < .001$) and in their perceptions of adolescents' risk of infection ($p < .01$), relative to their control group peers. *ARREST* participants also showed a significant decrease in negative attitudes about AIDS ($p < .05$).

In addition, on the role-play assessments of behavioral skills, teens who participated in the *ARREST* program demonstrated significantly greater skill in refusing to engage in risk-related activities ($p < .001$) and in proposing alternative lower-risk activities ($p < .001$), relative to their control group peers.

However, the two groups of teens did not differ on measures of self-efficacy or sexual behavior (e.g., number of sexual encounters, number of sexual partners, and condom use).

Summary

Overall, *ARREST* appeared to be effective in meeting its short-term objectives for improving teens' knowledge and behavioral skills, two important prerequisites for behavior change. Following their exposure to the three-session program, *ARREST* participants showed significant gains in their knowledge and attitudes about HIV transmission and prevention, perceived risk and appropriate concern about infection. Participation in the program was also associated with greater skill in discussing and negotiating HIV prevention and risk reduction, and in resisting coercive pressures to engage in unprotected sexual intercourse. Yet, program participation did not appear to have any impact on teens' perceived self-efficacy regarding preventive behaviors, or in reducing their involvement in unprotected sexual intercourse.

In interpreting the findings, the researchers suggested a number of reasons for the absence of any behavioral change among youths. First, teens' patterns of sexual activity were measured immediately after the intervention. This short period of time may have been insufficient for registering change. The relatively small sample size may also have hampered efforts to measure statistically significant outcomes. Finally, the brief duration of the *ARREST* intervention may have limited its effect on teens.

Moreover, the brief follow-up period made it difficult to attribute positive outcomes to participation in the program. The researchers recommended additional studies with longer follow-up periods to better understand the effectiveness of the intervention—not only on teens' knowledge, attitudes, and skills, but also on their risk-related behaviors.

ARREST IN THE COMMUNITY TODAY

In the past 3 years, *ARREST* has been implemented in communities in 5 states across the country.

NOTE

1. A full set of program materials, including curriculum manual, AIDS awareness form, evaluation materials, and more, is available for purchase from Sociometrics at http://www.socio.com/pasha.htm.

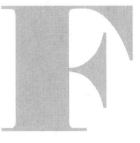

Programs Designed for Youth/Community Collaboration

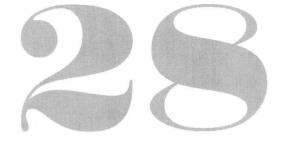

Focus on Kids: An Adolescent HIV Risk Prevention Program

Diana Dull Akers and Janette Mince

Original Program Developers and Evaluators

Bonita F. Stanton, MD
  Department of Pediatrics
  West Virginia University
  School of Medicine
  Morgantown, WV

Jennifer Galbraith, MA
Linda Kaljee, MA
Maureen Black, PhD
Susan Feigelman, MD
Xiaoming Li, PhD
Izabel Ricardo, PhD
  Department of Pediatrics
  University of Maryland Medical School
  Towson, MD

Focus on Kids was supported by contracts and grants from the National Institute of Mental Health, the National Institute of Child Health and Development, and the Agency for Health Care Policy and Research.

PROGRAM ABSTRACT

Summary

Focus on Kids is a culturally-based HIV-risk reduction intervention program directed toward high-risk urban youths. The program is designed for delivery in community center settings rather than schools or clinics in order to reach those with higher rates of truancy and lower use of health care services. The program targets "naturally-formed peer groups" through a series of eight 1.5-hour weekly sessions plus an optional 1-day retreat. The curriculum draws on Protection Motivation Theory and uses multiple delivery formats (lectures, video presentations, role playing, small group discussion) to present factual materials on HIV/AIDS, sexually transmitted infections (STIs), and contraception.

An evaluation of the curriculum was conducted in 1993 in nine recreation centers of three Baltimore public housing developments. The intervention group of 206 African American youths was compared with a control group of 177 African American youths at 6 and 12 months postintervention. Researchers found that at 6 months, condom-use rates were significantly higher among youths in the intervention group than the control group. Condom-use intention and perceptions about condom use were also positively affected. At 12 months, rates of condom use, condom use intention, and positive condom perceptions were no longer significantly higher among intervention than control subjects.

Focus

☐ Primary pregnancy prevention   ☐ Secondary pregnancy prevention   ☑ STI/HIV/AIDS prevention

Original Site

☐ School based   ☑ Community based   ☐ Clinic based

Suitable for Use In

The *Focus on Kids* program is designed for implementation in community/neighborhood settings (e.g., recreation centers, community centers) as opposed to school or clinic settings. The goal is to reach high-risk youths in the areas where they may be making decisions about high-risk behavior.

Approach

- ■ ☐ Abstinence
- ■ ☑ Behavioral skills development
- ■ ☑ Community outreach
- ■ ☑ Contraceptive access
- ■ ☑ Contraceptive education
- ■ ☑ Life option enhancement
- ■ ☑ Self-efficacy/self-esteem
- ■ ☑ Sexuality/HIV/AIDS/STD education

Original Intervention Sample

Age, gender   The original intervention sample included 383 youths ages 9 through 15; the median age of participants was 11.3 years at baseline. There were 206 youths in the intervention group and 177 youths in the control group; approximately half the sample (n = 213) was male.

Race/ethnicity   The original intervention sample population was 100% African American.

Program Components

- ■ ☑ Adult involvement
- ■ ☑ Case management
- ■ ☑ Group discussion
- ■ ☑ Lectures (parenting education)
- ■ ☑ Peer counseling/instruction
- ■ ☐ Public service announcements
- ■ ☑ Role play
- ■ ☑ Video
- ■ ☑ Other: One-day retreat at a rural campsite

Program Length

The intervention consists of eight sessions, including seven weekly, 90-minute meetings in participating recreation centers, and an optional 1-day session conducted in a rural campsite. There is some flexibility with the scheduling of the sessions. You may opt to meet twice a week instead; what is important is that the meeting times are regularly scheduled so that youths always know the time of the next meeting.

Staffing Requirements/Training

Program facilitators. At least two group leaders cofacilitate the weekly sessions; they bring diverse strengths to the intervention. Select facilitators who are from—or highly familiar with—the community where the intervention is conducted. Experience with education, HIV/AIDS prevention and/or child development is preferred. Minimally, facilitators should be able to model good communication and negotiation skills for youths. We recommend at least one initial staff training session to orient facilitators to the program's goals/logic.

Optional staff requirements. If you are including the 1-day retreat in your intervention, seek additional help from community members and/or parents to help coordinate and chaperone this event. Depending on the location of the retreat, one or more transportation drivers with appropriate licenses and driving records may be required.

BIBLIOGRAPHY

Centers for Disease Control and Prevention. (1993). *HIV/AIDS surveillance report. Morbidity and mortality weekly report, 5*, 10–11 (as cited in Stanton et al., 1996).

Centers for Disease Control and Prevention. (2007). *HIV/AIDS surveillance report, 2005* (Vol. 17, rev. ed.). Atlanta: U.S. Department of Health and Human Services, Centers for Disease Control and Prevention.

Institute of Medicine and National Academy of Sciences. (1986). *Confronting AIDS: Directions for public health, health care and research.* Washington, DC: National Academy Press.

Rogers, R. W. (1983). Cognitive and physiological processes in fear appeals and attitude change: A revised theory of protection motivation. In T. Caciopi & R. E. Petty (Eds.), *Social psychology* (pp. 153–176). New York: Guilford Press.

Stanton, B., Fang, X., Xiaoming, L., Feigelman, S., Galbraith, J., & Ricardo, I. (1997). Evolution of risk behaviors over 2 years among a cohort of urban African-American adolescents. *Archives of Pediatric & Adolescent Medicine, 151*(4), 398–406.

Stanton, B. F., Xiaoming, L., Ricardo, I., Galbraith, J., Feigelman, S., & Kaljee, L. (1996). A randomized, controlled effectiveness trial of an AIDS prevention program for low-income African-American youths. *Archives of Pediatric & Adolescent Medicine, 150*(4), 363–372.

University of Maryland, Department of Pediatrics. (1998). *Focus on Kids: Adolescent HIV Risk Prevention* (rev. 2005). Santa Cruz, CA: ETR Associates.

Related References by the Developers of *Focus on Kids*

Fang, X., Stanton, B. F., Li, X., Feigleman, S., & Baldwin, R. (1998). Similarities in sexual activity and condom use among friends within groups before and after a risk-reduction intervention. *Youth & Society, 29*(4), 431–450.

Li, X., Stanton, B. F., Cottrell, L., Burns, J. J., Pack, R., & Klajee, L. (2001). Patterns of initiation of sex and drug-related activities among urban low-income African-American adolescents. *Journal of Adolescent Health, 28*(1), 46–54.

Romer, D., Stanton, B. F., Galbraith, J., Feigleman, S., Black, M. M., & Li, X. (1999). Parental influence on adolescent sexual behavior in high-poverty settings. *Archives of Pediatric & Adolescent Medicine, 153*(10), 1055–1062.

Wu, Y., Burns, J. J., Li, X., Harris, C. V., Galbraith, J., & Wei, L. (2005). Influence of prior sexual risk experience on response to intervention targeting multiple risk behaviors among adolescents. *Journal of Adolescent Health, 36*(1), 56–63.

THE PROGRAM

Program Rationale and History

In the early 1990s, a team of researchers consisting of pediatricians, psychologists, health educators, and anthropologists were interested in addressing the numerous challenges faced, by urban youths—particularly the risks of acquiring and transmitting HIV/AIDS.[1] In designing the *Focus on Kids* program, the developers considered multidisciplinary perspectives and approaches to the challenge of educating youths about HIV/AIDS and reducing their rates of high-risk behaviors. They developed a curriculum based on Protection Motivation Theory, ethnographic and survey research, and community input that helped them ensure that their intervention was "developmentally and culturally grounded."

The developers also designed this intervention with a number of statistical concerns in mind. At the time (1993), the Centers for Disease Control and Prevention (CDC) was reporting that AIDS was the leading cause of death for African American men aged 25–34 years, and the second leading cause of death for women (CDC, 1993). In 2007, the CDC reported that although African Americans made up only about 13% of the U.S. population, they accounted for approximately 50% of the diagnosed cases of AIDS in 2005 (the most recent year for when complete data is available); the rate of diagnosis for African American men that same year was 10 times higher than the rate for white men; among women, the diagnosis rate for African Americans was nearly 23 times higher than the rate for whites (CDC, 2007).

The developers also noted that, given the long incubation period of AIDS, it was probable that many young adults contracted the virus in their teens. Finally, they understood a key finding from the AIDS intervention literature–that factual HIV interventions designed only to increase knowledge *had* increased knowledge, but did not guarantee behavior change. Behavioral change, including increases in effective, consistent condom use, was needed to help stem the epidemic (Institute of Medicine and National Academy of Sciences, 1986).

In response, the developers created *Focus on Kids*, designed as a culturally relevant, community-based AIDS-risk reduction intervention to be offered to urban, low-income African Americans in their preteen and early adolescent years. Because a key goal of the program was to reach higher-risk youths (e.g., those with higher rates of school truancy and absenteeism and lower use of health care services, etc.), it was designed to be delivered exclusively in community centers rather than schools or clinics. In an effort to increase attendance rates and reinforce educational messages, the program targeted "naturally formed (same gender) peer groups" through a series of eight 90-minute weekly sessions. (In the original implementation, a 1-day retreat was substituted for the standard presentation of Session 6 content. See below for more details.) The aim was to deliver the program to youths among their peers in neighborhood areas where they would actually be making decisions about high-risk activities.

An evaluation component was implemented to assess the effectiveness of the *Focus on Kids* program (see below). A second longitudinal study was later conducted to examine the evolution of a broader range of risk behaviors in the study cohort over a 2-year period

Theoretical Framework

Focus on Kids was guided by tenets of a social cognitive model, the protection motivation theory (PMT; Rogers, 1983). According to this model, environmental and personal factors can combine to pose a potential threat. When someone considers a maladaptive response to a threat, their choice is mediated by a balance between intrinsic and extrinsic rewards that accompany the behavior (e.g., personal pleasure, social approval), and the perceived severity of and vulnerability to the threat. These two appraisal pathways combine to shape one's "protection motivation," defined as one's intention to respond to a potential threat in either an adaptive or maladaptive manner.

Program Overview

The *Focus on Kids* program developers felt that when using this curriculum, "you and the youth should be having fun. People learn more quickly if they enjoy what they are doing. The curriculum includes factual information, but really emphasizes decision making, communication and negotiation" (University of Maryland, Department of Pediatrics, 1998, p. 4).

Core Elements of the Program

The core elements of the *Focus on Kids* program included:

1. The provision of an HIV intervention program to younger adolescents (ages 9–15) who were often overlooked in such programs.
2. Program recruitment and implementation in noninstitutional, community-based settings (e.g., recreation centers versus school/clinic settings) in order to address the needs and circumstances of high-risk youths.
3. Working with youths in their "natural friendship groups" in recognition that such groups influenced youths' behavioral choices, including commitment to attend the program.
4. An eight-session curriculum that drew on the theoretical tenets of PMT.

While the *Focus on Kids* program was originally designed for urban youths, ages 9–15 from predominantly low-income areas (all of whom were African American), the curriculum was relevant for other adolescent groups as well.

Program Schedule

The eight sessions of *Focus on Kids* covered the following topics, each rooted in a different PMT construct. In the field study, each group of 3 to 10 same-sex participants was led by two group leaders. Sessions were offered on a weekly basis.

Session 1: Trust Building and Group Cohesion. Following an introduction and overview, same-gender groups of up to nine participants engaged in group cohesion activities and established ground rules. They then proceeded to the "Family Tree" activity which addressed the social context of decision making, and the fact that decisions made while they were young could have an impact later in life. Youths were introduced to the anonymous questions box, which was used for the remaining sessions.

Session 2: Risks and Values. In Session 2, participants were introduced to the SODA model of decision making (stop, options, decide, act). Using worksheets, they learned STI and HIV facts (signs/symptoms, health and emotional consequences, ways to avoid infection/transmission, and testing). They reviewed a variety of sexual and nonsexual risk behaviors to learn about and determine levels of risk.

Session 3: Educate Yourself. Obtaining Information. Group leaders used age- and gender-appropriate vignettes followed by questions to encourage participants to practice step two (Options) of their SODA decision-making skills. Using the answers generated in the first activity, participants brainstormed how and where they might get information for each of the situations. Then, working in small groups, participants developed a list of sexuality-related questions, exchanged questions with the other groups, and found the answers, using worksheets.

Session 4: Educate Yourself: Examining Consequences. Youths practiced talking with an adult about something private by identifying an adult from their "Family Tree" (developed in Session 1), and role-playing talking about that issue with a partner. The group then played the "Numbers Game," to develop a more realistic understanding of HIV risk among people their age. This was followed by a condom demonstration, a condom card activity, and a condom race (for condom practice). Participants then practiced step three (Decide) of their SODA decision-making skills.

Session 5: Skills Building: Communication. After reviewing the first three steps of the SODA decision-making model, youths considered the fourth step: Action. The group leaders used age-appropriate thought questions to assist in this activity. From there, the session moved into discussions about communication (verbal, nonverbal, and mixed messages), and communication styles (aggressive, assertive, and nonassertive). Role plays were used for demonstration and practice. Finally, the group explored ways in which poor communication could result in misunderstandings, hurt feelings, or worse.

Session 6: Information About Sexual Health. Youths learned in this session that positive feelings usually associated with sexual intercourse could also be expressed without intercourse; they also learned that the largest pleasure organ was the brain. The group played the "HIV Transmission Game," to demonstrate how quickly/easily STIs and HIV could spread or be prevented. They also learned about various forms of contraception, including condoms and emergency contraception.

In the field study of *Focus on Kids*, Session 6 was conducted as a day-long retreat at a local rural park area, close to but outside of the city where the intervention was being given. Only participants who had attended at least three sessions of the program went on the retreat. Session 6 components were alternated with other recreational activities (relays, tug-of-war, hikes, etc.). There was a presentation by an outside speaker. The retreat offered boys' and girls' groups an opportunity to work together. The ratio of chaperones to youths was one to four.

Session 7: Attitudes and Skills for Sexual Health. In this session, participants learned about short- and long-term goal-setting, including both support and obstacles. They used the "I Can Do It!" worksheet to explore their interests and options, gather information about those interests, implement a plan to become more involved, and take action. Through role play, they learned and practiced saying no or asking to use a condom.

Session 8: Review and Community Project. Through the "Knowledge Feud" game, participants reviewed their STI/HIV prevention knowledge as well as the steps in the SODA model for decision making. The group then engaged in the "Pat on the Back" activity in which each participant wrote at least one positive thing they had learned about or with the help of each of the other participants. Finally, using a list of possible community projects (prepared in advance by the group leaders), the group selected a project to work on in their community, and used the "Activity Planning Sheet" to flesh out the project (e.g., goals, target audience, main message, etc.).

Each session included between five and nine activities or lessons devoted to that session's theme. The original *Focus on Kids* pilot program offered Session 6 as an all-day retreat, an incentive for youths who had attended three or more sessions.

Program Objectives

There were three main objectives for participants who completed the *Focus on Kids* program. By the end of the program, participants would be able to

- state correct information about HIV/AIDS and other STIs including modes of transmission and prevention;
- state their own personal values and understand how these related to pressures to engage in sexual risk behaviors;
- be skilled in decision making, communicating and negotiating with other youths regarding sexual topics and drug topics, and be able to use a condom correctly.

Program Implementation

Planning and Implementation

As you prepare to implement the *Focus on Kids* program, collaborate with interested community members who may want to be involved in this effort.

In the field study, community involvement occurred on many different levels. Parents served on planning committees or as chaperones for the all-day retreat. Recreation club directors served as consultants or facilitators. Local restaurants donated food for the program's retreat and closing graduation ceremony. Print shops donated supplies or duplication services for needed curricular materials. Educators, social service workers, and other community professionals served on an advisory board for the program. This was a community-based program, so community "buy-in" for the program was important each step of the way.

Training

All of the above topic points were covered in an initial training session for group leaders before the program began. If you design your own training, include (a) discussions of implementation issues, (b) modeling of program content and teaching strategies, and (c) practice for effective implementation.

PROGRAM EVALUATION

The Original Evaluation

In 1993, the effectiveness of the pilot *Focus on Kids* program was evaluated through a randomized, controlled trial of this community-based intervention. Study participants were recruited from the nine recreation centers in the area. Eligible groups consisted of 3–10 same gender friends, all between 9 and 15 years of age. Young people who volunteered for the study were randomly assigned within their naturally formed friendship groups to either the intervention or control condition.

The intervention group youths attended the eight-session intervention with their natural friendship-group members. The program was delivered using a variety of learning strategies, including role playing, lectures, video, interactive exercises, and community projects. The sessions were delivered to single-gender groups, although males and females were combined for the retreat session. Control group youths were invited to attend weekly factual sessions on AIDS and AIDS risk behaviors. Attendance was not required, and individuals could attend with or without friends. The key differences between the intervention and control groups were that the former youths received facts in the context of decision making based on PMT principles, and while in the company of their natural friendship group peers.

At the completion of the intervention, each peer group had the option of either working one-on-one as peer educators with community members, or working as a group to produce a product that would deliver an HIV prevention message to a particular population.

All participants in the study were given a computer-based pretest at baseline and a posttest 6 and 12 months after the beginning of the intervention. Evaluators sought to determine whether the intervention would impact self-reported condom use among sexually active participants when compared to a control group receiving 6 weeks of standard HIV/AIDS education. Evaluators also assessed condom use intention and perceptions of condoms.

Participant Recruitment and Final Sample Composition

Research staff conducted three introductory sessions at each of the nine Baltimore recreation centers to describe the purpose, design and enrollment criteria to potentially eligible youths. Eligible youths had to be part of a naturally formed "friendship group" comprised of 3 to 10 same-gender friends who were within 3 years of age of each other. Interested youths were provided with written materials and consent forms. The final sample was made up of 76 naturally formed peer groups consisting of 383 youths, ages 9–15, all African American. The median age of participants was 11.3 years at baseline. Approximately half the sample (n = 213) was male. The groups were then randomized to receive (n = 38 groups, 206 youths) or not receive (n = 38 groups, 177 youths) the intervention.

Evaluation Questions

The evaluation was designed to include both *process measures* (e.g., attendance rates, program delivery concerns) and *outcome measures* to assess the effects of the program on participating youths. Youths in all 76 friendship-groups completed a baseline, multicomponent risk assessment questionnaire called the Youth Health Risk Behavioral Inventory (YHRBI). The instrument measured actual risk behaviors, perceptions of risk behaviors, and intentions. Question formats included multiple-choice, five-point Likert scales, and true-false. The questionnaire utilized "local terms" to ensure comprehension. Questions that assess perceptions were organized around the seven constructs of the guiding PMT model.

Questionnaires were administered and completed in private using a "talking" Macintosh computer and headsets. Youths each received modest stipends ($5 to $10) for completion of the baseline, 6-month, and 12-month measures.

In conducting the evaluation of the *Focus on Kids* pilot program, evaluators attempted to answer one central question in particular: Can a theoretically and culturally based, AIDS-risk reduction intervention delivered to naturally formed peer groups increase self-reported condom use among African American early adolescents at 6 and 12 months of follow-up? The intervention's impact on self-reported condom use was the primary study outcome of interest (also assessed by age and gender subgroups). However, intervention impact was also assessed for three secondary outcomes: intention to use a condom the next time the youths engaged in coitus (a hypothetical question for virgins), perception of condoms, and knowledge regarding AIDS.

Evaluation Results

The results indicate that the *Focus on Kids* curriculum had significant or positive effects in several areas, particularly self-reported condom use. Effects were analyzed at both the 6-month and 12-month follow-up points. Results have been listed below.

Self-Reported Condom Use

- At baseline, condom-use rates did not differ significantly between the intervention and control subjects. At the 6-month follow-up, rates were significantly higher among the intervention group than the control group (85% vs. 61%, $p < .05$).
- The intervention was especially effective for boys (85% vs. 57%, $p < .05$) and for teens ages 13–15 (95% vs. 60%, $p < .01$).
- By the time of the 12-month assessment, rates of condom use were no longer significantly higher among intervention than control subjects.
- When comparing intervention subjects who attended less than five sessions ("low attenders") with those who attended five or more sessions ("high attenders"), self-reported condom use was significantly higher among higher attenders at 6 months ($p < .01$). However, by 12 months, this "dose effect" was no longer significant.

Condom Use Intention

- Intervention and control youths did not differ significantly in their intentions to use condoms at baseline. At 6 months, intervention subjects were significantly more likely to report condom use intention than control subjects.
- By the time of the 12-month assessment, rates of condom use intention were no longer significantly higher among intervention than control subjects.

Condom-Related Perceptions

- At 6 months, intervention subjects exhibited a significantly greater perception of peer use of condoms than control subjects did, and a significantly greater perception of themselves as vulnerable to HIV than control subjects did.
- By the time of the 12-month assessment, the differences between intervention and control subjects regarding condom-related perceptions were no longer significant.

Researchers concluded that this theoretically and culturally based HIV/AIDS prevention program can significantly increase or improve self-reported condom use, condom-related perceptions and condom use intentions among participants at 6 months. However, "booster" sessions may be needed for these changes to be sustained beyond this 6-month period.

Summary

The results of the study indicated that this theoretically and culturally based HIV/AIDS prevention intervention *can* significantly increase or improve self-reported condom use, condom-related perceptions, and condom use intentions among participants at 6 months. The study also supported the idea that programs that build on existing community resources and use naturally formed social networks offer considerable promise. Finally, the study provided support for the approach that community-based interventions may be a productive avenue for reaching high-risk youths that are sometimes missed in school-based interventions due to higher rates of truancy, absenteeism, and dropouts.

The study also showed that short-term improvements in behaviors and intentions were followed by some relapse over longer periods of time. As the researchers concluded, the fact that the significant outcomes were not sustained over time underscores the importance of providing ongoing HIV/AIDS prevention education and support to youths, particularly those in high-risk categories.

AWARDS AND RECOGNITION

Focus on Kids has received the following awards and honors:

- *Focus on Kids* has been designated as one of the Center for Disease Control's Department of Adolescent School Health's "Programs that Work."
- *Focus on Kids* has been chosen as a promising program in the Center for Substance Abuse Prevention (CSAP)'s *Prevention Science Decision Support System,* an initiative to identify and promote effective prevention programs.
- *Focus on Kids'* derivative program entitled *My Future! My Choice!*—developed for Namibia—is one of Africa's "Best Practices" programs.

FOCUS ON KIDS IN THE COMMUNITY TODAY

In the past 3 years, *Focus on Kids* has been implemented in communities in 3 states: California, Ohio, and Wyoming.

NOTE

1. A full set of program materials, including facilitator's manual, video, evaluation materials, and more, is available for purchase from Sociometrics at http://www.socio.com/pasha.htm.

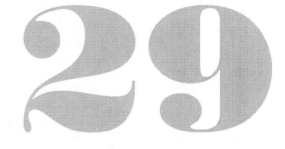

Poder Latino: A Community AIDS Prevention Program for Inner-City Latino Youths

Anne Belden, Starr Niego, and Janette Mince

Original Program Developers and Evaluators

Deborah E. Sellers, PhD
Sarah A. McGraw, PhD
John B. McKinlay, MA
Kevin W. Smith, MA
New England Research Institutes
Watertown, MA

Jose Duran, Executive Director
Heriberto Crespo, Program Director
Hispanic Office of Planning and Evaluation (HOPE)
Roxbury, MA

PROGRAM ABSTRACT

Summary

This multifaceted community-based intervention targets Latino youths at elevated
risk for HIV/AIDS. One goal of the program is to increase awareness of the disease

---

Poder Latino: A Community AIDS Prevention Program for Inner-City Latino Youths was supported by
grants from the National Institute of Child Health and Human Development (RO1 HD25026).

by saturating target neighborhoods with public service announcements broadcasting risk-reduction messages. In addition, the program aims to reduce HIV infection rates by encouraging sexually active teens to use condoms. Project messages are reinforced through ongoing activities conducted by specially trained peer leaders. These activities include: workshops in schools, community organizations, and health centers; group discussions in local residents' homes; presentations at community centers; and door-to-door canvassing. At all activities, condoms are available, along with pamphlets explaining their correct use.

In a field study of the intervention in Boston, Massachusetts, researchers compared the sexual behavior of teens in the target community with that of teens in a similar community not exposed to the program. At the 18-month follow-up assessment, the program appeared to reduce the number of partners among sexually active females and delay the onset of sexual activity among males who were not sexually active when the program began.

Focus

☐ Primary pregnancy prevention ☐ Secondary pregnancy prevention ☑ STI/HIV/AIDS prevention

Original Site

☐ School based ☑ Community based ☐ Clinic based

Suitable for Use In

Poder Latino was specially designed for an inner-city Latino community. However, the structure and content of the program might be adapted for use with other groups at high risk for HIV infection.

Approach

- ☐ Abstinence
- ☑ Behavioral skills development
- ☑ Community outreach
- ☑ Contraceptive access
- ☑ Contraceptive education
- ☐ Life option enhancement
- ☑ Self-efficacy/self-esteem
- ☑ Sexuality/HIV/STI education

Original Intervention Sample

Age/gender   During the field study, the intervention targeted an entire community; evaluation of the program included 586 youths, who ranged in age from 14 to 20 years.

Race/ethnicity   100% Latino, nearly all Puerto Rican.

Program Components

- ☑ Adult involvement
- ☐ Case management
- ☑ Group discussion
- ☑ Lectures
- ☑ Peer counseling/instruction
- ☑ Public service announcements
- ☑ Role play

■ ☐ Video
■ ☐ Other

Program Length

There is no requisite length for the program; the field study was implemented over an 18-month period.

Staffing Requirements/Training

Program activities are led by peer leaders who take part in an extensive training program. Staff who lead this training should be knowledgeable about HIV/AIDS, Latino culture, and group process skills. Additionally, staff and peer leaders should be able to communicate both in English and Spanish.

BIBLIOGRAPHY

Centers for Disease Control and Prevention. (2007). CDC HIV/AIDS fact sheet: HIV/AIDS among Hispanics/Latinos. Retrieved October 11, 2007, from http://www.cdc.gov/hiv/resources/factsheets/ PDF/hispanic.pdf

McGraw, S. A., Smith, K. W., Crawford, S. L., Costa, L. A., McKinlay, J. B., & Bullock, K. (2002). *The effectiveness of Poder Latino: A community-based AIDS prevention program for inner-city Latino youth.* Unpublished manuscript.

Sellers, D. E., McGraw, S. A., & McKinlay, J. B. (1994). Does the promotion and distribution of condoms increase teen sexual activity? Evidence from an HIV prevention program for Latino youth. *American Journal of Public Health, 84*(12), 1952–1959.

Related References by the Developers of *Poder Latino*

Neff, J. A., & Crawford, S. L. (1998). The health belief model and HIV risk behaviours: A causal model analysis among Anglos, African Americans and Mexican-Americans. *Ethnicity & Health, 3*(4), 283–299.

Smith, K. W., McGraw, S. A., Costa, L. A., & McKinlay, J. B. (1996). A self-efficacy scale for HIV risk behaviors: Development and evaluation. *AIDS Education & Prevention, 8*(2), 97–105.

THE PROGRAM

Program Rationale and History

Throughout the United States, Latino neighborhoods have shown elevated rates of HIV infection.[1] The Hispanic population has been disproportionately represented in the HIV/AIDS epidemic in this country. As recently as 2005, Hispanics accounted for approximately 13% of the U.S. population, yet they accounted for 19% of the new HIV/AIDS diagnoses that same year. In 2004, AIDS was the fourth leading cause of death among Hispanic men and women between the ages of 35 and 44 (CDC 2007).

Poder Latino sought to address that disparity. The program was a multifaceted intervention designed to raise the entire community's awareness of HIV/AIDS through involving and engaging the community. It also sought to reduce the risk of infection among Hispanic/Latino inner city youths by increasing the use of condoms among sexually active teens.

In 1990, the New England Research Institutes (NERI) launched this community-based intervention in an inner-city Latino neighborhood in Boston, Massachusetts. NERI enlisted a local organization, the Hispanic Office of Planning and Evaluation (HOPE), to develop the intervention materials. NERI staff, in conjunction with HOPE personnel, began by conducting interviews and focus groups to investigate local residents' opinions, attitudes, beliefs, and behaviors related to AIDS. The results of the study helped shape both the structure and content of the program. In particular, *Poder Latino* was designed to (a) provide explicit, factual information in language that was comprehensible to teens; (b) offer educational activities appealing and relevant to the Latino community; (c) enhance feelings of pride and self-esteem; and (d) empower residents to take healthy action for their own lives and for their community.

During the field study of the program, much of HOPE's efforts focused on recruiting, training, and supervising peer educators, who were Latino teens in the target community. The peer educators then took responsibility for educating their community through a variety of activities. To promote *Poder Latino*'s HIV prevention messages, the youths created and displayed posters; wrote teen newsletters; broadcasted public service announcements; held community workshops; attended health fairs; and led home-based *charlas,* or chats. HOPE staff also trained parents to serve as Community Health Educators; the adults, too, held *charlas* with other adults, as well as with adolescents and adults together.

Theoretical Framework

The lack of research on factors related to HIV transmission in Latino communities required the program developers to use innovative methods to develop appropriate educational strategies. Using ethnographic research methods, they sought to understand local residents' opinions, attitudes, beliefs and behaviors related to AIDS. An anthropologist from NERI conducted focus groups and interviews with 44 parents, caretakers, adolescents, church leaders, teachers, and counselors in the target community. The following principles emerged from these conversations:

1. The intervention would be community-based.
2. The intervention would target a broad age range.
3. The intervention would involve community outreach.
4. The intervention would be factual and explicit in presenting AIDS information, yet address teens in ways that they can understand.
5. The intervention would instill in Latino teens a sense of cultural pride and a sense of history.
6. The intervention would be bilingual.
7. The intervention would facilitate a sense of empowerment among Latino teens.
8. The intervention would utilize peer leaders or forums facilitated by teens.
9. The intervention would seek to involve the parents of adolescents.

Guided by the principles listed above, the program developers engaged local adolescent and adult residents to serve as persuasive and appealing opinion leaders. After completing a training program, the leaders were charged with promoting program messages in a variety of social settings. The training followed a "health circles" approach, patterned after the successful literacy campaigns organized by Paulo Freire in Brazil. In the *Poder Latino* program, trainers and trainees took part in activities designed to discover, create, and promote the most effective and relevant prevention messages for the target community. The success of this method required that the trainers enter into a continuing dialogue with the trainees so that ownership over the process would be shared; from this process the *Poder Latino* curriculum emerged and evolved.

Program Goals

As an HIV/AIDS prevention program, *Poder Latino* aimed to achieve three goals:

1. Increase awareness of HIV/AIDS by saturating the community with risk-reduction messages
2. Reduce HIV infection by encouraging sexually active teens to use condoms
3. Increase communication between parents and teens about sexuality and HIV/AIDS

Program Components

Three program components—each encompassing multiple activities—were implemented during the field study of *Poder Latino*. You might follow a similar structure in your own community, or modify components to fit local residents' interests, needs, and values.

Peer Educators

Based on the premise that youths could most effectively convince their peers to refrain from risky behaviors, HOPE staff members recruited and trained Latino teens to serve as peer educators/leaders in their local community. Sixteen youths (ages 14–19) were recruited to participate in an intensive program teaching basic information about HIV/AIDS, the importance of practicing safer sex and community resources for diagnosis, testing, and treatment. In addition, group exercises helped develop and strengthen participants' self-esteem and pride in Latino culture, as well as decision-making skills. To prepare the teens for assuming educational leadership roles in their community, the training also included discussion and repeated practice in conveying health education information to youths.

After completing the training program, the youths were charged with creating and conducting AIDS awareness activities with their peers. To reach adolescents in a wide variety of settings, the peer educators

- developed posters promoting the use of condoms for HIV prevention and posted them at local businesses and public transit facilities;
- wrote "Teen View" newsletters and distributed them throughout the neighborhood;
- wrote public service announcements promoting condom use for local radio and television stations;
- conducted workshops in neighborhoods, community centers, and schools to talk about HIV/AIDS, sexuality and the importance of using condoms for safer sex;
- staffed booths at health fairs and handed out condom packets;
- canvassed the neighborhood to educate local residents about HIV/AIDS transmission and prevention;
- distributed on street corners, door-to-door, and at all program activities kits of condoms and instructions on how to use them;
- visited residents' homes to conduct a series of *charlas* (chats) encouraging teens and parents to discuss sexuality.

Parent Training

Parents were recruited and trained to serve as volunteer community health educators. Participating parents learned basic information about HIV/AIDS, as well as techniques to enhance their communications skills. As community health educators, the parents conducted *charlas* (chats) with other adults and teens in home settings.

Community Advancement Collaboration

HOPE staff members organized a network of seven community-based Latino agencies, called *Proyecto Luces*. The network was designed to

1. encourage collaboration among community-based Latino agencies in shaping and delivering HIV prevention messages;
2. act as a catalyst and resource, enabling the community to mobilize itself;
3. ensure that HIV education and prevention would continue once the field study of *Poder Latino* concluded.

Within the target community, participating agencies helped organize cultural festivals, health fairs, and workshops at which condoms were distributed and AIDS awareness messages promoted. Individual community members also got involved. Latino/Latina artists, for example, designed materials to promote program messages that had originally been developed by the peer educators.

Training Schedule

The primary focus of *Poder Latino* was to train peer educators/leaders, who then created and implemented a variety of program activities promoting HIV prevention messages.

Peer Educator Training

During the field study of the program, training sessions were held both during the school year and summer, during which the teens were paid. An overview of the 7-week summer program (with three or four sessions per week, each lasting about 3 hours) is presented below.

Week 1: Introduction to the Program. During the first week of the training program, the leaders strived to build rapport between themselves and the teens. Discussions were designed to clarify roles and expectations for the teens' work as peer educators, particularly the importance of educating others about risky behaviors and how to avoid them. Toward that end, the teens identified situations in which they could pass on prevention messages to their peers. At various points during the sessions, youths facilitated the discussion so that they could begin developing and practicing leadership and communication skills.

Week 2: Cultural Identity, Personal Growth, and Development. During the second week of the training program, activities helped teens develop pride in Latino culture and better understand the strength and beauty of the diverse nationalities and ethnic origins of Latinos. In one exercise, for example, participants wrote their autobiographies, describing how long they (or their parents) had lived in the United States, a typical day in their life and their future aspirations. The disproportionate impact of AIDS on the Latino community was also discussed. Then, as a group, teens shared what they have liked, or found difficult, about growing up as a member of a particular ethnic minority (e.g., Puerto Rican). Finally, the focus shifted to pressures teens faced in school, at home and from peers. Role-play exercises helped practice resisting peer pressure.

Week 3: Building Self-Esteem, Skills in Decision Making, and Conflict Resolution. The first session of the week began with a group discussion of teens' personal accomplishments. The trainers highlighted the importance of self-esteem and striving to reach one's potential. The remainder of the week focused on the development of decision-making skills, especially as they related to conflict resolution and HIV prevention. The field study of the program also included a field trip to the Massachusetts State House, during which the teens were introduced to elected officials and invited to share their thoughts and feelings about leadership.

Week 4: AIDS 101: Counseling & Testing, and Impact Upon Family and Friends. During this set of sessions, youths learned basic facts about HIV/AIDS, including transmission, prevention, treatment and testing. Group discussions explored loss and other feelings that a person with AIDS/HIV might have experienced. The youths also learned a process for assisting someone with the "to test or not to test" decision.

Week 5: AIDS and Substance Abuse. Focusing on risky behaviors and their relationship to HIV infection, teens defined substance abuse and identified signs and symptoms of abuse among their peers. The first session of the week began with an icebreaker exercise in which the youths explored their own values and beliefs about drugs and drug abuse. Additional discussion focused on the impact of the media on teens' perceptions of drugs. The field study of the program also featured a presentation offering a community perspective on substance use and abuse. Finally, the group took part in a series of role-play exercises to practice resisting pressures to use alcohol and other drugs.

Week 6: How to Serve as a Peer Educator/Leader. The final 2 weeks of the training program prepared teens to serve as HIV prevention peer educators and leaders. The trainers helped the youths identify and practice basic communication and self-presentation skills, including listening, facilitating group discussions, open questioning to promote dialogue, and assertiveness. The youths also learned problem-solving skills they would need as they began planning and leading educational activities in their community. To apply these skills, the youths used the third and fourth days of the week to begin working on a newsletter, contest, or other prevention activity committee. Each committee created a plan for its first project, including a budget, timeline and outline for promotion, recruitment, production, and evaluation of their work.

Week 7: Linking With Community Resources and Summary. During the final segment of the training program, the teens spent about 4 days working with their committees to finalize their project plans. Throughout the sessions, the trainers emphasized the importance of the teens' work and encouraged them to involve others in their efforts, including community leaders and representatives from social service agencies. Guest speakers were invited to visit the group and offer additional suggestions for community education activities.

Optional Week: Sexual Identity, Healthy Lifestyles, and the Risk of Sexually Transmitted Infections (STIs). During the original field study, an additional set of sessions was designed to improve teens' understanding of sexual orientation, sexual identity and STIs. The group learned basic facts about puberty, reproductive development and the impact of teen pregnancy/parenting on adolescents' lives. The trainers emphasized the benefits of delaying pregnancy until one was emotionally ready to meet the challenges. Treatment and prevention of STIs were also discussed. You may want to organize a similar set of sessions for your intervention.

Parent Training

The *Poder Latino* program developers also created a two-session training curriculum to provide Latino parents and community members with basic information about HIV as it pertained to the Latino community. The curriculum encouraged the development of communication skills needed to serve as a Community Health Educator.

The parent training program contains three modules or units:

1. HIV—The Facts
2. Listening and Communications Skills
3. Home-Based Education Sessions

In the field study, the training was delivered over a 2-day period, with 3- to 3.5-hour sessions offered each day, as described below.

Day 1: HIV—The Facts. The first training session provides adults with basic information about AIDS: what causes AIDS, how HIV differs from other viruses, how HIV is transmitted, and how it could be prevented. During the field study, adults also completed a short, 20-item test of their understanding of HIV/AIDS.

Day 2: Listening and Communication Skills and Home-Based Education Sessions. The second day of the program was designed to enhance participants' confidence, knowledge and skills in presenting AIDS risk-reduction messages as they pertained to the Latino community. The participants completed a series of exercises to practice their listening and communication skills. The trainers then distributed a copy of the *Poder Latino Home-Based Education Sessions Manual* and *HIV—Basic Facts Presentation Packet* to each adult and discussed the concepts and objectives of the home-based sessions.

Program Implementation

Your implementation of *Poder Latino* will benefit greatly from active support and participation across all segments of the community, including community-based organizations, church representatives, teachers and educational administrators, civic leaders, parents and especially, teenagers. Moreover, it is helpful to begin building support for your work before the peer and parent training programs begin.

During the field study of the program, the ethnographic research was used as an opportunity to introduce residents to the goals and objectives of the program. Project staff wrote and distributed an open letter describing their work and requesting residents' participation in the focus groups and interviews. Local organizations and community leaders proved helpful in identifying and recruiting teens and adults to participate in the training programs. Following the training, they invited the peer educators to lead sessions at local events and activities.

PROGRAM EVALUATION

The Original Evaluation

Design

NERI evaluated a field study of *Poder Latino* conducted in Boston, Massachusetts, between June 1990 and December 1991. The researchers compared Latino youths in the intervention city (Boston) with their peers in a comparison city (Hartford, Connecticut) on measures of AIDS-related knowledge and attitudes, as well as patterns of sexual activity. To measure the impact of the program over time, interviews were conducted with teens at two points:

- Time 1: before the start of the program (baseline)
- Time 2: following the conclusion of the program (follow-up)

Evaluation Question

Opponents of condom distribution to teens asserted that promoting the use of condoms could encourage increased sexual activity and promiscuity. NERI's study was designed to test those assertions—and assess the effectiveness of the *Poder Latino* program. To that end, the evaluators addressed three questions.

1. Were adolescents who had not initiated sexual activity prior to the start of *Poder Latino* more likely to become sexually active as a result of the intervention?

2. Were adolescents who were sexually active at the end of *Poder Latino* more likely to have had multiple partners as a result of the intervention?
3. Were adolescents who were sexually active at the end of *Poder Latino* having sex more frequently as a result of the intervention?

Data Collection Procedures

Because the program was designed to reach the entire adolescent population in the target neighborhood of Boston, the researchers gathered data from representative community samples, rather than groups of students or teens who actually participated in program activities. The researchers first identified census blocks in Boston in which at least 20% of the population was of Hispanic origin. They then used standard block sampling and household enumeration procedures to identify eligible Latino adolescents in these target neighborhoods.

Following the same sampling procedures, the researchers constructed the comparison group of teens in Hartford, Connecticut. Hartford was chosen as the comparison community because its Latino population is similar, in many ways, to that of Boston. At the same time, the researchers reasoned that the 100-mile distance between the two cities would make it difficult for the intervention activities to spill over into the comparison population.

Trained, bilingual staff conducted the two sets of interviews with teens. Within each city, interviewers were paired with participants of the same sex. The interviews, which were held in private places to protect teens' confidentiality, included sociodemographic questions, along with items about AIDS-related knowledge and attitudes, patterns of sexual activity and condom use. To minimize any potential biases among respondents, a separate project title and research team were used throughout the evaluation. In addition, the survey was presented as an investigation of adolescent health, rather than HIV/AIDS.

To minimize attrition over the 18-month study period, the researchers recontacted participants at 3-month intervals. They distributed a one-page flyer, *Para La Salud*, which was designed, in part, to update teens about project activities. Included in the mailing was a stamped postcard on which the teens were requested to write their address and phone number, even if they had not moved.

Research Sample

Baseline interviews were completed with 586 Latino adolescents, who ranged in age from 14 to 20. Of this group, nearly all (94%) were Puerto Rican. At the Time 2 assessment, interviews were completed with 536 adolescents, yielding a follow-up rate of 91%. The attrition rate was 7.2% in Boston, the intervention city, and 9.3% in Hartford, the comparison city.

Evaluation Results

Initiation of Sexual Activity

In order to measure the impact of the program on the initiation of sexual activity, the researchers focused on the subset of teens who had not yet become sexually active when the intervention began. At the Time 1 assessment, nearly half of the adolescents (47.8%) had not had intercourse, and of this group, 227 (88.7%) provided complete data for all of the interview questions.

After statistically adjusting for baseline differences between the treatment and comparison groups, the evaluators found that males in the intervention community were less likely to become sexually active than were their peers in the comparison community ($p < .012$). For females, the intervention neither increased nor decreased their chances of becoming sexually active ($p = .692$).

Number of Sexual Partners

In order to measure the impact of the program on the number of sexual partners, the researchers looked at the group of teens who were sexually active at the follow-up assessment period. In the Time 2 interviews, 433 respondents (80.8%) reported sexual activity, and 403 teens (93.1%) provided complete data. Again, statistical methods were used to control for baseline differences between the two groups of youths.

For female adolescents in the target community, the intervention appeared to reduce the incidence of multiple sexual partners ($p < .006$). There was no corresponding effect for males, who neither increased nor decreased their number of partners ($p = .790$).

Frequency of Sexual Activity

Focusing again on the subset of teens who were sexually active at Time 2, the researchers found that *Poder Latino* had no impact on the frequency of sexual activity among either males or females.

Summary

Evaluation of *Poder Latino* showed that the intervention delayed the onset of males' sexual activity and reduced the number of sex partners among females. Both of these effects are valuable HIV risk reduction outcomes. Together, this evidence suggested that the program was an effective HIV risk reduction intervention for inner-city Latino youths. Moreover, since only 75% of adolescents interviewed for the study had actually been exposed to intervention activities or messages, the results may have offered a conservative picture of the program's effectiveness.

The findings also offered no evidence that the promotion and distribution of condoms as part of an HIV education and prevention program encouraged sexual activity or promiscuity in the target population of Latino adolescents. Teens in the intervention city who were not sexually active prior to the intervention were no more likely to become sexually active than those in the comparison city. In fact, males in the intervention city were less likely than those in the comparison city to begin having sexual intercourse.

In interpreting the evaluation data, the researchers offered a few caveats. To begin, they noted that the small size of the treatment and comparison groups, and particularly the subgroups used in their analyses, made it difficult to detect significant differences. In addition, because only one intervention and one comparison city were included in the investigation, the findings were not generalizable to Latino teens in other parts of the country. Moreover, the exclusive focus on Latino youths made it impossible to generalize the findings to youths from other ethnic groups. Yet, the data from this study suggested that future investigations in other cities and with other groups of teens would be valuable.

AWARDS AND RECOGNITION

Poder Latino received a Youth Advocacy Award from the Children's Advocacy Network in May 1991. Additionally, the Boston Initiative for Teen Pregnancy Prevention gave *Poder Latino* a first-place award for its newsletter and a runner-up award for its poster in the 1991 "Positive Images of Teens" Media Contest.

PODER LATINO IN THE COMMUNITY TODAY

In the past 3 years, *Poder Latino* has been implemented in communities in 3 states—Massachusetts, New York, and Ohio.

NOTE

1. A full set of program materials, including peer educator training guide, parent training guide, home-based education sessions manual, activity materials, evaluation materials, and more, is available for purchase from Sociometrics at http://www.socio.com/pasha.htm.

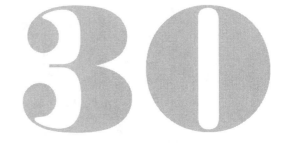

Safer Choices: A High School-Based Program to Prevent STIs, HIV, and Pregnancy

Tabitha A. Benner

Original Program Developers and Evaluators

ETR Associates
  Scotts Valley, CA

Center for Health Promotion Research and Development,
  Health Science Center
  University of Texas—Houston

PROGRAM ABSTRACT

Summary

Safer Choices is a comprehensive intervention to reduce the number of students engaging in unprotected sexual intercourse by reducing the number of students who initiate or have sex during their high school years, and by increasing the use of latex condoms and other birth control methods among those students who do have sex.

The program incorporates five primary components:

1. *School organization:* a broad-based School Health Promotion Council supports and coordinates *Safer Choices* activities.

Safer Choices was supported by a contract from the Centers for Disease Control and Prevention (#200–91–0938).

2. *Curriculum and staff development:* There are 10 classroom lessons for 9th and 10th graders (for a total of 20). Sessions are sequential in nature; activities in each class build on those from prior classes. In-class peer leaders receive training to assist with specific activities. Teacher training prepares educators to implement the curriculum completely, and to provide a feedback loop at the end of the school year.
3. *Peer resources and school environment:* A student peer resource team/club conducts activities such as publishing articles in the school newspaper, conducting opinion polls and organizing public speakers throughout the school year.
4. *Parent education:* Newsletters are sent to parents three times a year to help increase parent-child communication in the areas of sexuality, HIV, and other sexually transmitted infections (STIs).
5. *School community linkages:* Homework assignments require students to develop information on and/or visit local health service providers.

Safer Choices was originally delivered during the 1993–1994 and 1994–1995 school years. The randomized trial involved 20 high schools—10 each in Texas and California. Five schools from each state were randomized into either the experimental condition or a standard, knowledge-based HIV prevention curriculum.

Baseline data were collected from all participants (n = 3,869) in fall 1993. Follow-up data were collected at three additional time points: 7 months after baseline, 19 months after baseline, and 31 months after baseline.

The evaluation of the intervention revealed that it reduced the frequency of sex without a condom ($p = .02$), reduced the number of sexual partners in the last 3 months with whom a condom was not used ($p = .04$), increased condom use during last sex among those who had sex in the last 3 months ($p = .02$), and marginally increased contraceptive use among those who had sex in the last 3 months ($p = .07$).

Focus

☑ Primary pregnancy prevention   ☐ Secondary pregnancy prevention   ☑ STI/HIV/AIDS prevention

Original Site

☑ School based   ☐ Community based   ☐ Clinic based

Suitable for Use In

Safer Choices is suitable for use in standard high school class settings, as well as in STI-related clinics and other community-based organizations that offer reproductive health services to youths.

Approach

- ☑ Abstinence
- ☑ Behavioral skills development
- ☑ Community outreach
- ☐ Contraceptive access
- ☑ Contraceptive education
- ☑ Life option enhancement
- ☑ Self-efficacy/self-esteem
- ☑ Sexuality/HIV/AIDS/STI education

Original Intervention

Age, gender   The original intervention sample consisted of 3,869 students who were 14–15 years old at baseline; 53% were female.

Race/ethnicity   31% self identified as White, 27% as Hispanic, 18% as Asian or Pacific Islander; 17% as African American, <1% as American Indian or Alaskan Native, and 7% as Other.

Program Components

- ☑ Adult involvement
- ☐ Case management
- ☑ Group discussion
- ☑ Lectures
- ☐ Peer counseling/instruction
- ☐ Public service announcements
- ☑ Role play
- ☑ Video
- ☑ Other: Site visits in the community, guest speaker who is HIV-positive, peer club leading school-wide activities

Program Length

As part of the curriculum and staff development component, students receive 10 lessons in the 9th grade and 10 lessons in the 10th grade. Each lesson is designed for presentation in a standard 45-minute classroom period. The activities and participation by members of the other program components are not reflected here.

Staffing Requirements/Training

Training is needed for all groups involved with the program—teachers, peer team/club members, and members of the School Health Promotion Council. In addition, there is specific training for the in-class peer leaders for both intervention years. This training will require approximately 3 hours.

Because the goal of the curriculum implementation is to reach a majority of students in the targeted grade levels, the curriculum should be implemented in a required class rather than in an elective class. Teachers selected to implement the program should have knowledge of the content areas covered in the curriculum, be comfortable discussing the material, have experience teaching a skills-based program, and be interested in and committed to the goals of the program.

BIBLIOGRAPHY

Basen-Enquist, K., Parcel, G., Harrist, R., Kirby, D., Coyle, K., Banspach, S., et al. (1997). The Safer Choices project: Methodological issues in school-based health promotion intervention research. *Journal of School Health, 67*(9), 365–371.

Coyle, K., Basen-Enquist, K., Kirby, D., Parcel, G., Banspach, S., Collins, J., et al. (2001). Safer Choices: Reducing teen pregnancy, HIV, and STIs. *Public Health Reports, 116* (Suppl.), 82–93.

Coyle, K., Basen-Enquist, K., Kirby, D., Parcel, G., Banspach, S., Harrist, R., et al. (1999). Short-term impact of Safer Choices: A multicomponent, school-based HIV, other STI, and pregnancy prevention program. *Journal of School Health, 69*(5), 181–188.

Coyle, K., Kirby, D., Parcel, G., Basen-Enquist, K., Banspach, S., Rugg, D., et al. (1996). Safer Choices: A multicomponent school-based HIV/STI and pregnancy prevention program for adolescents. *Journal of School Health, 66*(3), 89–94.

Kirby, D., Baumler, E., Coyle, K., Basen-Enquist, K., Parcel, G., Harrist, R., et al. (2004). The Safer Choices intervention: Its impact on the sexual behaviors of different subgroups of high school students. *Society for Adolescent Medicine, 35*(6), 442–453.

THE PROGRAM

Program Rationale and History

Over the last several years, many teen STI/HIV and pregnancy prevention programs have been developed and implemented in school settings across the country.[1] These programs have demonstrated varying effects on teens' knowledge and behaviors. However, most positive effects have been shorter-term in nature. The *Safer Choices* research team sought to develop and implement an intervention focused on school-wide environmental change. By involving teachers, parents, community members and students, the program was designed to have a positive influence on teens' decisions regarding sex, and help them feel supported in making the safest choice.

The 20-session intervention was first offered during the 1993–1994 and 1994–1995 school years. Unlike many other school-based interventions, however, *Safer Choices* was a multicomponent intervention, with the following five key features:

1. *School organization:* The *School Health Promotion Council,* made up of teachers, students, parents, community representatives and school administrators, planned and conducted *Safer Choices* program activities. A site coordinator played a central role in coordinating the Council's efforts.
2. *Curriculum and staff development: Safer Choices* was designed for presentation in the classroom beginning in 9th grade. There were 10 sessions each for 9th and 10th graders. Sessions were sequential in nature, activities in each class building on those from prior classes. In-class peer leaders (chosen by their classmates) received training in advance to help with certain activities. Teacher training prepared educators to implement the curriculum completely, and to provide a feedback loop at the end of the school year.
3. *School–community linkages:* Homework assignments required students to gather information about local community services and resources. A "Resource Guide" developed by the Council (see #1, above) listed local resources related to HIV/STI and pregnancy prevention. In addition, Level 2 included a lesson involving an HIV-positive speaker.
4. *Peer resources and school environment:* Drawing from the full student body and with the support of an adult peer coordinator, the Peer Resource Team/Club planned and hosted a variety of school-wide activities designed to alter the normative culture of the school. These activities included scheduling guest speakers for assemblies; creating, stocking, and staffing an information booth or kiosk with HIV/AIDS-related brochures; hosting opinion surveys; and conducting poster contests.
5. *Parent education:* Newsletters sent to parents about three times a year, provided parents with information about the *Safer Choices* program, including background knowledge on HIV/AIDS and tips for communicating with their teens. The curriculum (see #2, above) included homework assignments that required parental participation. Parents also served on the Council (see #1, above).

Theoretical Framework

The primary theoretical underpinnings of the intervention were social cognitive theory, social influence models, and models of school change. Consistent with these models and recognizing that information alone was insufficient to effect sustained behavior change, *Safer Choices* lessons addressed functional knowledge, attitudes and beliefs (including self-efficacy), social skills (in particular, refusal and negotiation skills), social and media influences, peer norms, and parent/child communication.

Program Overview

As originally designed, the first year (10 sessions) of the *Safer Choices* curriculum was presented in 9th grade. The second year of the program (10 sessions) was presented in 10th grade. Meanwhile, school-wide activities were going on outside the classroom, helping to reinforce the intervention's message.

Program Design

The program had seven main goals:

1. Increase knowledge about STIs/HIV
2. Promote more positive attitudes about choosing not to have sex, and using latex condoms if having sex
3. Promote more positive peer norms regarding not having sex and using condoms if having sex
4. Increase students' belief in their ability to refuse sexual intercourse or unprotected sexual intercourse, use a condom, and communicate about safer sexual practices
5. Decrease perceived barriers to condom use
6. Align students' perceptions of STI/HIV risk based on their risk behaviors
7. Increase communication with parents

The curriculum included a broad spectrum of experiential activities, such as role plays, games, small-group activities, guided discussion, and question-and-answer sessions. In addition to the in-class curriculum, the School Health Promotion Council and the Peer Resources Team/Club conducted other school-wide activities in support of the *Safer Choices* program and its goals.

Program Implementation

Program Planning

Before delivering *Safer Choices* in your setting, you may want to revisit your school district's philosophy regarding STI/HIV and pregnancy prevention to ensure that the curriculum adheres to any guidelines.

During the original field study of the program, the research team found it helpful to have an established School Health Promotion Council that had met at least once to begin activity planning. In addition, prior to implementing the program, parents received written notification describing the goals of the intervention and the content. Parents were given the option of excluding their children from participating in the classroom curriculum.

Level 1 (9th Grade)

Each session was designed to be taught in a standard 45-minute class period. The program developers conducted all 10 class sessions within a 3- to-4-week period to maximize retention, and minimize the time needed to review the previous class's material.

Class 1: Not Everybody's Having Sex. Students brainstormed reasons teens would choose *not* to have or *to* have sex. Groups compared and contrasted reasons. Students generated a list of possible influences on personal decisions, and identified ways to show love and affection without having sex. Student/parent homework was assigned.

Class 2: The Safest Choice: Deciding Not to Have Sex. The concept of a "norm" and its influence on personal decisions was presented. Students' perceptions of the number of 9th graders who had not had sex were compared with actual percentages (based on the most recent Youth Risk Behavior Survey information, available at http://www.cdc.gov/healthyyouth/yrbs/). Verbal and nonverbal refusal skills were introduced and demonstrated through scripted role plays. Discussion and practice using a half-scripted role play helped students distinguish between ineffective and effective statements and actions.

Class 3: Saying No to Having Sex. Two new refusal skills—alternative actions and delay tactics—were introduced and modeled. Students practiced three refusal skills in small groups using a half-scripted role plays. Students also responded to pressure to have sexual intercourse by using clear "no" statements, alternative actions and delay tactics. They then identified the refusal skills used in the role-play activities.

Class 4: Understanding STIs and HIV. Students worked in small groups to examine facts and create posters about STIs. They discussed commonalities among STIs, brainstormed reasons why teens might not get tested, and identified ways to address those barriers. As homework, volunteers called hotlines for answers to student-generated questions that were not answered in class.

Class 5: Examining the Risk of Unsafe Choices. Students who had volunteered in Class 4 to call hotlines related their experiences in making the calls. Class members shared what they had learned from the Class 1 student/parent homework. Students personalized their vulnerability to HIV, and personalized the impact of a pregnancy on their lives.

Class 6: Teens With HIV: A Reality. Students viewed the video *Teen AIDS in Focus,* which presented personal experiences of teens and adults infected with HIV. Discussion focused on the physical, social, and emotional impact of HIV on the individuals' daily lives and future goals. HIV transmission was clarified, and students completed a worksheet to personalize their risk. Students also examined their attitudes toward people with HIV.

Class 7: Practicing the Safest Choice. After a review of refusal skills, student groups wrote refusals for typical pressure lines, using clear verbal and nonverbal "no" statements, alternative actions and delay tactics. Selected groups performed their lines and refusals for the class. Students practiced ways to say "no" and still maintain relationships, using a half-scripted role play. They completed a worksheet to personalize the advantages of not having sex and the use of refusal skills.

Class 8: Safer Choices: Using Protection—Part I. Methods of protection from STIs and/or pregnancy commonly used by teens were presented and discussed. A small group activity helped students differentiate between methods that offered little or no protection, those that protected from pregnancy only, and those that protected from STI/HIV and pregnancy. As homework, students went to local stores to research which protective products were available and readily accessible to teens.

Class 9: Safer Choices: Using Protection—Part II. After the teacher demonstrated the proper use of condoms, student pairs examined condom packages to identify characteristics, and then practiced using condoms, rolling them down on two fingers or using a penis proxy. Barriers to getting and using protection and ways to overcome these barriers were discussed. Students practiced responding to typical pressure lines in role-play situations in which young people were being pressured to have unprotected sex.

Class 10: Knowing What You Can Do. To conclude the Level 1 *Safer Choices* classes, students reviewed homework assignments, summarizing what they had learned from talking with their parents/guardians (or other adults) regarding ways to prevent STI/HIV/pregnancy. Students created a list identifying locations where they could obtain products to protect themselves. They then completed a worksheet about what they would say or do if they wanted to delay having sex or keep from having unprotected sex.

Level 2 (10th Grade)

Like Level 1, Level 2 comprised 10 sessions, delivered in standard 45-minute class settings. Unlike Level 1, there was an HIV-positive guest speaker who participated in Class 3 of Level 2.

Class 1: Making Safer Choices. To reinforce *Safer Choices,* the class reviewed *unsafe, safer,* and *safest* choices. In small groups, students identified positive and negative consequences resulting from telling a partner they were not ready to have sex, choosing to have sex before they were ready, telling a partner they would not have sex again without protection, and having sex without protection. The discussion focused on the benefits of choosing not to have sex, the safest choice, or choosing to use latex condoms correctly every time. Students identified factors that made it difficult for teens to refuse to have sex and/or use protection. Student/parent homework was assigned.

Class 2: The Safer Choices Challenge. The *Safer Choices* Challenge game reviewed information and skills from Level 1 lessons. As a homework assignment, students called or visited a nearby clinic to obtain information about how the clinic operated and the available services. Students also completed a worksheet in preparation for the HIV-positive guest speaker scheduled for Class 3.

Class 3: Talking With a Person Infected With HIV. A guest speaker visited the class and talked about his/her experience living with HIV or AIDS. The talk was followed by a question and answer period. Students created a list of behaviors that put people at risk for becoming infected with HIV. As a homework assignment, they examined how their feelings and attitudes had changed as a result of the presentation.

Class 4: Personalizing the Risk for Pregnancy. The homework review focused on students' attitudes toward people living with HIV and AIDS. After discussing the concept of risk, students participated in a pregnancy risk activity to personalize their vulnerability to pregnancy. They completed a worksheet that examined the immediate impact of a pregnancy on their lives by scheduling baby-related activities into their Saturday routine.

Class 5: Avoiding Unsafe Choices. Students discussed what made it difficult to talk with parents/guardians or other adults about sensitive issues, using the homework assignment from Class 1 as a basis. They review and discuss three steps for avoiding unsafe choices; think about their own limits regarding sexual behavior; then work in small groups to identify situations that might challenge specific personal limits, and identify ways to stick to their limits.

Class 6: Sticking With Your Decision. Students reviewed refusal skills, including clear "no" statements, alternative actions and delay tactics, and then practiced using them with half-scripted and unscripted role plays.

Class 7: Using Condoms Consistently and Correctly. Students completed the role-play demonstrations from Class 6 ("Real Situations"). Peer leaders and the teacher demonstrated the proper use of condoms, using a penis proxy, and students worked in pairs to practice—both describing and demonstrating the skill. In small groups, students identified challenges to condom use and came up with solutions.

Class 8: Resources. Working in small groups, students examined issues around STI/HIV and pregnancy testing. They identified basic information regarding the tests themselves, including confidentiality and when/where to get tested. Students listed resources and discussed how to use available resources to locate selected health services. The homework assignment from Class 2 (visit or call a clinic) was reviewed. Discussion focused on available services, students' experiences calling or visiting the clinics, and whether students would have recommended the clinic to their friends. A student/parent homework exercise ("What Do You Think?") was assigned.

Class 9: Media Influences. Students discussed media influences on sexual behaviors, and then worked in small groups to develop media messages that promoted ways teens could protect themselves from STI/HIV and pregnancy.

Class 10: Making a Commitment. Students summarized the benefits of talking with their parents/guardians (or other adults) about ways to prevent STI/HIV/pregnancy, using the homework assignment from Class 8 as a basis. Students presented their media messages from Class 9. Students made a commitment to protect themselves from STI/HIV/pregnancy, using colored dots to represent their choices. The activity was completed anonymously to protect students' privacy and minimize potential peer influence.

While the curriculum was being taught in 9th and 10th grades, the Peer Resources Team/Club was conducting other *Safer Choices*–related activities schoolwide that they had developed with guidance from the School Health Promotion Council.

PROGRAM EVALUATION

The Original Evaluation

Study Design

The research team hypothesized that teens who received the *Safer Choices* curriculum would initiate sexual intercourse at a slower rate than a comparison group. They also hypothesized that intervention teens who had already initiated sexual intercourse would have less unprotected sex and sex with fewer partners than their control group counterparts. Finally, the team hypothesized that intervention students would be more likely to report condom use at first intercourse (for those who reported sexual initiation during the follow-up period), greater contraceptive use at last intercourse, less alcohol (and other substance) use prior to intercourse, and more frequent testing for STI/HIV, and fewer sexual partners.

The evaluation used a randomized controlled trial involving 10 public high schools in an urban area of California and 10 in a suburban area of Texas. Five schools in each state were randomized into the *Safer Choices* program. The remaining 5 in each state received a standard, knowledge-based HIV prevention curriculum.

Active parental consent was required for survey participation. Approximately 80% of all possible participants (n = 6,488) had consent to participate. However, many of these students left school during the first year of the study, and did not reenroll in the school for 10th grade, so were lost to the study.

In the fall of the 1993–1994 school year, all 9th graders with parental consent completed paper-and-pencil self-report surveys, immediately before the intervention (n = 3,869). Follow-up surveys were conducted an average of 7 months post-intervention, in spring 1994 (n = 3,677, or 95% of the baseline sample); in spring 1995, 19 months postintervention (n = 3,211, or 83%); and 31 months postintervention (n = 3,057, or 77%).

Study Population

Schools in the study were chosen because they served a diverse population. Baseline demographics confirm this: approximately 17% self-identified as African American, 18% as Asian or Pacific Islander, 27% as Hispanic, 31% as White, <1% as American Indian or Alaskan Native, and 7% as Other. Approximately 71% of the students reported not yet having initiated sexual intercourse. Of those who had, 60% had had sex in the last 3 months, and about 56% used a condom at first sex.

Evaluation Questions and Outcome Measures

The survey instrument consisted of items assessing demographic characteristics, sexuality-related psychosocial factors, sexual behaviors, and program exposure.

The survey measured three primary behavioral outcomes:

1. Whether intervention participants delayed initiation of sexual intercourse
2. Among students reporting intercourse, the number of times they had sex without a condom in the last 3 months
3. Among students reporting intercourse, the number of sexual partners with whom students had intercourse without a condom during the last 3 months

In addition, the survey assessed a series of secondary behavioral outcomes.

- Use of a condom at first intercourse among students who initiated sexual intercourse following baseline
- Use of protection at last intercourse
- Number of sexual partners in the last 3 months
- Use of alcohol or other substances before sexual intercourse in the last 3 months
- Being tested for STIs or HIV

Several psychosocial scales were also included:

- HIV and other STI knowledge;
- attitudes about sexual intercourse;
- attitudes about condoms;
- normative beliefs about sexual intercourse;
- normative beliefs about condoms;

- self-efficacy in refusing sex, using condoms, and communicating with partners;
- barriers to condom use;
- HIV and other STI risk perception;
- communication with parents.

Evaluation Results

Behavioral Factors: Primary Behavioral Outcomes

Among the primary outcomes listed above, at the 31-month follow-up, all three were in the desired direction, and two were statistically significant. Sexually experienced students in the intervention schools reported having unprotected sex fewer times than their control school counterparts ($p = .05$) by a 0.63 ratio. Intervention students also reported having fewer partners with whom they had sex without a condom than did their sexually experienced counterparts ($p = .02$); the ratio of adjusted means was 0.73.

Although there was no statistical difference between intervention and control students in the incidence of sexual initiation, the trend was in the desired direction (odds ratio = .83), but not significant ($p = .39$).

Behavioral Factors: Secondary Behavioral Outcomes

Safer Choices students who reported sexual intercourse in the last 3 months were 1.68 times more likely to have used condoms ($p = .04$) and 1.76 times more likely to use an effective pregnancy prevention method (birth control pills, birth control pills plus condoms, or condoms alone) ($p = .05$) than were control students.

The evaluation revealed no significant differences between the two groups at final follow-up on any other secondary behavioral outcomes, although mean differences between the two groups were in the desired direction for five of the six remaining outcomes.

Psychosocial Factors

Intervention students scored significantly higher than their control counterparts on the HIV and other STI knowledge scales (by an adjusted mean difference of 11 and 9 percentage points); expressed significantly more positive attitudes about condoms ($p = .01$); and reported greater condom-use self-efficacy ($p = .04$), fewer barriers to condom use ($p = .01$), and higher levels of perceived risk for HIV ($p = .02$) and other STIs ($p = .04$). *Safer Choices* students also reported greater normative beliefs about condom use and more communication with parents than did the control group students.

There were no significant differences between students in the two groups in their attitudes toward sexual intercourse ($p = .95$), normative beliefs regarding sexual intercourse ($p = .79$), self-efficacy to refuse sex ($p = .10$), or self-efficacy to communicate with a partner about sexual limits ($p = .60$).

Summary

Safer Choices was successful in changing four of five outcomes addressing condom use and other protective behaviors. The program also enhanced numerous behavioral determinants, particularly those related to condom use. These positive effects lasted over a 31-month period. This study indicated that theory-driven, school-based, multicomponent programs with a clear message enhanced psychosocial variables and reduced sexual risk behaviors related to HIV, other STIs, and pregnancy prevention among high school students.

SAFER CHOICES IN THE COMMUNITY TODAY

Since the release of the replication kit in 2006, *Safer Choices* has been implemented in communities in 6 states across the country.

NOTE

1. A full set of program materials, including implementation manual, peer leader training guide, curriculum manuals, brochures, posters, activity cards, evaluation materials, and more, is available for purchase from Sociometrics at http://www.socio.com/pasha.htm.

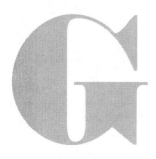

Programs Designed for Gay/Lesbian/Bisexual/ Transgender Youths

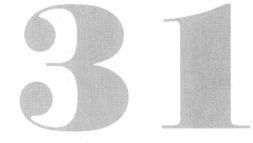

Adolescents Living Safely: AIDS Awareness, Attitudes, and Actions for Gay, Lesbian, and Bisexual Teens

Anne Belden, M. Jane Park, and Janette Mince

Original Program Developers and Evaluators

Sutherland Miller, PhD
Joyce Hunter, DSW
    HIV Center for Clinical & Behavioral Studies
    New York Psychiatric Institute
    New York, NY

Mary Jane Rotheram-Borus, PhD
Helen Reid, MA
Margaret Rosario, PhD
    UCLA Health Risk Reduction Project
    University of California, Los Angeles
    Los Angeles, CA

Adolescents Living Safely: AIDS Awareness, Attitudes, and Actions for Gay, Lesbian, and Bisexual Teens was supported by grants from the National Institute of Mental Health (Grant #1P50 MH 43520) and the William T. Grant Foundation.

PROGRAM ABSTRACT

Summary

Adolescents Living Safely: AIDS Awareness, Attitudes, and Actions for Gay, Lesbian, and Bisexual Teens (ALS II) is specially designed to provide education, social, and medical services and peer support to gay, lesbian, and bisexual youths between 14 and 19 years of age. It combines case management, comprehensive health care and risk assessment counseling with 25 small-group discussion sessions. During the group sessions, transmission and prevention of HIV/AIDS are investigated through video and art workshops in which teens review commercially available videos and create their own materials, such as soap operas and raps on HIV/AIDS and safer sex. Participants learn how to cope with high-risk situations, such as when the HIV status of a potential partner is unknown. The sessions also address such topics as coming out, stigma and self-acceptance, which are particularly important to teens confronting sexual identity issues. The case management and counseling components are designed to identify individual needs and provide participants with appropriate services (e.g., legal, medical, vocational).

A field study of the intervention was conducted with 138 males at a community-based agency serving gay youths in New York City. The impact of the program was found to vary over time and across racial/ethnic groups. Among sexually active participants (70% of the sample), African American and White teens showed a significant decrease in unprotected anal intercourse at the 3-month follow-up assessment; at 6 months the decrease was significant only among Whites. On measures of unprotected oral intercourse, White and Hispanic youths engaged in fewer risk acts through the 12-month assessment; among African Americans, the decrease was maintained until 6 months following the intervention.

Focus

☐ Primary pregnancy prevention   ☐ Secondary pregnancy prevention   ☑ STI/HIV/AIDS prevention

Original Site

☐ School based   ☑ Community based   ☐ Clinic based

Suitable for Use In

ALS II can be implemented in a variety of community-based and/or clinic-based settings serving youths at high risk for contracting HIV/AIDS, provided that case management and counseling services are available. This program is also suitable for implementation in residential drug treatment programs. Although it was field tested with a group of adolescent males, the curriculum was designed for use with females, as well.

Approach

- ■ ☐ Abstinence
- ■ ☑ Behavioral skills development
- ■ ☐ Community outreach
- ■ ☑ Contraceptive access
- ■ ☑ Contraceptive education
- ■ ☐ Life option enhancement
- ■ ☑ Self-efficacy/self-esteem
- ■ ☑ Sexuality/HIV/STI education

Original Intervention Sample

Age, gender   The original sample included 138 gay males, ages 14 to 19 years (average = 16.7).

Race/ethnicity   51% Hispanic, 31% African American, 12% White, 6% Other.

Program Components

- ■ ☐ Adult involvement
- ■ ☑ Case management
- ■ ☑ Group discussion
- ■ ☐ Lectures
- ■ ☐ Peer counseling/instruction
- ■ ☐ Public service announcements
- ■ ☑ Role play
- ■ ☐ Video
- ■ ☑ Other: Video and art workshops

Program Length

The full intervention consists of 25 group sessions in addition to regular counseling and case management services. It is recommended that two to four sessions be scheduled per week, over a 7- to 10-week period. Each session lasts approximately 90 to 120 minutes.

Staffing Requirements/Training

Group sessions (with approximately 10 youths) are facilitated by two leaders, selected for their sensitivity to issues of cultural and sexual diversity. Training should include cognitive-behavioral risk reduction strategies, coping with clinical crises and group process skills. Other professionals (e.g., lawyers, vocational counselors) should be on call to provide other specialized services as needed.

BIBLIOGRAPHY

Rotheram-Borus, M. J., Reid, H., & Rosario, M. (1994). Factors mediating changes in sexual HIV risk behaviors among gay and bi-sexual male adolescents. *American Journal of Public Health, 84*(12), 1938–1946.

Related References by the Developers of *ALS II*

Rotheram-Borus, M. J., Mahler, K. A., & Rosario, M. (1995). AIDS prevention with adolescents. *AIDS Education & Prevention, 7*(4), 320–336.

Rotheram-Borus, M. J., Murphy, D. A., Kennedy, M., Stanton, A., & Kulkinsky, M. (2001). Health and risk behaviors over time among youth living with HIV. *Journal of Adolescence, 24*(6), 791–802.

Stein, J. A., Rotheram-Borus, M. J., Swendeman, D., & Milburn, G. (2005). Predictors of sexual transmission risk behaviors among HIV-positive young men. *AIDS Care, 17*(4), 433–442.

THE PROGRAM

Program Rationale and History

ALS II was a comprehensive program developed to meet the needs of gay and bisexual male adolescents, who were at high risk for contracting HIV.[1] Although the program was originally implemented with gay and bisexual males, the curriculum was equally appropriate for use with lesbian and bisexual females. At the time this program was conceptualized, transgenderism had not yet surfaced as an important issue. While the original materials do not specifically address this issue, the topics covered are sufficiently broad to include all teens who may be questioning or developing their sexual identities.

The original program developers recognized that teens often know the safest alternatives for sexual situations, but they lack the social skills to implement their knowledge. Thus, in designing the *ALS II* curriculum, they adapted key components from programs that had been successful in changing sexual risk behaviors in runaways and adult gay men and in changing other adolescent health-risk behaviors. These components included social skills training, behavioral self-management, and group and social support from peers. Issues especially pertinent to gay, lesbian, and bisexual teens (e.g., coming out, stigma, shame, self-acceptance) were covered as well. The program also addressed teenagers' needs for comprehensive health care.

A field study of the program was conducted with 138 gay and bisexual males, predominantly African American and Hispanic. The study took place at the Hetrick Martin Institute, a community-based agency that provided recreational and social services to gay youths in New York City.

Theoretical Framework

ALS II was guided by a cognitive-behavioral approach to health promotion, which relies heavily on social learning theory. Bandura's social learning theory elaborates the processes through which intentions can be translated into behavioral change among teens. Bandura asserts that learning occurs through practice and observation of social models; it is mediated by internal beliefs about one's ability to succeed, and anticipated rewards and consequences of one's actions and others' evaluation of one's performance. *ALS II* emphasized the importance of practicing, observing, and modeling as vehicles for learning new skills and improving old ones.

The cognitive-behavioral method yields a practical and theoretically grounded approach for helping adolescents that can be tailored to suit the needs of the client population, institutional setting, and community. The program aimed to increase adolescents' awareness and understanding of their own feelings before trying to increase knowledge, attitudes, or behavioral skills. If teens could not talk about and understand their own feelings, they would be unable to communicate with potential partners about safer sexual practices. Such self-understanding was particularly critical for teens confronting questions of sexual identity. Research has revealed that youths who felt comfortable with their bisexuality or homosexuality were less likely to engage in risky social and sexual behaviors.

Program Model

ALS II was based on the following model of human behavior:

People will continue to behave in a certain way if

1. they expect something good to result from their behavior;
2. something that they want does occur;
3. something good happens often;
4. any negative consequences occur a long time after the positive ones.

People will behave effectively in their best interests if

1. they know what is in their best interest;
2. they have the skills;
3. they have opportunities to learn skills in many ways: through observing, imitating and practicing;
4. they believe they have effective tools and can use them effectively;
5. they fit into the environment in which they live and the environment supports them.

Program Goals

The overall aim of the program was to reduce high-risk behavior among adolescents. Specifically, the intervention was designed to help participants

- abstain from sex and unsafe behavior if they had not yet had sexual intercourse;
- use a condom or dental dam when engaging in sexual activities where an exchange of body fluids was possible;
- screen potential partners and avoid sex with those who were risky or of questionable HIV status;
- refrain from getting high on alcohol or drugs before having sex.

Educational Objectives

In addition, the program developers defined 11 educational objectives for teens who participate in the *ALS II* program:

1. Acquire general knowledge about HIV/AIDS: definitions, consequences, routes of transmission, high-risk behaviors, prevention strategies, and testing
2. Believe that they could get AIDS, they could prevent themselves from getting AIDS, and they could change their own behavior
3. Label, assess, and control the intensity of their feelings in high- risk situations
4. Reward themselves with positive feedback for thought and behavior patterns that were likely to reduce the risk of infection
5. Use self-talk to guide themselves successfully through situations that were sexually risky
6. Identify and change dysfunctional thoughts
7. Solve interpersonal problems through clarifying goals; identifying risks, costs and opportunities; evaluating alternative strategies for fixing the situation; trying out alternatives and analyzing success
8. Express their needs assertively, say "no" in risky situations, and communicate with confidence
9. Determine the advantages and disadvantages of being tested for HIV
10. Identify community resources and use these resources as needed, particularly free condoms, dental dams, and health and mental health care
11. Deal with being gay, lesbian, or bisexual by defining themselves positively; coming out to themselves and others; improving relationships with friends and lovers and coping with stigma

Hypothesized Outcomes

It was hypothesized that this intensive, community-based intervention, accompanied by case management, counseling services and health care, would enable teens to

- decrease their sexual risk acts, such as unprotected anal, vaginal, or oral sex;
- increase their use of condoms and dental dams when engaging in sexual activity.

Program Content

ALS II sessions included five main components.

1. *Knowledge.* Facts about HIV were communicated through two types of activities. First, teenagers participated in video and art workshops to develop soap opera dramatizations, public service announcements, commercials and raps about HIV prevention. Second, they reviewed commercial HIV prevention videos.
2. *Coping skills.* Participants received training to address unrealistic expectations about their ability to cope in high-risk situations. They learned to identify personal cues or triggers that placed them at potential risk for HIV transmission and to identify and practice behavioral and cognitive coping responses to such situations.
3. *Health care.* Participants made at least one visit to a community-based agency that provided vocational and educational counseling, recreational opportunities and referrals for comprehensive health and mental health care, as well as legal aid.
4. *Individual barriers.* Through private counseling sessions, participants reviewed their individual barriers to safer sex, especially negative attitudes.
5. *Attitudes.* Participants and group leaders discussed prejudice against gays. It was believed that positive feelings and attitudes toward coming out improved teens' attitudes toward safer sex.

Program Schedule

ALS II consisted of 25 group sessions, plus one individual counseling session. Each group session shared the following six strategies:

1. Positive behaviors were reinforced, particularly by giving teens small tokens of colored paper as a symbol of their contributions to the group discussion.
2. Participants were encouraged to assess, monitor and label their feelings through the use of a "Feeling Thermometer." This thermometer, printed on a sheet of paper, showed a scale ranging from 0 to 100. Throughout the program sessions, teens "took their temperature" by assessing their position on the scale—from 0, indicating that one felt very, very comfortable, to 100, representing a high level of discomfort.
3. Talk was used to diminish group members' anxiety concerning taboo topics.
4. After group leaders modeled effective coping skills, participants practiced through role plays.
5. Concern was continually raised regarding unsafe sexual behaviors, involvement in risky situations and with risky partners.
6. Group cohesion was established through active participation and appreciation of each person's contribution.

Description of Program Sessions

Session 1: What Will Adolescents Living Safely Do for Me? The leaders and participants introduced themselves at the start of the first session. The topic of safer sex was explored by inviting teens to consider sexual behaviors on a continuum, from low-risk to high-risk activities. After discussing reasons why people engaged in unsafe acts, even if they knew better, the group identified strategies that could help people practice safe sex. The session continued with a brief review of the goals and ground rules of the program and discussion of the first homework assignment. Homework activities were used in all program sessions to link the curriculum material to teens' everyday experiences. Finally, the leaders encouraged participants to recognize at the end of each session fellow group members whose contributions they appreciated.

Session 2: What Is It Like Being a Gay or Lesbian Adolescent? This lesson was designed to help participants confront negative stereotypes about gay and lesbian people and to begin to define positive identities for themselves. After exploring the concept of the "self," individuals shared with the group their most outstanding quality. In the original field study, two men and two women, chosen to represent positive role models of gay and lesbian identity, were invited to describe their lives. The group also discussed famous gay and lesbian figures and their contributions to society. The facilitators ended the session by inviting participants to express their appreciation for their peers' contributions to the meeting.

Session 3: Coming Out to Myself. To reinforce the lessons of the previous session, teens shared with the group something brave that they had done. Then the focus shifted to a discussion of coming out, first to oneself and then to others. The leaders emphasized that self-acceptance was required before one could take the necessary steps to reduce one's risk of HIV infection (or if one was HIV-positive, to lead a high-quality life). A series of exercises was used to help group members think about the complex feelings involved in coming out. In the original field study, each participant was presented with a certificate "for being themselves."

Session 4: Coming Out to Others. The focus of this lesson was a step-by-step approach teens could use in coming out about their sexual identity to others. The model presented a series of questions prompting reflection about why one wanted to come out and how to proceed. Exercises provided group members with practice in confronting reactions they may have faced from family and friends.

Session 5: How to Recognize My Feelings. This session was designed to help participants identify their personal levels of comfort and discomfort in social situations. After a discussion of the importance of feelings to safer sexual behavior, the group engaged in a series of exercises using the feeling thermometer. Breathing exercises for relaxation in tense situations were also introduced; similar exercises would be used in several later program sessions.

Session 6: How Serious Is the Threat to Me? This lesson provided teens with a clearer understanding of the threats posed by HIV and AIDS, especially death. In one exercise, teens pretended that they are at a party. Each "guest" wore a name tag, and some of the tags had small flowers on them. During a brief mingling period, participants introduced themselves to one another and decided which guests they would want to have sex with. When the mingling ended, the facilitators explained that guests whose name tags had flowers are HIV-positive. If, in real life, the teens had decided to have sex with such people, they would have put themselves at risk for HIV infection. A second exercise was designed to encourage participants to think of death in relation to their hopes and dreams for the future—what they hoped to accomplish before they died. For homework, participants thought of one step they could take toward their personal lifetime goals.

Session 7: What Do I Need to Know About HIV/AIDS? Basic facts and terminology about HIV/AIDS were discussed in this session. In the original field study, the teens viewed a video describing the AIDS antibody test and discussed reasons why it might be important to take the test. You may want to hold a similar discussion with your own teens. Toward the end of the session, participants identified myths and misunderstandings they believed their peers had about AIDS; for homework, each teen educated two friends about the virus that caused AIDS.

Session 8: What Are My High-Risk Situations? Learning how to recognize and avoid high-risk situations was the goal of this session. Through role plays, discussions and games, the group leaders helped participants identify the particular situations they were likely to face. Additional exercises encouraged group members to think of ways they could get out of such situations without resorting to commonly-used rationalizations for unsafe activities.

Session 9: When Is My Sexual Behavior Safe? To address participants' confusion about the safety of particular activities, this session focused on sex as a continuum of behaviors. In one exercise teens thought about the safety level of various friends' sexual practices; each was evaluated as "safe," "possibly safe," or "definitely un-safe." During the next exercise, group members looked at their own personal be-haviors, again considering the safety of their actions. At the close of the session a group profile of safe sex behaviors was compiled.

Session 10: How to Use a Condom and Dental Dam. The proper use of condoms and dental dams was taught during this session, and humor was recommended as a tension-reducing strategy. The facilitators emphasized the importance of latex con-doms, along with appropriate lubricants. As a group, participants first practiced putting a condom on their hand or a penile proxy (e.g., banana, zucchini) and then practiced using a dental dam. For homework, participants located a local store where they could purchase condoms.

Session 11: How to Spread the Word About Safer Sex. At the start of the meeting, the group leaders emphasized the importance of condoms by explaining that participants would be asked to show that they were carrying condoms with them at all future ses-sions. Participants divided into three teams and each created a media message (e.g., TV commercial, rap or newscast) about ways to protect oneself from HIV. Each team spent about 20 minutes creating their skit, then performed the piece for the rest of the group. For homework, participants evaluated messages about HIV that they encoun-tered as they watched TV, listened to the radio or read a newspaper or magazine.

Session 12: Tell Me More About Sex. Through role-play exercises and discussion, the group explored feelings about sexual activity, sex education and communication in intimate relationships. During the second half of the session, the group split into male and female teams, and each met privately with a same-sex leader. Participants wrote any questions they had about sex on an index card, and the leader addressed them. During the field study, the leaders were given a booklet summarizing ques-tions frequently asked by teens.

Session 13: How to Cope With Trouble. This session introduced participants to strate-gies for coping in difficult situations. In a role-play exercise, participants illustrated each of eight possible strategies, from "seek support" to "escape the scene." The group leaders emphasized problem-solving as one of the best coping techniques. Using a problem analysis form, participants learned how to define, assess and con-structively confront a problem situation. Techniques for relaxing in such situations were rehearsed.

Session 14: Coping With My Use of Drugs and Alcohol. The relationship of drug and alcohol use to HIV infection was explored in this session. Through observation, role play, and discussion, participants evaluated the effects of drugs and alcohol on their lives and especially, the risk level of their behaviors. An exercise critiquing the behaviors of various actors involved in risky situations showed participants how to gain a sense of control over their lives. An additional exercise helped participants identify the emotional triggers that led them to get high. Finally, the group leaders demonstrated the proper procedure for cleaning intravenous drug needles with bleach.

Session 15: Dealing With Pressures to Use Drugs/Alcohol. Through a series of exercises on communication skills, gaining confidence, role-play scenarios and "I statements," participants learned how to deliver effective refusals and requests in risky situations. Participants also reviewed the previously learned coping techniques for taking control when pressured to use drugs or engage in unsafe sex.

Session 16: Friends and Lovers. This lesson was based on the premise that experimentation and observation were key ways to learn about adult sexual and social relationships. In one exercise, participants identified group members they would like to know better. They introduced themselves and then reported on their experiences. Techniques for starting conversations and coping with relationship issues were also discussed.

Session 17: How to Handle Thoughts That Don't Help Me. Shifting to cognitive strategies for promoting safer sex, the group leaders helped participants distinguish self-defeating from self-enhancing thoughts. Working with a partner, each teen wrote down self-defeating thoughts that they had used a lot in their lives; next to each thought they devised a self-supporting thought that could be used instead. The group continued this exercise together, focusing on thoughts that occurred during sexual situations. For homework, participants were asked to catch themselves in the middle of unhelpful thoughts, yell "Stop!" to themselves and come up with self-affirming thoughts.

Session 18: Visiting a Person With AIDS. To reduce teens' stereotypes about people with AIDS, and reinforce the point that HIV was not transmitted in everyday social encounters, this session enabled students to meet and talk with HIV-positive individuals. The facilitators encouraged participants to ask questions, show respect and share their own feelings. Typically, the visit included an informal meal. The visit was followed by a debriefing session in which group members discussed their feelings and reactions to the meeting.

Session 19: Should I Be Tested for HIV? The "HIV Antibody Test Sheet" was used to engage participants in a discussion of the test and the meaning of the results, whether positive or negative. Working in pairs, the teens explored their own possible reactions to a positive test result. Then group members raised and explored the question of whether they would be tested. The facilitators gave group members a list of local agencies, first where they could get tested and second, where they could receive treatment. (You may wish to prepare a comparable guide of resources in your own community.)

Session 20: Using Self-Talk to Practice Safer Sex. The group leaders promoted the idea that teens could feel better about themselves by giving themselves compliments and rewards. An exercise encouraged group members to practice using self-talk, or talking to themselves, in tough situations. Finally, the group split up by gender to participate in an activity that involved rewriting negative self-talk in a rap song.

Session 21: How to Choose Safe Friends. This session was designed to help participants assess the risks posed by their friends and sexual partners. In an introductory exercise, the teens learned that they often do not know which friends are HIV-positive. This exercise highlighted two points: first, that that there was no way to tell if someone was HIV-positive just by looking at him or her, and second, it was what people did, not who they were that led to HIV infection. For these reasons, the leaders emphasized, safe sex was essential. In a second exercise boys and girls met separately to create lists of the qualities they liked in partners. Strategies for starting and ending relationships were also explored, and the group practiced screening partners through discussion and role playing.

Session 22: Looking Over a Community Resource. The goal of this session was to introduce group members to community case management agencies that provided services to gay, lesbian, bisexual, and transgender youths. A list of other local resources was also given to participants. (You may wish to prepare such a list for participants in your setting.)

Session 23: Dealing With Stigma. This session was designed to improve teens' skill in coping with social stigma, harassment, and violence. In the first part of the lesson, the leaders discussed ways in which various groups were stigmatized. Role-play exercises helped the teens think about what they could do when harassed.

A personal counseling session. In addition to the group discussion sessions, each teen had an individual counseling session with a trained professional. The counselor first determined whether the adolescent was sexually active and then designed a plan to overcome barriers to practicing safer sex or maintaining abstinence. The counselor also addressed any questions the teen had regarding sex and HIV/AIDS.

Session 24: Making a Soap Opera on HIV/AIDS. To integrate the lessons of the previous sessions, the group created an original soap opera on HIV/AIDS. The leaders first encouraged the group to devise a story and choose script writers, a director, camera men or women, actors and editors. Once the story was complete, the skit was performed, videotaped and viewed.

Session 25: The End and the Beginning. During the final session, group members shared their feelings about the program. Members explored their hopes for the future by creating postcards that they would mail to their peers in 5 years. A relaxation technique was used to help group members feel good as they offered their good-byes.

PROGRAM EVALUATION

The Original Evaluation

Design

The effectiveness of the *ALS II* program was investigated in a field study conducted between 1988 and 1991 in New York City. The researchers recruited 138 male youths, ages 14 to 19, who sought services at the Hetrick-Martin Institute, a community-based agency providing recreational and social services to gay youths.

At the time of the study, there was only one site serving New York City's gay and bisexual youths, and the researchers feared that a comparison group selected from the same site would threaten validity. Moreover, given the scarcity of services for gay and bisexual youths, the researchers felt that it would be unethical to withhold the program and its related services from a group of teens. For these reasons, no comparison group was used.

The study focused on measures of high-risk sex acts, including the frequency of intercourse, number of partners and number of unprotected acts of oral and anal intercourse. To assess these behaviors, interviews were conducted with the gay males at four points:

- Time 1: before the start of the study (baseline)
- Time 2: 3 months following the baseline assessment (posttest)
- Time 3: 6 months following the baseline assessment (6-month follow-up)
- Time 4: 12 months following the baseline assessment (12-month follow-up)

Data Collection Procedures

Following their regular intake interview for the institute, the youths were invited to participate in the field study. They were asked to complete an informed consent form and the baseline assessment interview. Participants received $2 for taking part in the baseline interview, and $20 to $25 for each of the follow-up assessments.

All interviews were conducted by three highly skilled master's-level research assistants, under the supervision of a master's-level research psychologist. Of the original group of participants, 88% took part in at least one follow-up assessment, 79% completed two assessments, and 52% completed all four assessments.

Sample

Among the 138 males originally recruited for the study, 51% were Hispanic, 31% were African American, 12% were White, and the remaining 6% were classified as Other. Sixty-six percent labeled themselves as gay, 25% bisexual, 3% straight, and 6% refused to identify with any of these labels.

Evaluation Questions

The researchers investigated whether program participation was associated with

- a reduction in the number of unprotected active and receptive anal acts;
- a reduction in the number of unprotected active and receptive oral acts;
- abstinence from anal sex;
- a reduction in the total number of sexual partners.

Evaluation Results

At the baseline assessment, most of the participating gay and bisexual males (89%) had engaged in sex in the course of their lives, and 70% said they had been sexually active during the previous 3 months. On measures of high-risk sex acts, about half (53%) had engaged in anal sex during the previous 3 months, and 60% of these youths had used a condom. Similarly, 61% of the teens had participated in oral sex during the previous 3 months, but only 28% had used a condom for protection. In addition, sexually active youths reported a median of 2.0 partners, and 7% of the sample had engaged in commercial sex. The researchers found no differences in the behaviors as a function of racial or ethnic background or age.

Following the program, the researchers measured significant reductions in a number of high-risk sex acts among participants. They also examined outcomes across racial and ethnic groups, as well as by involvement in commercial sexual activity, as explained below.

Anal Sex Acts

At the 3-month follow-up assessment, program participation was associated with a decrease in unprotected anal sex for all but the Hispanic youths. At 6 months, the researchers found a positive association between the number of sessions attended and a reduction in risk acts, for White teens only. In contrast, both African American and Hispanic teens showed an increase in unprotected anal sex acts at the 6-month assessment. At the 12-month follow-up, no significant outcomes were observed for any ethnic group.

Oral Sex Acts

There was a significant rise in the number of protected oral sex acts over the course of the field study. In particular, the mean proportion of protected oral sex acts rose from 28% at baseline to 45% at 12 months. At 12 months, among White and Hispanic teens, the frequency of risk activity decreased as the number of intervention sessions increased (when previous risk activity and commercial sexual activity were controlled). African Americans significantly reduced their risk acts at 3 and 6 months, but not at the 12-month follow-up.

Abstinence

Attending the *ALS II* program was not associated with significant increases in abstinence from anal sex.

Sexual Partners

Program participants significantly reduced the number of sexual partners following the intervention. In the 3 months prior to the baseline interview, the youths had an average of 2.2 partners. At the follow-up assessments, the average number of partners in the previous 3 months decreased to about 1.5 (3 months = 1.3, $p < .01$; 6 months = 1.6, $p < .05$; 12 months = 1.6, $p < .01$). This reduction was maintained through the 12-month follow-up. However, the researchers found that program participation was not associated with any significant changes in the number of partners for oral or anal sex acts.

Ethnicity

Focusing on patterns of sexual activity across racial/ethnic groups, the researchers found that African American teens showed significant and substantial reductions in both anal and oral risk acts over the study period. The proportion of protected anal acts rose from 36% at baseline to 80% at 3 months, 67% at 6 months, and 84% at 12 months. Hispanic youths had somewhat higher percentages of protected sex at baseline (anal, 67%; oral, 31%) and these increased through 6 months (anal, 88%; oral, 31%). At 1 year, levels of protection returned toward baseline levels (anal, 72%; oral, 40%). Whites, Asian, and Native American participants also showed positive shifts in their HIV risk acts, but the numbers were too small for significance testing.

Commercial Sexual Activity

The researchers found that gay and bisexual teens who engaged in commercial sexual activity increased their anal and oral sex risk acts over time, despite participation in the program.

Summary

The *ALS II* program, combining group discussions, behavioral skill development, peer support, personal counseling, and case management, was associated with a number of positive changes in the sexual risk behaviors of teenage gay and bisexual males. In particular, the researchers measured a reduction in the number of unprotected acts of oral and anal sex, as well as a reduction in the number of sexual partners, among participating teens.

Overall, the researchers observed more positive outcomes for teens who had engaged in fewer risky acts prior to the study. In contrast, teens who had participated in commercial sexual activity showed an increase in the number of high-risk sex acts following the program. The findings also varied by ethnicity, with African Americans showing the most dramatic reductions in unprotected anal and oral sex over the 1-year follow-up period.

In interpreting their results, the evaluators noted that the best predictor of future sexual behavior appeared to be past behavior, and thus urged early intervention for HIV prevention. They also cautioned that without a comparison group, it was impossible to attribute positive changes to the effects of the program. Finally, because there were no measures of the dosage of specific components, the researchers could not determine which components held the most promise for adolescent for risk reduction.

ALS II IN THE COMMUNITY TODAY

In the past 3 years, *ALS II* has been implemented in communities in Pennsylvania.

NOTE

1. A full set of program materials, including curriculum manual, activity packets, evaluation materials, and more, is available for purchase from Sociometrics at http://www.socio.com/pasha.htm.

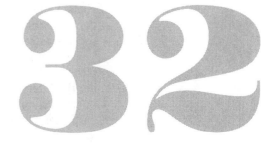

Youth and AIDS Project's HIV Prevention Program: An STI/HIV/AIDS Prevention Program for Young Gay Men

J. Barry Gurdin, Starr Niego, and Janette Mince

Original Program Developer and Evaluator

Gary Remafedi, MD, MPH
  Department of Pediatrics
  University of Minnesota
  Minneapolis, MN

PROGRAM ABSTRACT

Summary

A community, clinic, and university collaborative launched this program to provide education, peer support, counseling and case management to gay and bisexual male adolescents between 13 and 21 years of age, who are at high risk for HIV/AIDS. The program begins with an interview for individualized HIV/AIDS risk assessment and risk reduction counseling. Youths then participate in an interactive peer education program designed to provide clear, factual information in an atmosphere of mutual support. The program's lessons are reinforced in an educational

Youth and AIDS Project's HIV Prevention Program was supported by grants from the Minnesota Department of Health (MNDOH/12500–29679–01), and the Maternal and Child Health Program, Health Resources and Services Administration, Department of Health and Human Services (BRH/PO5053 and MCJ000985–111).

video. Optional peer support groups meet weekly, if youths wish to attend. Finally, there is a follow-up visit for reassessment and referrals, as needed, to medical and social services.

A field study of the program was conducted with a predominantly white sample of males, ages 13–21, who identified themselves as gay or bisexual. Following the intervention, the 139 participants reported less frequent unprotected anal intercourse and more frequent use of condoms. A reduction in substance abuse, particularly amphetamines and amyl nitrate, was also recorded.

Focus

☐ Primary pregnancy prevention ☐ Secondary pregnancy prevention ☑ STI/HIV/AIDS prevention

Original Site

☐ School based ☑ Community based ☑ Clinic based

Suitable for Use In

This program can be implemented by a variety of clinics and community-based organizations serving gay, bisexual, and transgender teens, providing that necessary medical and social services are available for referrals.

Approach

- ■ ☐ Abstinence
- ■ ☑ Behavioral skills development
- ■ ☐ Community outreach
- ■ ☐ Contraceptive access
- ■ ☑ Contraceptive education
- ■ ☐ Life option enhancement
- ■ ☑ Self-efficacy/self-esteem
- ■ ☑ Sexuality/HIV/STI education

Original Intervention Sample

Age, gender   The original sample included 139 males, ages 13 to 21 years (average = 19.3 years).

Race/ethnicity   75% White, 14% African American, 4% Asian American, 3% Latino, 3% Native American

Program Components

- ■ ☐ Adult involvement
- ■ ☑ Case management
- ■ ☑ Group discussion
- ■ ☑ Lectures
- ■ ☑ Peer counseling/instruction
- ■ ☐ Public service announcements
- ■ ☑ Role play
- ■ ☑ Video
- ■ ☑ Other: Optional peer support groups

Program Length

The basic program includes 5–6 hours of activities, beginning with a 2.5-hour risk assessment interview and a 1.5-hour peer education session. Meetings of the peer support groups follow the education sessions; participation in these groups is optional.

Staffing Requirements/Training

One peer educator (18 to 22 years old) is recommended for every four teens; these educators must be well informed about issues pertinent to gay, bisexual and transgender youths. Training includes background information on HIV/AIDS, as well as practice in facilitating group discussions. A psychologist, physician, or social worker is needed to perform the risk assessments. Additional professional staff (e.g., physicians, vocational counselors) should be on call to provide necessary services.

BIBLIOGRAPHY

Centers for Disease Control and Prevention. (2007). *HIV/AIDS surveillance in adolescents and young adults (through 2005)*. Retrieved October 13, 2007, from http://www.cdc.gov/hiv/topics/surveillance/resources/slides/adolescents/index.htm

Remafedi, G. (1994). Cognitive and behavioral adaptations to HIV/AIDS among gay and bisexual adolescents. *Journal of Adolescent Health, 15*(2), 142–148.

Related References by the Developers of the *Youth and AIDS Project's HIV Prevention Program*

Guenther-Grey, C. A., Varnell, S., Weiser, J. I., Mathy, R. M., O'Donnell, L., Steuve, A., et al. (2005). Trends in sexual risk-taking among urban young men who have sex with men, 1999–2002. *Journal of the National Medical Association, 97*(7 Suppl.), 38–43.

Remafedi, G. (1998). The University of Minnesota Youth and AIDS Projects' Adolescent Early Intervention Program: A model to link HIV-seropositive youth with care. *Journal of Adolescent Health, 23*(2 Suppl.), 115–121.

Remafedi, G. (2001). Linking HIV-seropositive youth with health care: Evaluation of an intervention. *AIDS Patient Care & STDs, 15*(3), 147–151.

Shew, M. L., Remafedi, G. J., Bearinger, H. L., Faulkner, B. L., Taylor B. A., Potthoff, S. J., et al. (1997). The validity of self-reported condom use among adolescents. *Sexually Transmitted Diseases, 24*(9), 503–510.

THE PROGRAM

Program Rationale and History

The *Youth and AIDS Project's HIV Prevention Program (YAPHPP)* was a combined educational, counseling, case management and peer support intervention.[1] It was specially designed for young males who believed they may have been gay or bisexual, self-identified as gay or bisexual or had sex with other men. (Note: When *YAPHPP* was first developed, the issue of adolescent transgenderism had not yet entered the vernacular as an important issue in adolescent sexual health. Thus, no mention was made of transgender youths. However, the program content was sufficiently broad so as to apply to all youths, regardless of gender or sexual identity.)

At the start of the program, a physician or social worker conducted an individual interview to assess the HIV-risk level of each participant. The professional then counseled the youth about ways to reduce his risk of infection and provided referrals to specialized services, as needed. Afterward, participants attended a peer education session; they also took part in optional peer support groups for gay and bisexual youths. A final counseling session was held to correct any remaining misinformation the youth might have had and to stress HIV/AIDS prevention goals. At that time, if the young person needed additional medical, mental health or social services, referrals and assistance with scheduling, finances and transportation were provided.

A field study of the program was conducted between 1989 and 1991 in Minnesota. A group of 139 gay and bisexual male adolescents ages 13 to 21 participated.

Theoretical Framework

YAPHPP was based on the finding that gay and bisexual youths—ages 13 to 21— were at elevated risk of exposure to HIV. Their risk is compounded by the practice of anal intercourse, psychosocial problems that fuel risky behavior and few preventive services. Although preventive services and overall awareness have increased since the development of this program, HIV/AIDS among adolescent males remains a significant public health issue. As recently as 2007, the Centers for Disease Control and Prevention (CDC) reported that among the cases of HIV/AIDS reported between 2001 and 2005 for young men ages 13–19, the method of transmission in 77% of those cases was unprotected male-to-male sex; among young men ages 20–24, 75% reported transmission through unprotected male-to-male sex (Centers for Disease Control and Prevention, 2007).

The original program developers recognized that gay, lesbian and bisexual youths often struggled to arrive at a positive image of their sexual orientation. At the same time, youths who had established a comfortable identity as a gay, lesbian or bisexual teenager were less likely to engage in high-risk behaviors.

In the absence of a proven model for facilitating HIV risk reduction among this population of teens, the program developers sought to understand short-term changes in gay and bisexual male youths' HIV-related knowledge, attitudes and behaviors. Education, peer support, counseling and case management were selected as strategies to improve youths' understanding of homosexuality and HIV/AIDS, overcome feelings of isolation and reduce high-risk behaviors.

Program Objectives

As a sexually transmitted infection (STI)/HIV/AIDS risk reduction program, *YAPHPP* was designed to

1. broaden participants' knowledge of adolescent homosexuality;
2. deepen participants' understanding of the psychosocial and emotional problems faced by gay and lesbian teens;
3. counsel and support participants;
4. educate participants about HIV/AIDS, including transmission and prevention;
5. enhance participants' understanding of the adverse effect of alcohol and drugs on HIV risk reduction;
6. link participants to any needed medical, mental health or social services.

Hypothesized Outcomes

Following their participation in the program, it was predicted that teens would

1. be able to distinguish facts from myths about HIV disease;
2. avoid the use of alcohol and drugs in sexual situations;
3. communicate clearly with sexual partners about risk reduction;
4. employ risk-reduction strategies in all relationships;
5. use condoms consistently during oral, vaginal or anal intercourse;

6. replace high-risk sexual practices with lower-risk behaviors;
7. use HIV antibody counseling and testing, as appropriate.

Program Content

YAPHPP combined education, peer support, counseling and case management to increase gay and bisexual males' self-esteem, knowledge about homosexuality and HIV/AIDS-preventive behaviors. Program sessions reinforced the message that, in the United States and elsewhere worldwide, most HIV infections among both adolescent and adult men had been transmitted through unsafe sex between men. (Among both adolescent and adult women, the most frequent transmission route is through unprotected sex with an infected male partner.)

Counseling and peer education sessions encouraged youths to practice safe sex by using latex condoms lubricated with water-based lubricants for anal, vaginal or oral intercourse. (Originally, the program recommended the use of spermicides containing nonoxynol-9. However, more recent research has revealed that nonoxynol-9 can irritate vaginal—or anal—linings and cause microscopic tears which leave the individual more susceptible to infection.) Teens were further encouraged not to share any intravenous drug equipment ("works"), or to clean them with bleach if no other alternatives were available, and to avoid exposure to another person's blood, semen or vaginal fluids.

In addition, the program included group activities to help participants develop new skills for communicating clearly and forcefully in real-life romantic situations. Participants participated in two exercises, one which depicted how rapidly HIV spread through a tightly knit community of sexually active individuals, and the other which identified the levels of risk associated with various sexual and drug-use behaviors.

Program Components

The program was divided into three components, ranging in length from 1.5 to 2.5 hours. In the original field study of the intervention, a fourth component—peer support meetings for gay and bisexual youths—was available if the youths wished to participate. You may want to organize a similar activity for your teens.

A brief overview of each component is provided below.

Initial Risk Assessment Interview and Counseling Session

The initial interview was designed to elicit a detailed evaluation of the youth's HIV-related knowledge, attitudes and behaviors, along with his psychosocial well-being and substance use. Once the assessment had been made, the counselor/case manager conducted individualized education and risk-reduction counseling. Finally, the professional provided referrals, as appropriate, for housing, medical care, further counseling and/or social support groups. The full interview and counseling session typically required about 2.5 hours to complete.

Peer Education Session

Following the risk assessment and counseling session, groups of up to four youth met for a single 90-minute peer education session. Group members viewed the video *Surviving AIDS*, learned about the correct use of condoms, and participated in two group exercises. In the first exercise, participants considered their personal values about engaging in various sexual and risk-taking behaviors. In the second exercise, teens practiced negotiating safer sex in several different situations. During the final part of the session, youths had an opportunity to ask any questions they may have had about HIV and to set personal prevention goals. For example, gay youths often raised practical questions, such as "How risky is oral sex?" The peer educators were trained to offer relevant and factual responses.

Final Counseling Session

After the peer education session, the counselor/case manager met again with each subject to correct any remaining misinformation and to reinforce HIV/AIDS prevention goals. Additionally, if the young person was considered in need of additional medical, mental health or social services, the professional referred him to the appropriate agency and helped arrange appointments, finances and transportation, if requested.

Optional Social Support Group

In the field study, a social support group for gay and lesbian young people was available to all program participants. The youths decided whether they wished to take part. In addition to reinforcing program messages about HIV/AIDS prevention, the group provided opportunities for friendship and support. In particular, teens helped one another cope with the homophobia they experienced in anti-gay comments, jokes and negative stereotypes, as well as the typical stressors of adolescence. The group also provided connections to such organizations as PFLAG. (Originally, PFLAG was a support organization made up of Parents and Friends of Lesbians and Gays. However, with advances in awareness, the organization has grown to include parents of bisexual and transgender people as well.)

Program Implementation

In the original field study of the program, the peer educators' training included background information on HIV/AIDS, as well as practice leading group discussions. The educators were gay and bisexual males, ages 18 to 22, who had been nominated by members of the University of Minnesota Youth and AIDS Project's social support groups. These youths were selected for their sensitivity to issues concerning adolescence, homosexuality and HIV/AIDS.

Obtaining Necessary Support

The subject matter of *YAPHPP* was controversial when first implemented. Before implementing this program—or any STI/HIV/AIDS prevention initiative—ensure that you understand and apply all policies and mandates relevant to your clinic or community organization.

Establishing Ground Rules

Ground rules were established at the start of the intervention and followed by all physicians, caseworkers, counselors, peer educators and youths involved in the program activities. This created an atmosphere of trust and comfort in which participants were free to discuss sexuality and protection from STIs.

The procedures listed below were adapted from recommendations drafted by PFLAG:

1. Do not act surprised when someone tells you they think they may be gay, lesbian, bisexual, or transgender. The person has decided that you can be trusted and helpful. Do not let him or her down.
2. Respect confidentiality. Gay, lesbian, bisexual, and transgender teenagers who share their identity with you have established a sacred trust that must be respected.

3. Be supportive. Let gay, lesbian, bisexual, or transgender teenagers know that they are "okay." Explain that many people have struggled with the issues of homosexuality and sexual identity. Acknowledge that dealing with one's sexuality is difficult. Keep the door open for further conversations and assistance.
4. Assess his or her understanding of homosexuality and sexual identity. Replace misinformation with accurate knowledge. Don't assume that gay, lesbian, bisexual, and transgender teens know a lot about human sexuality. We have all been exposed to myths and stereotypes, so it is very helpful to provide clarification.
5. Read reliable references and talk to qualified persons. Know the community resources available to provide gay, lesbian, bisexual or transgender youths with social support and information.
6. Deal with feelings first. Most gay, lesbian, bisexual, and transgender teenagers feel alone, afraid, and guilty. You can help by listening and allowing them to unburden uncomfortable feelings and thoughts.
7. Examine your own biases so that you can remain a neutral source of information and support to the youths.
8. Use nonjudgmental, all-inclusive language in your discussion. Pay attention to verbal and nonverbal cues. Do not label or categorize.
9. Anticipate some confusion. Many gay, lesbian, bisexual, and transgender teenagers are sure of their sexual orientation by the time they enter high school. Others will be confused and unsure.

PROGRAM EVALUATION

The Original Evaluation

Design

The effectiveness of the original *YAPHPP* program was investigated in a field study conducted in Minnesota between 1989 and 1991. A group of 139 male adolescents, ages 13 to 21, participated; all identified themselves as gay or bisexual.

The evaluators used a diverse set of measures to study changes in the teens' knowledge, beliefs, attitudes and behaviors over time. Questionnaires were administered to all teens twice during the study period:

Time 1: at the initial assessment interview (pretest)

Time 2: 3 to 6 months following the initial interview (posttest)

Evaluation Questions

The researchers investigated whether program participation was associated with changes in the youths'

- friendship patterns;
- knowledge of and attitudes toward HIV/AIDS;
- patterns of sexual activity, especially high-risk behaviors;
- use of condoms;
- substance use/abuse.

Data Collection Procedures

Several strategies were employed to recruit participants for the study. The researchers placed advertisements in gay publications and businesses, spoke at social and community meetings and sought referrals from school and health professionals and previous participants in the University of Minnesota Youth and AIDS Project activities. Eligible youths were male, between the ages of 13 and 21, who either identified themselves as gay or bisexual, regardless of their sexual behavior, or reported having sexual intercourse with men.

Because no comparison group was used in the study, all participants received the same intervention. That is, they took part in individualized risk assessment, small-group peer education, and counseling/case management sessions. Youths with special needs were referred to appropriate medical and/or psychosocial services and assisted with scheduling and transportation arrangements.

Participation in the study and the program was voluntary and confidential. The youths provided verbal and written consent for each component, but parental consent was not required. At their initial risk assessment interview, a number of instruments were administered to the youths, consisting of both self-report surveys and structured interview questions. These measures were re-administered at the follow-up assessment session, which took place between 3 and 6 months later. On average, 4.75 months elapsed between the Time 1 and Time 2 assessments.

Youths received $20 for attending the initial risk assessment interview and peer education session and $10 for the follow-up interview; they were also eligible to receive a $5 bonus for each friend referred for an interview.

Sample

Of the 239 youths who took part in the initial assessment interview, 41 were unable to complete the Time 2 measures. Of this group, 24 had moved out of state and the remaining 17 entered the program too late to allow for a follow-up assessment. Complete data were available for 139 teens, ages 13 to 21 years. The great majority of the sample (91%) identified themselves as gay, and the rest as bisexual. At the time of the study, the typical youth was 19.3 years old and had completed 12th grade. About 75% of the participants were currently enrolled as students. The evaluators found no significant differences in background characteristics or frequency of sexual intercourse between those teens who did and did not take part in the two assessments.

Reflecting the demographic characteristics of the region in which the program was located, the final sample was largely White (75%). Other racial/ethnic groups represented in the study included African American (14%), Asian American (4%), Hispanic (3%), and Native American (2%).

Evaluation Results

Participation in *YAPHPP* was associated with a number of positive outcomes, including reductions in HIV risk behaviors.

Effects on Knowledge and Attitudes

Participants scored well on measures of basic HIV etiology and transmission at both assessment periods. At Time 2, the youths were more likely to know that "AIDS causes other diseases" and that the HIV antibody test is not "a test for AIDS." Additionally, both before and after the intervention, participants generally reported realistic beliefs about the risk levels of various sexual behaviors.

Effects on Friendship

YAPHPP was designed, in part, to reduce feelings of isolation and alienation among gay and bisexual youths. Following the intervention, teens reported an increase in the proportion of their friends who were bisexual and homosexual, and nearly half (43%) had revealed their own orientation to more friends. Additionally, a larger number of participants were living with another bisexual or homosexual person, but the percentage of teens who were involved in a steady relationship was unchanged.

Effects on Substance Use

A summary measure of the severity of teens' substance abuse showed significant improvement following the program ($p < .001$). Although the youths did not significantly modify their use of alcohol, marijuana, or binge drinking, their use of amphetamines ($p < .011$) and amyl nitrites was significantly lower at the Time 2 assessment ($p < .05$).

Effect on Sexual Behavior

Overall, the researchers found that bisexual behavior diminished over time, while homosexual behavior remained relatively steady. Among participants who were sexually active at both assessment periods, there were no significant changes in the number of sexual partners. However, at the Time 2 assessment, more than one-third of the teens showed a significant drop in their rates of insertive and receptive anal intercourse with male partners ($p < .0001$).

Use of Condoms

Changes in teens' use of condoms varied for different forms of intercourse. At the Time 2 assessment, teens reported more consistent use of condoms during anal intercourse; in fact, the rate of unprotected anal intercourse dropped by 60%, and 78% of the youths reported consistent use of condoms during anal intercourse with new partners ($p < .005$). Yet, no change was recorded in the use of condoms during oral sex, and the trend for vaginal intercourse fell short of significance ($p < .07$).

Effect on Ongoing HIV Risk

"High risk" for HIV transmission was defined as any unprotected anal intercourse or shared use of uncleaned needles or syringes with any partner since Time 1. Overall, 35 participants (25% of the sample) were found to be at high risk during the follow-up. These included all persons who continued, started or relapsed into risky behaviors, notably receptive and insertive anal intercourse without condoms and shared use of uncleaned needles or syringes.

The high-risk teens differed significantly from the rest of the sample on a number of characteristics. In particular, they were less likely to be enrolled in school and reported that a larger proportion of their friends were gay. They also reported engaging in more frequent anal intercourse with a greater number of partners than their lower risk peers.

Summary

Findings from the field study document short-term changes associated with participation in *YAPHPP*. In particular, youths showed significant reductions in their frequency of high-risk sexual behaviors, including insertive and receptive anal intercourse with male partners, and unprotected anal intercourse. Teens' severity of substance abuse also declined.

Overall, the researchers found that anal intercourse, and to a lesser extent, oral sex, were the two practices youths were mostly likely to change. Moreover, the teens employed both risk-avoidance and risk-reduction strategies. Some teens used condoms to prevent HIV transmission during anal intercourse, while others abstained from this sexual behavior. Alternatively, they practiced oral sex in place of other, more dangerous behaviors.

Nevertheless, 25% of the participants remained at high risk for HIV transmission at the follow-up assessment. It appeared that youths who were most in need of condoms were the ones least likely to use them.

In interpreting their findings, the researchers noted that the absence of a comparison group prevented any causal attribution about their program. In other words, they were unable to determine whether the observed outcomes were due to program participation, or other factors (e.g., maturation, information the teens received from other sources).

NOTE

1. A full set of program materials, including handbook, peer education session, videotape, brochure, evaluation materials, and more, is available for purchase from Sociometrics at http://www.socio.com/pasha.htm.

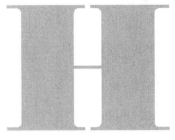

Programs Designed for Runaway Youths

33

Adolescents Living Safely: AIDS Awareness, Attitudes, and Actions

Anne Belden, William S. Ferrell, Starr Niego, and Janette Mince

Original Program Developers and Evaluators

Mary Jane Rotheram-Borus, PhD
Helen Reid, MA
Margaret Rosario, PhD
   UCLA Health Risk Reduction Project
   University of California, Los Angeles
   Los Angeles, CA

Sutherland Miller, PhD
Cheryl Koopman, PhD
Clara Haignere, PhD
Calvin Selfridge
   HIV Center for Clinical & Behavioral Studies
   New York Psychiatric Institute
   New York, NY

Adolescents Living Safely: AIDS Awareness, Attitudes, and Actions was supported by grants from the National Institute of Mental Health (Grant #1P50 MH 43520), the National Institute on Drug Abuse, and the William T. Grant Foundation.

PROGRAM ABSTRACT

Summary

Originally designed to meet the comprehensive needs of runaway youths, *Adolescents Living Safely: AIDS Awareness, Attitudes, and Actions (ALS I)* combines 20 small-group discussion sessions with one private counseling session. The group meetings provide general instruction about HIV/AIDS through video, role plays and other activities in which youths both review professionally produced educational materials and create their own skits, commercials and videos. Several exercises encourage the teens to think about the ways in which high-risk sexual behaviors might prevent them from accomplishing all that they hope for in their lives. Participants also practice strategies for coping with high-risk situations involving drug and alcohol use. The counseling component is designed to identify individual needs and provide youths with appropriate resources.

A field study of the program was conducted at two shelters serving predominantly Hispanic and African American runaways between 11 and 18 years of age in New York City. The 20-session sequence was offered continuously over a 2-year period, but youths joined the program at various points, and their levels of participation varied. For teens who attended at least fifteen sessions, the high-risk pattern of sexual behavior (50% or less condom use combined with 10 or more sexual encounters and/or sex with 3 or more partners) dropped in frequency from 20% to zero over a 6-month period. In addition, consistent condom use rose from 33% to 63% at the 6-month evaluation. At the 2-year follow-up assessment, program effects remained strongest for male and African American participants.

Focus

- ☐ Primary pregnancy prevention
- ☐ Secondary pregnancy prevention
- ☑ STI/HIV/AIDS prevention

Original Site

- ☐ School based
- ☑ Community based
- ☐ Clinic based

Suitable for Use In

This program can be implemented in a variety of community-based settings serving high-risk youths, especially runaways, providing that case management and counseling services are available. It is also appropriate for residential treatment programs.

Approach

- ☐ Abstinence
- ☑ Behavioral skills development
- ☐ Community outreach
- ☑ Contraceptive access
- ☑ Contraceptive education
- ☐ Life option enhancement
- ☑ Self-efficacy/self-esteem
- ☑ Sexuality/HIV/STI education

Original Intervention Sample

Age, gender   The original sample included 78 runaway youths, ages 11 to 18 (average = 15.5 years); 64% were female.

Race/ethnicity   63% African American, 22% Latino, 8% White, 7% Other.

Program Components

- ☐ Adult involvement
- ☑ Case management
- ☑ Group discussion
- ☐ Lectures
- ☐ Peer counseling/instruction
- ☐ Public service announcements
- ☑ Role play
- ☑ Video
- ☑ Other: Video and art workshops

Program Length

In addition to ongoing counseling and case management services, the full intervention includes 20 group sessions, held over a 3-week period. Each session is designed to last 90 to 120 minutes.

Staffing Requirements/Training

Group sessions (with approximately 6 to 10 youths) are facilitated by two leaders, preferably one male and one female, who are from diverse backgrounds. Participating teens may also split into male and female groups, with same-sex leaders, as warranted. Other professional staff (e.g., lawyers, vocational counselors) should be on call to provide necessary services.

Training should include cognitive and behavioral risk reduction strategies (e.g., turning negative into self-affirming thoughts, avoiding risky situations), coping with clinical crises and group process skills. Although staff may be familiar with social support and therapy groups, a structured, cognitive-based intervention may at first be challenging for them. It is important to discuss the ways in which this program differs from group therapy.

BIBLIOGRAPHY

Reid, H. M., Rotheram-Borus, M. J., Rosario, M., & Gwadz, M. (1993, June). *Effectiveness of HIV prevention with homeless youth over two years.* Paper presented at the 9th International Conference on AIDS, Berlin.

Rotheram-Borus, M. J., Feldman, J., Rosario, M., & Dunne, E. (1994). Preventing HIV among runaways: Victims and victimization. In R. J. DiClemente & J. L. Peterson (Eds.), *Preventing AIDS: Theories and methods of behavioral intervention* (pp. 175–188). New York: Plenum Press.

Rotheram-Borus, M. J., Koopman, C., & Bradley, J. S. (1990). Barriers to successful AIDS prevention programs with runaway youth. In J. O. Woodruff, D. Dougherty, & J. G. Athery (Eds.), *Troubled adolescents and HIV infection: Issues in prevention and treatment* (pp. 37–55). Washington, DC: CASSP Technical Assistance Center.

Rotheram-Borus, M. J., Koopman, C., & Ehrhardt, A. A. (1991). Homeless youths and HIV infection. *American Psychologist, 26*(1), 118–119.

Rotheram-Borus, M. J., Koopman, C., Haignere, C., & Davies, M. (1991). Reducing HIV sexual risk behaviors among runaway adolescents. *Journal of the American Medical Association, 266*(9), 1237–1241.

Related References by the Developers of *ALS I*

Rotheram-Borus, M. J., Mahler, K. A., & Rosario, M. (1995). AIDS prevention with adolescents. *AIDS Education & Prevention, 7*(4), 320–336.

Rotheram-Borus, M. J., Murphy, D. A., Kennedy, M., Stanton, A., & Kulkinsky, M. (2001). Health and risk behaviors over time among youth living with HIV. *Journal of Adolescence, 24*(6), 791–802.

Stein, J. A., Rotheram-Borus, M. J., Swendeman, D., & Milburn, G. (2005). Predictors of sexual transmission risk behaviors among HIV-positive young men. *AIDS Care, 17*(4), 433–442.

THE PROGRAM

Program Rationale and History

ALS I was an HIV risk-reduction program originally designed to meet the comprehensive needs of runaway youths, who were at high risk for STI/HIV/AIDS.[1] Based on a cognitive-behavioral model that had guided several previous health promotion efforts with adolescents, the program encouraged skill building and self-efficacy in an environment of peer support. The importance of safe sex was emphasized throughout all of the lessons. The curriculum for this companion program included additional sessions focused on the particular needs of teens who self-identified as gay, lesbian or bisexual, as well as youths who were unsure of their sexual orientation. Although the original implementation of *ALS I* did not specifically address transgenderism, the intervention content was sufficiently broad to apply to all runaway youths, regardless of sexual orientation or gender identity.

Twenty group discussion sessions form the core of *ALS I.* In these sessions youths received basic information about HIV/AIDS and learned strategies for practicing safe sex. In addition, participants completed exercises in sexual assertion, refusal skills, partner negotiation, self-management, problem-solving, risk recognition and correct condom and dental dam use. Finally, a personal counseling session was included to ensure that the individual needs of each youths were addressed.

The program was developed by researchers at Columbia University and the HIV Center for Clinical and Behavioral Studies and Division of Child Psychiatry at the New York State Psychiatric Institute. Between 1988 and 1990 a field study was conducted with runaway teens recruited from two publicly funded shelters in New York City.

Theoretical Framework

ALS I was guided by a cognitive-behavioral approach to health promotion, which relies heavily on social learning theory.

Bandura's social learning theory elaborates the processes through which intentions can be translated into behavioral change among teens. Bandura asserts that learning occurs through practice and observation of social models; it is mediated by internal beliefs about one's ability to succeed, anticipated rewards and consequences of one's actions and others' evaluation of one's performance. *ALS I* emphasized the importance of practicing, observing and modeling as vehicles for learning new skills and improving old ones.

The cognitive-behavioral method yielded a practical and theoretically grounded approach for helping adolescents that could be tailored to suit the needs of the client population, institutional setting and community. The program aimed to increase adolescents' awareness and understanding of their own feelings before trying to increase knowledge, attitudes or behavioral skills. If teens could not talk about and understand their own feelings, they would be unable to communicate with potential partners about safer sexual practices.

Program Model

ALS I is based on the following model of human behavior:

People will continue to behave in a certain way if

1. they expect something good to result from their behavior;
2. something that they want does occur;
3. something good happens often;
4. any negative consequences occur a long time after the positive ones.

People will behave effectively in their best interests if

1. they know what is in their best interest;
2. they have the skills;
3. they have opportunities to learn skills in many ways: through observing, imitating and practicing;
4. they believe they have effective tools and can use them effectively; and
5. they fit into the environment in which they live and the environment supports them.

The program developers expanded on this model of behavior to develop a set of principles for the *ALS I* sessions.

Program Goals

The overall aim of the program was to reduce high-risk sexual behaviors among adolescents. Specifically, the intervention was designed to help participants

- abstain from sex and unsafe behavior if they have not yet had sexual intercourse;
- use a condom or dental dam when engaging in sexual activities where an exchange of body fluids was possible;
- screen potential partners and avoid sex with those who were risky or of questionable HIV status;
- refrain from getting high on alcohol or drugs before having sex.

Program Objectives

To meet the goal of reducing sexually risky behavior, the program developers defined 10 behavioral objectives for teens who participated in the *ALS I* program:

1. Acquire general knowledge about HIV/AIDS: definitions, consequences, routes of transmission, high-risk behaviors, prevention strategies, and testing
2. Believe they could get AIDS, they could prevent themselves from getting AIDS, and they could change their own behavior
3. Label, assess, and control the intensity of their feelings in high-risk situations
4. Reward themselves with positive feedback for thought and behavior patterns that were likely to reduce the risk of infection
5. Use self-talk to guide themselves successfully through situations that were sexually risky
6. Identify and change dysfunctional thoughts
7. Solve interpersonal problems through clarifying goals; identifying risks, costs, and opportunities; evaluating alternative strategies for fixing the situation; trying out alternatives and analyzing success
8. Express their needs assertively, say "no" in risky situations, and communicate with confidence
9. Determine the advantages and disadvantages of being tested for HIV
10. Identify community resources and use these resources as needed, particularly free condoms, dental dams and health and mental health care

Hypothesized Outcomes

It was hypothesized that an intensive community-based intervention program, accompanied by case management, counseling services and health care, would enable youths to

- decrease their sexual risk acts, such as unprotected anal, vaginal, or oral sex;
- increase their use of condoms and dental dams when engaging in sexual activity.

Program Content

ALS I sessions included four main components:

1. *Knowledge.* Facts about HIV were communicated through two types of activities. First, teenagers participated in video and art workshops to develop soap opera dramatizations, public service announcements, commercials and raps about HIV prevention. In the original field study, they also reviewed commercial HIV prevention videos.
2. *Coping skills.* Participants received training to address unrealistic expectations about their ability to cope in high-risk situations. They learned to identify personal cues or triggers that placed them at potential risk for HIV transmission and to identify and practice behavioral and cognitive coping responses to such situations.
3. *Health care.* In the field study of the program, participants made at least one visit to a community-based agency providing vocational and educational counseling, recreational opportunities and referrals for comprehensive health and mental health care and legal aid.
4. *Individual barriers.* Through private counseling sessions, participants reviewed their individual barriers to safer sex, especially negative attitudes.

Program Schedule

ALS I consisted of 20 group sessions lasting approximately 90–120 minutes that were held approximately four times a week over a 3- to 5-week period. All meetings were facilitated by two trained professionals. In addition, an individual counseling session was held with each participant.

Each group session shared the following seven elements:

1. Positive behaviors were reinforced, particularly by giving teens small tokens of colored paper as a symbol of their contributions to the group discussion.
2. Participants were encouraged to assess, monitor and label their feelings through the use of a "Feeling Thermometer."
3. Talk was used as a strategy to diminish group members' anxiety concerning taboo topics.
4. After group leaders modeled effective coping skills, participants practiced through role plays.
5. Self-esteem was promoted through positive interaction and esteem-building exercises. Self-efficacy was promoted by enabling the teens to demonstrate newly acquired skills and receive feedback from group leaders.
6. Concern was continually raised regarding unsafe sexual behaviors and involvement in risky situations and with risky partners.
7. Group cohesion was established through active participation and appreciation of each person's contributions.

Description of Program Sessions

Session 1: What Will Adolescents Living Safely Do for Me? The leaders and participants introduced themselves at the start of this session. The topic of safer sex was explored by inviting teens to consider sexual behaviors on a continuum, from low-risk to high-risk activities. After discussing reasons why people engaged in unsafe acts, even if they knew better, the group identified strategies that could help people practice safe sex. The session continued with a brief review of the goals and ground rules of the program and discussion of the first homework assignment. Throughout the program, homework activities were used to carry over into the teens' real lives the material presented during group discussions. Finally, the leaders encouraged participants to recognize at the end of each session fellow group members whose contributions they had appreciated.

Session 2: How to Recognize My Feelings. This session was designed to help participants identify their personal levels of comfort and discomfort in social situations. After a discussion of the importance of feelings to safer sexual behavior, the group engaged in a series of exercises using the "Feeling Thermometer." This thermometer, printed on a sheet of paper, showed a scale ranging from 0 to 100. Throughout the program sessions, teens to "took their temperature" by assessing their position on the scale—from 0, indicating very, very comfortable, to 100, representing a high level of discomfort. Breathing exercises for relaxation in tense situations were also introduced, both here and later, during many of the sessions. The facilitators ended the session by inviting participants to express their appreciation for their peers' contributions to the meeting.

Session 3: How Serious Is the Threat to Me? This lesson provided teens with a clearer understanding of the threats posed by HIV and AIDS, especially death. In one exercise, teens pretended that they were at a party. Each guest wore a nametag, and some of the tags had small flowers on them. During a brief mingling period, participants were asked to introduce themselves to one another and decide which guests they would want to have sex with. When the mingling ended, the facilitators explained that guests whose name tags had flowers were HIV-positive. If, in real life, the teens had had sex with such people, they would have put themselves at risk for HIV infection. A second exercise was designed to encourage participants to think of death in relation to their hopes and dreams for the future—what they hoped to accomplish before they died. For homework, participants considered one step they could take toward their personal lifetime goals.

Session 4: What Do I Need to Know About HIV/AIDS? Basic facts and terminology about HIV/AIDS were discussed in Session 4. In the original field study, the teens viewed a video describing the AIDS antibody test and discussed reasons why it might be important to take the test. (You may want to hold a similar discussion with your own teens.) Toward the end of the session, participants identified myths and misunderstandings they believed their peers had about AIDS; for homework, each person was asked to educate two friends about the virus that caused AIDS.

Session 5: What Are My High-Risk Situations? Learning how to recognize and avoid high-risk situations was the goal of Session 5. Through role plays, discussions, and games, the group leaders helped participants identify the particular situations they were likely to face. Additional exercises encouraged group members to think of ways they could get out of such situations and argue against commonly used rationalizations for unsafe activities.

Session 6: When Is My Sexual Behavior Safe? To address participants' confusion about the safety of particular activities, this session focused on sex as a continuum of behaviors. In one exercise teens considered the safety level of various friends' sexual practices; each was evaluated as "safe," "possibly safe," or "definitely unsafe." During the next exercise, group members examined their own personal behaviors, again considering the safety of their actions. At the close of the session, a group profile of safe sex behaviors was compiled.

Session 7: How to Use a Condom and Dental Dam. The proper use of condoms and dental dams was taught during this session, and humor was recommended as a tension-reducing strategy. The facilitators emphasized the importance of latex condoms, along with appropriate lubricants and spermicides. (At the time *ALS I* was developed, it was common practice to recommend the use of spermicides containing nonoxynol-9. More recent research has revealed, however, that the use of nonoxynol-9 can irritate the vaginal and/or anal membranes, causing microscopic tears that leave the user more susceptible to becoming infected.) As a group, participants first practiced putting a condom on their hand or a penile model (e.g., banana, zucchini) and then practiced using a dental dam. For homework, participants were asked to locate a local store where they could purchase condoms.

Session 8: How to Spread the Word About Safer Sex. At the start of the meeting, the group leaders emphasized the importance of condoms by explaining that participants would be asked to show that they were carrying condoms with them at all future sessions. Participants divided into three teams and each created a media message (e.g., TV commercial, rap, or newscast) about ways to protect oneself from HIV. Each team spent about 20 minutes creating their skit and then performed the piece for the rest of the group. For homework, participants evaluated messages about HIV that they encountered as they watched TV, listened to the radio or read a newspaper or magazine.

Session 9: Tell Me More About Sex. Through role-play exercises and group discussion the group explored feelings about sexual activity, sex education and communication in intimate relationships. During the second half of the session, the group split into male and female teams, and each met privately with a same-sex leader. Participants wrote any questions they had about sex on an index card, and the leader addressed them. In the field, each facilitator was given a guide for discussing questions commonly asked by teens. (You may want to put together such a guide for your own group leaders.)

Session 10: How to Cope With Trouble. This session introduced participants to strategies for coping in difficult situations. In a role-play exercise, participants illustrated each of eight possible strategies, from "seek support" to "escape the scene." The group leaders emphasized problem solving as one of the best coping techniques. Using a problem analysis form, participants learned how to define, assess and constructively confront a problem situation. Techniques for relaxing in such situations were rehearsed.

Session 11: Coping With My Use of Drugs and Alcohol. The relationship of drug and alcohol use to HIV infection was explored in this session. Through observation, role play, and discussion, participants evaluated the effects of drugs and alcohol on their lives and especially, the risk level of their behaviors. An exercise critiquing the behaviors of various actors involved in risky situations showed participants how to gain a sense of control over their lives. An additional exercise helped participants identify the emotional triggers that could lead them to get high. The leaders helped the youths see that they had choices other than using drugs. Finally, the group leaders demonstrated the proper procedure for cleaning intravenous drug needles with bleach.

Session 12: Dealing With Pressures to Use Drugs/Alcohol. Through a series of exercises on communication skills, gaining confidence, role-play scenarios and "I statements," participants learned how to deliver effective refusals and requests in risky situations. Participants also reviewed previously learned coping techniques for taking control when pressured to use drugs or engage in unsafe sex. These activities were designed to enhance teens' self-confidence in coping with high-risk situations, which was also linked to their self-esteem and self-efficacy.

Session 13: How to Handle Thoughts That Don't Help Me. Shifting to cognitive strategies for promoting safer sex, the group leaders helped participants distinguish self-defeating from self-enhancing thoughts. Working with a partner, each teen wrote down self-defeating thoughts that they used a lot in their lives; next to each thought they devised a self-supporting thought that could be used instead. The group continued this exercise together, focusing on thoughts that occurred during sexual situations. For homework, participants were asked to catch themselves in the middle of unhelpful thoughts, yell "Stop!" to themselves, and come up with self-affirming thoughts.

Session 14: Visiting a Person With AIDS. To reduce teens' stereotypes about people with AIDS, Session 14 was designed to enable students to meet individuals with the virus. The facilitators encouraged participants to ask questions, show respect, and share their own feelings. Typically, the visit included an informal meal, which served to promote feelings of intimacy and reduce myths about catching HIV through normal human contact. The visit was followed by a debriefing session in which group members discussed their feelings and reactions to the meeting.

Session 15: Should I Be Tested for HIV? The "HIV Antibody Test Sheet" was used to engage participants in a discussion of the test and the meaning of the results, whether positive or negative. The facilitators gave group members a list of local agencies, first where they could get tested and second, where they could receive treatment. Working in pairs, the teens then explored their own possible reactions to a positive test result. Finally, group members explored the question of whether they should be tested.

Session 16: Using Self-Talk to Practice Safer Sex. The group leaders promoted the idea that teens could feel better about themselves by giving themselves compliments and rewards. An exercise encouraged group members to practice using self-talk, or talking to themselves, in tough situations. Finally, the group split up by gender to participate in an activity that involved rewriting negative self-talk in a rap song.

Session 17: How to Choose Safe Friends. This session was designed to help participants assess the risks posed by their friends and sexual partners. In an introductory exercise, the teens learned that they often did not know which friends were HIV-positive. This exercise highlighted two points: first, that it was not possible to tell if someone was HIV-positive just by looking at them, and second, what led to HIV infection was what the person did, not who the person was. For these reasons, the leaders emphasized, safe sex was essential. In a second exercise boys and girls met separately to create lists of the qualities they liked in partners. Strategies for starting and ending relationships were also explored. The group practiced screening partners through discussion and role playing.

Session 18: Looking Over a Community Resource. The goal of Session 18 was to introduce group members to community case management agencies that provided services to runaway youths. You may wish to prepare a similar list for your milieu.

A personal counseling session. In addition to the group discussion sessions, each teen had an individual counseling session with a trained professional. The counselor first determined whether the adolescent was sexually active and then designed a plan to overcome barriers to practicing safer sex or maintaining abstinence. The counselor also addressed any questions the teen had regarding sex and HIV/AIDS.

Session 19: Making a Soap Opera on HIV/AIDS. To integrate the lessons of the previous sessions, the group created an original soap opera on HIV/AIDS. The leaders encouraged the group to devise a story and select scriptwriters, a director, cameramen or women, actors and editors. Once the story was complete, the skit was performed, videotaped and viewed. In the field study of the program, the teens particularly enjoyed creating and acting out humorous scripts.

Session 20: The End and the Beginning. During the final session, group members were asked to share their feelings about the program. Members explored their hopes for the future by creating postcards that they would mail to their peers in 5 years. A relaxation technique was used to help group members feel good as they offered their good-byes.

PROGRAM EVALUATION

The Original Evaluation

Design

In a field trial, researchers compared the sexual risk and STI protective behaviors of *ALS I* participants to those of a comparison group of runaway teens.

The study was conducted between 1988 and 1990 at the only two publicly funded shelters for runaway youths in New York City. At one shelter, volunteers were recruited into the *ALS I* program; at the second shelter, volunteers joined the comparison group. The comparison group received no intervention other than the usual counseling and informal education provided by staff. However, condoms were also available to this group.

All data were gathered with semistructured interviews. Three interviews were held with each participant during the study period:

- Time 1: At the start of the intervention (pretest)
- Time 2: 3 months following the intervention (3-month follow-up)
- Time 3: 6 months following the intervention (6-month follow-up)

Additionally, the researchers recontacted many of the participants for an additional follow-up assessment 2 years following the intervention.

Evaluation Questions

Three empirical questions guided the field study:

1. Did participation in the *ALS I* program lead to lower rates of high-risk sex acts?
2. Did program participants use STI protection more effectively than members of the comparison group?
3. Did program participants show lower rates of sexual activity relative to their peers?

Data Collection Procedures

After providing informed consent, each participant completed the baseline interview—a semistructured protocol assessing sexual activities during the prior 3 months. Youths participating in the *ALS I* program then joined the discussion groups and completed additional interviews at 3- and 6-month intervals. Comparison group members were recontacted for follow-up assessments at the appropriate times. Participants received $2.00 for completion of the baseline interview, and $20 to $25 for each of the follow-up assessments.

The three interviews were identical in format. Questions were combined to form three measures of sexual risk.

1. *Abstinence:* having no sexual partners in the past 3 months.
2. *High-risk pattern of sexual behavior:* infrequent condom use (use during less than 50% of sexual encounters) combined with 10 or more sexual encounters and/or three or more sexual partners.
3. *Consistent condom use:* use of a condom during every instance of oral, vaginal, or anal sex.

Because few encounters with same-sex partners were reported, only heterosexual activities were considered in the analyses. Demographic measures were also recorded, including age, gender, ethnicity, length of time since living at home, number of days at the shelter, and number of group sessions attended (for program participants only).

Sample

The researchers observed that teens moved in and out of the shelters as other housing arrangements became available, and the levels of participation varied. The final sample comprised 78 *ALS I* participants and 67 comparison group members. The youths ranged in age from 11 to 18 years (average = 15.5 years); 64% were female and the majority were African American or Hispanic. None of the teens had symptoms of HIV infection or AIDS at the time of the study.

At the start of the investigation, the researchers found no significant differences in patterns of sexual behavior between program participants and members of the comparison group. Also, the teens who stayed longer at the shelters did not differ from others on any of the demographic or behavioral measures. At both shelters, follow-up contact was more likely to be maintained with females than with males.

Evaluation Results

The impact of the program was found to vary with the number of discussion sessions attended. Fifteen sessions emerged as a significant "cutting point." That is, the 21 youths who attended at least 15 sessions showed significant improvements on two of the three behavioral outcomes, as explained below.

High-Risk Sexual Behavior

For program participants attending at least 15 group discussion sessions, the incidence of high-risk sexual behaviors dropped from 20% at baseline to zero at the 3- and 6-month follow-up assessments.

Condom Use

For runaways participating in 15 or more sessions, condom use rose from 33% at baseline to 57% at 3 months and 63% at 6 months after the intervention.

Abstinence

The program appeared to have no significant impact on abstinence among teens. Regardless of the level of participation in the *ALS I* program, no differences were found in self-reported abstinence between program and comparison group teens.

In addition, at the 3- and 6-month follow-up assessments, the researchers found no significant differences on any of the outcome measures as a function of youths' ethnicity, age, gender or time of entry into the program.

When contacted again for a 2-year follow-up assessment, program participants continued to show significant reductions in HIV risk-related behaviors. However, different patterns emerged at this point across ethnic group and gender. Overall, program participation was most effective for African American teens and males.

Summary

The empirical results demonstrated that *ALS I* could produce significant, positive changes in the sexual behaviors of runaway adolescents. Compared to a comparison group of their peers, the 21 teens who attended at least 15 group discussion sessions showed more effective use of condoms and a reduction in the number of high-risk sex acts at the 3- and 6-month follow-up assessments. These effects remained significant even 2 years following the intervention.

On the other hand, no change was observed in the levels of abstinence recorded among program participants. Although *ALS I* did not discourage sexual activity, it did promote safer sexual practices among this group of high-risk youths. Additionally, it was possible that self-selection played a role in the behavioral outcomes. The researchers found that the 21 youths who attended at least 15 sessions did not differ from the rest of the sample on demographic or sexual risk behavior measures at baseline. Still, these youths may have differed in other significant ways from their peers who participated less regularly in the *ALS I* program.

ALS I IN THE COMMUNITY TODAY

In the past 3 years, *ALS I* has been implemented in communities in 5 states, primarily in the south-central portion of the country.

NOTE

1. A full set of program materials, including curriculum manual, activity packets, evaluation materials, and more, is available for purchase from Sociometrics at http://www.socio.com/pasha.htm.

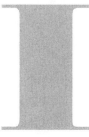

Programs Designed for Use by Primary Caregivers

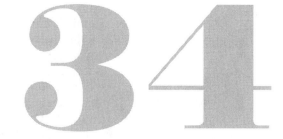

ASSESS: For Adolescent Risk Reduction

Diana Dull Akers

Original Program Developers and Evaluators

Bradley O. Boekeloo, PhD, MS
Kathy O'Connor, MPH
Lisa Schamus, MPH
Samuel J. Simmens, PhD
   George Washington University Medical Center
   Department of Health Care Science
   Washington, DC

Tina L. Cheng, MD, MPH
Lawrence D'Angelo, MD, MPH
   Children's National Medical Center
   Department of General Pediatrics & Adolescent Medicine
   Washington, DC

PROGRAM ABSTRACT

Summary

The *ASSESS* (Awareness, Skills, Self-Efficacy/Esteem, and Social Support) program provides tools to enhance risk-reduction communication between health

ASSESS was supported by grants from the National Institute of Child Health and Human Development (#R01 HD32572) and the Health Resources and Services Administration (#5U69PE00105).

care providers and teens while in a physician's office or clinic setting. A randomized controlled behavioral intervention trial of the program was conducted in the metropolitan Washington, DC, area between 1995 and 1997. The trial involved 19 physicians at five primary-care pediatric practices and 215 teens, aged 12–15.

After obtaining consent from both the teen and parent(s), researchers randomly assigned the teen to either the intervention (n = 105) or the control group (n = 114). Control group teens received their usual-care health examination. Intervention group teens listened to a 14-minute audiotape (wearing headphones for privacy) and answered 11 risk-related questions on the *ASSESS* Answer Sheet (that did not contain the questions). With the parent out of the room, the physician used program materials (answer sheets, pamphlets, and an *ASSESS* Pyramid icebreaker) to encourage the teen to discuss risk behaviors and their answers on the Answer Sheet. The physician used role-play strategies to encourage the teen to practice refusing risky behaviors.

All participants were given a face-to-face exit interview following their checkup to determine how many sexual topics they had discussed with their health care provider. Telephone follow-up interviews were conducted at 3 months and 9 months.

Study findings showed that *ASSESS* program materials had a positive impact on adolescent-reported discussion with the physician about sex. More intervention teens reported discussion on sexual topics with their physicians than did their control group counterparts. The program also had a positive impact on young adolescent knowledge about HIV transmission and attitudes towards condom use. At 3-month follow-up, more sexually active teens reported condom use in the intervention group than the control group. While more vaginal intercourse was also reported in the intervention group than the control group, this was not true of overall sexual intercourse (including anal and oral). At 9 months, there were no group differences in sexual behavior; however, more signs of sexually transmitted infections (STIs) were reported by the control than the intervention group.

Focus

☐ Primary pregnancy prevention   ☐ Secondary pregnancy prevention   ☑ STI/HIV/AIDS prevention

Original Site

☐ School based   ☐ Community based   ☑ Clinic based

Suitable for Use In

ASSESS is suitable for use in physician and clinic offices (for routine general health examinations or annual physical exams as required for participation in sports), as well as school and STI-related clinics.

Approach

- ☑ Abstinence
- ☑ Behavioral skills development
- ☐ Community outreach
- ☑ Contraceptive access
- ☑ Contraceptive education
- ☐ Life option enhancement
- ☑ Self-efficacy/self-esteem
- ☑ Sexuality/HIV/AIDS/STI education

Original Intervention Sample

Age, gender   The original intervention sample of 215 young adolescents aged 12–15 included 107 males and 108 females.

Race/ethnicity   More than half of the participants (65%) were African American, 19% were White, 7% were Hispanic, and 13% were Other.

Program Components

- ☑ Adult involvement
- ☐ Case management
- ☐ Group discussion
- ☐ Lectures
- ☐ Peer counseling/instruction
- ☐ Public service announcements
- ☑ Role play
- ☐ Video
- ☑ Other: Audio cassette, individual discussion

Program Length

This single-session, two-component intervention is designed to be offered while participants wait for their scheduled general health check up, and then continued in the physician's office without a parent present. The first part of the intervention involves the participant listening to a 14-minute audiotape and answering personal risk-related questions. The physician uses the color-coded responses to the questions to guide the private discussion that follows.

Staffing Requirements/Training

Although the original intervention focused on primary care physicians to deliver the intervention, you may choose to include physician assistants, nurse practitioners and other health professionals among those who administer *ASSESS* in your setting.

BIBLIOGRAPHY

Boekeloo, B. O., Schamus, L. A., Cheng, T. L., & Simmens, S. J. (1996). Young adolescents' comfort with discussion about sexual problems with their physician. *Archives of Pediatric & Adolescent Medicine, 150,* 1146–1152.

Boekeloo, B. O., Schamus, L. A., & O'Connor, K. (1998). The effect of patient-education tools on physicians' discussions with young adolescents about sex. *Academic Medicine, 73*(10), s84–s87.

Boekeloo, B. O., Schamus, L. A., Simmens, S. J., & Cheng, T. L. (1996). Tailoring STD/HIV prevention messages for young adolescents. *Academic Medicine, 71*(10), s97–s99.

Boekeloo, B. O., Schamus, L. A., Simmens, S. J., & Cheng, T. L. (1998). Ability to measure sensitive adolescent behaviors via telephone. *American Journal of Preventive Medicine, 14*(3), 209–216.

Boekeloo, B. O., Schamus, L. A., Simmens, S. J., Cheng, T. L., O'Connor, K., and D'Angelo, L. J. (1999). A STD/HIV prevention trial among adolescents in managed care. *Pediatrics, 103*(1), 107–115.

Related References by the Developers of *ASSESS*

Boekeloo, B. O., Bobbin, M. P., Lee, W. I., Worrell, K. D., Hamburger, E. K., & Russek-Cohen, E. (2003). Effect of patient priming and primary care provider prompting on adolescent-provider communication about alcohol. *Archives of Pediatric & Adolescent Medicine, 157*(5), 433–439.

Boekeloo, B. O., Jerry, J., Lee-Ougo, W. I., Worrell, K. D., Hamburger, E. K., Russek-Cohen, E., et al. (2004). Randomized trial of brief office-based interventions to reduce adolescent alcohol use. *Archives of Pediatric & Adolescent Medicine, 158*(7), 635–642.

Boekeloo, B. O., Snyder, M. H., Bobbin, M., Burstein, G. R., Conley, D., Quinn, T. C., et al. (2002). Provider willingness to screen all sexually active adolescents for chlamydia. *Sexually Transmitted Infections, 78*(5), 369–373.

THE PROGRAM

Program Rationale and History

At the time the *ASSESS* program was developed and tested in the late 1990s, most STI/HIV prevention research had focused on adults and older teens.[1] There was little such research on young adolescents, in spite of the vulnerability of this group to STIs. The *ASSESS* program also observed that while primary care providers had a unique opportunity to engage young adolescents in discussions about sexual awareness, activity, and risk reduction strategies, these opportunities were often missed. Research documented physicians citing a variety of barriers to discussing sexuality and sexual health with adolescents. These barriers included confidentiality issues, lack of time, and concerns over risk reduction methods.

The *ASSESS* program was designed with the goals of reducing barriers to physician/adolescent communication around sexual health and sexual risk reduction topics. The program presumed that in order for adolescents to make responsible decisions, they needed first to be aware of risks and risk behaviors and how to reduce those risks. They then needed to develop the skills necessary to avoid and/or confront risky situations. Finally, they needed to possess a sense of self-efficacy that they could resist peer pressure, and self-esteem or a positive self-image to motivate them to use risk reduction skills. *ASSESS* program developers felt the achievement of these goals should be supported not only by parents, but also by health care provider(s) who had the potential to be influential sources of such information.

The *ASSESS* program was created as a single-session intervention that provided both health care providers and adolescents with communication tools to begin a one-on-one discussion about sexuality. The program was developed in the mid-1990s with focus group input from teens, parents and health care providers. The major message of the program was that unprotected intercourse was unsafe, that condom-protected intercourse was safer, and abstinence (including no physical contact, dry kissing, and nonpenetrative physical contact) was the safest behavior. Rather than specifying that only abstinence or condom use was an acceptable option, the materials describe the potential for STI and HIV infection from vaginal, oral, and anal sexual behaviors and explained how to lower risks through barrier protection or abstinence.

A randomized intervention trial with 3- and 9-month follow-ups was conducted between August 1995 and June 1997. The study took place in five managed care sites in the metropolitan Washington, DC, area; a total of 19 physicians (pediatricians) participated in the trial. The goal of the study was to determine if STI risk assessment and educational tools provided as part of office-based primary care would (a) increase physician-adolescent discussion about sexual issues; and (b) improve adolescents' STI knowledge and attitudes, and delay or decrease sexual activity (or increase condom use) at 3- and 9-month follow-ups.

Theoretical Framework

The primary theoretical underpinning of the intervention is social cognitive theory, which emphasizes the development of confidence regarding the execution and outcome of specific skills. The intervention is also informed by the theory of reasoned action as it relates to increasing adolescents' perception of the physician's expectations.

Program Overview

As originally designed, *ASSESS* was offered as a one-time intervention in a physician's office during a routine physical examination. The intervention could be offered, however, by other members of a doctor's staff such as nurse practitioners, or physician's assistants, or by a school or clinic nurse.

Program Design

The program had four main goals:

1. Overcome barriers to discussion of sex and drugs between health care providers and early adolescents
2. Improve STI/HIV risk assessment skills of providers
3. Improve STI/HIV risk reduction skills of providers
4. Identify, to providers, adolescents, and parents, locally available resources for support, counseling, testing, referral, and follow-up

To meet those goals, the development team created specific tools for both the physician and the patient. These tools included physician training and demonstration materials (a program manual and videotape of a sample doctor/patient interaction for the physician), a risk assessment audiotape and answer sheet for use by the patient, an *ASSESS* Pyramid "ice-breaker" for use by both physician and patient in their discussion, and brochures for use by patients and their parents. The development team's research had shown that when only the adolescent patient or the physician had the tools, risk-related discussions tended to not take place. However, when both had the tools, the discussions were much more likely to occur.

The program was designed to address the objectives and recommendations of the Department of Health and Human Services, as well as the American Medical Association's "Guidelines for Adolescent Preventive Services."

Program Implementation

Program Planning

Before delivering *ASSESS* in your setting, you may want to revisit or develop a written confidentiality policy. Understanding that concerns over confidentiality could be a barrier to adolescent health care was the first step in improving service delivery to this high-risk group. In the field study of *ASSESS*, clinicians were prepared to discuss the confidentiality policy with the parent present, before either the parent or teen asked about it.

The research team prepared a letter of consent or other information about the *ASSESS* program that parents received in advance of the visit. The letter informed parents that all of the adolescent patients were given the same intervention format, customized to the patient's age and sexual maturity, each time he or she came to the office for a routine physical examination. It was important that both parents and teens understood that they were not being singled out for any reason.

Suggested Structure

The developers of the *ASSESS* program suggested a seven-step structure for incorporating the program into routine office visits:

1. Establish rapport and trust.
2. Conduct an initial health history with the parent present.

3. Discuss confidentiality with both adolescent and parent present.
4. Assess specific sexual and drug risks without parent present.
5. Conduct the physical exam of the adolescent.
6. Discuss the *ASSESS* Pyramid (once the adolescent was dressed).
7. Discuss the brochures and conduct role play to develop risk reduction skills

The Intervention

Upon arrival at the doctor's office, the teen listened to the previsit "Audio Risk Assessment" audiotape that addressed awareness and perceived susceptibility to STIs. The audiotape was administered in private, either with headphones or in a private location. In the audiotape, two doctors (a man and a woman) explained the importance of discussing sexual concerns with a physician. The teen then answered the 11 closed-ended risk assessment questions on the tape, using the color-coded answer sheet that contained responses only. Questions on the tape addressed such issues as feelings of sexual attraction, history of kissing, history of sexual intercourse (vaginal, oral or anal), and use of street drugs or alcohol. Red-coded responses signified that the teen had engaged in unsafe behaviors, yellow coded-responses signified safer behaviors, and green-coded responses signified safest behaviors.

The audiotape stressed the importance of selecting latex condoms lubricated with a spermicide containing nonoxynol-9. Research conducted since the development of the intervention has revealed that women can experience adverse reactions to nonoxynol-9. Specifically, nonoxynol-9 can irritate the vaginal and/or anal membranes, resulting in microscopic tears which leave the user more susceptible to infection.

During the initial portion of the consultation, a parent was present. The physician explained that he or she was the *teen's* doctor, and that anything the teen said would remain confidential (unless it was life-threatening). The parent was then given a copy of two brochures ("Drugs: Talking With Your Teen" and "HIV: Talking With Your Teen") and asked to read them over while in the waiting room.

Following the physical exam and after the teen is dressed, the physician reviewed the teen's answer sheet with the teen, paying particular attention to any red items. The physician then used the three-dimensional *ASSESS* Pyramid to encourage the teen to guide the direction of the risk-reduction conversation that followed. During the focus group research and trials of the *ASSESS* intervention, many teens indicated that they liked holding the Pyramid, and that it helped them with their nervousness at discussing sexual issues.

There were three brochures for the doctor to give to the teen. Two of these ("How to Use Condoms the Right Way, Every Time" and "101 Ways to Say No to Sex") could be used for role play or cognitive rehearsal during the visit. For example, the doctor would say, "What if your boyfriend/girlfriend said, 'I don't want to use a condom.' How might you respond? Take a look at the brochure and find a response you like, and say it aloud to me."

PROGRAM EVALUATION

The Original Evaluation

Study Design

The randomized, controlled behavioral intervention trial of the *ASSESS* program was conducted between August 1995 and June 1997 in five primary care sites in the Washington, DC, area. Nineteen pediatricians (13 women, 6 men) participated in the study. Adolescents aged 12–15 were recruited from the five participating offices and randomly assigned to one of two groups. The intervention group (n = 101) received a general health exam plus the *ASSESS* intervention. The usual care control group received the general health exam only. All participants completed a face-to-face exit interview (baseline). Additionally, 93% (n = 200) completed the 3-month telephone follow-up, and 92% (n = 197) completed the 9-month telephone follow-up.

Study Population

All of the adolescent study participants were culled from five offices of a major health maintenance organization in the metropolitan Washington, DC, area. The study group was 48% female, 65% African American, 19% White, 13% Other, and 3% Hispanic. All participants were between 12 and 15 years of age. There were no significant demographic differences between the intervention and control groups at baseline or at the 3- and 9-month follow-up periods.

Evaluation Questions and Outcome Measures

The research team sought to determine if educational tools provided as part of a single-session educational intervention in a primary-care setting would increase physician-adolescent discussion about sexual issues; reduce adolescent-reported STIs, HIV, and other sexually risky behaviors; and increase condom use.

Evaluation Results

Knowledge and Beliefs

At baseline, intervention adolescents reported significantly more discussion with the physician about 11 of 13 topics regarding sexuality than control group adolescents. Discussion was also greater among females than males, and among sexually experienced adolescents and older adolescents. Intervention group participants were also more likely than their control group counterparts to know how HIV was transmitted, more likely to believe that they should use condoms during intercourse; and more likely to believe that they could refuse to have sex with a partner who refused to use a condom.

Sexual Behaviors

All sexual and other risk behaviors were self-reported at baseline (researcher-assisted pencil-and-paper survey) and at 3- and 9-month intervals (telephone surveys).

Bivariate analyses revealed no statistically significant differences between the two groups regarding intercourse (vaginal, oral, or anal) in the last 3 months or in one's lifetime at any of the interview points. There were also no bivariate differences between the groups in the number of vaginal intercourse partners or the frequency of vaginal intercourse at any of the three interview points. However, a trend suggested that the rate of vaginal intercourse during the last 3 months was higher in the intervention group at the 3-month interval. A mixed model regression controlling for baseline sexual experience and physician indicated that the likelihood of vaginal intercourse was higher in the intervention than control group (odds ratio [OR] = 2.46, 95% confidence interval [CI] = 1.04–5.84) at the 3-month follow-up, but not at baseline or the 9-month follow-up.

With regard to condom use at last intercourse among teens who were sexually active at baseline, bivariate analysis revealed no statistically significant differences between the two groups at baseline and the 9-month follow-up. The rate of condom use at last intercourse was greater among sexually active intervention than control group participants at the 3-month follow-up (χ^2 $p \le .01$). The rate of unprotected intercourse at 3 months was 0.8% in the intervention group compared with 43% in the control group. This finding was confirmed by a mixed model regression controlling for baseline sexual experience and physician (OR = 1.55, 95% CI = 1.27–256.03).

Sexual Outcomes

At the 3-month follow-up, there were no differences between the groups in their reported STI diagnoses, genital signs of possible STIs, STI treatments or pregnancies during the preceding 3 months. At 9 months, there were no group differences in sexual behaviors. However, more control (7/103) than intervention (0/94) teens reported seeing signs of possible STI infection in the preceding 6 months.

Although the positive impact on self-reported condom use at 3 months had dissipated by 9 months, reported STI outcomes suggested a positive program impact at 9 months.

In sum, the *ASSESS* study materials had a positive impact on adolescent-reported discussions with the physician about sex, on their knowledge about HIV transmission, their attitudes toward condom use and their self-reported STI outcomes. Although the positive impact on adolescent-reported condom use at 3 months dissipated by 9 months, adolescent reported STI outcomes suggested a positive program impact at 9 months. The developers noted that while the program could facilitate STI/HIV prevention education among young adolescents, it was likely that repeated follow-up efforts were needed for long-term impact on sexual risk behaviors.

ASSESS IN THE COMMUNITY TODAY

In the past 3 years, *ASSESS* has been implemented in communities in 3 clinic settings in the metropolitan New York City area.

NOTE

1. A full set of program materials, including program manual, audiotape, videotape, brochures, evaluation materials, and more, is available for purchase from Sociometrics at http://www.socio.com/pasha.htm.

Index